Patricia J. Bush, PhD
Deanna J. Trakas, PhD
Emilio J. Sanz, MD, PhD
Rolf L. Wirsing, PhD
Tuula Vaskilampi, PhD
Alan Prout, PhD
Editors

Children, Medicines, and Culture

Pre-publication
REVIEWS,
COMMENTARIES,
EVALUATIONS . . .

"**T**his book is essential reading for professionals interested in the interface of children and medicine. The multicultural perspectives, the diversity of theoretical and clinical approaches, the description of multinational health care systems, and the richness of the data will reward all readers."

Roger Bibace, PhD
Professor of Psychology,
Clark University;
Professor, Department of Obstetrics
and Gynecology,
UMass Medical School

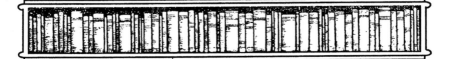

"**T**his book is truly unique. It is one of the first books in medical anthropology that makes an attempt to cover Europe and treat it as one cultural area while respecting the magnitude of its cultural differences even within allegedly similar cultures like the Nordic ones.

Anthropological studies are often evaluated according to the degree to which researchers made their objects visible and feelable. In this study the authors reached their goal, because the children (and their opinions) have truly been made visible in this book. They have been studied as a tribe in their own right!

When anthropology connected with psychology in the fifties many studies were written on children, on socialization, on education and so forth, but in most of these studies children have remained hidden behind those who spoke for them, those who had produced them.

Another piece of research that was so widely neglected in medical anthropology is on the lay belief models of fever in western societies. This addition to the ethnography of disease concerning fever is found in Chapter 6, in which the reaction to fever is studied within five different cultures. While a vast body of literature is quoted, substantial empirical data are presented. This chapter, like many others, makes this book truly an anthropological adventure. I recommend this work strongly."

Beatrix Pfleiderer, PhD
Psychotherapist;
Professor Affiliate of Anthropology,
University of Hawaii

"**F**or scholars who study patient medication behavior, this book is a must read. It is written by a team of scholars who have explored the foundations of medication use in children. It's scope is international and it provides new knowledge for the study of patient care."

Bernard Sorofman, PhD
Associate Professor,
College of Pharmacy,
University of Iowa

"**C**hildren, Medicines, and Culture is not only a comparative study on medicine use in children in the industrialized world, but it also leads us into the still enduring, profound discussion of the pros and cons of qualitative vs. quantitative research. Furthermore, it tells us the story of an international, multidisciplinary and multicentered research team of scientists from ten countries– still an unusual undertaking. It is an agreeable feature of the book, that the 'human factor of science' becomes visible on both the researchers' and the research subjects' side.

The authors intended to provide anyone concerned with the use of drugs in children with a basis for working more effectively. According to their careful scientific design they did not present a synthesis of different theoretical principles and methodologies or a complete, applicable set of rules, but they give access to a wealth of interesting and detailed information that is relevant to professional needs. The The reader is able to discover another perspective of medicine use, beyond the one of pharmacoepidemiological data. The book is indeed, as formulated by the project leader Deanna J. Trakas, '. . . a concert, wherein each musician performs under the direction of a conductor.' In other words: lively science."

Christine Tuschinsky, PhD
Medical Anthropologist,
University of Hamburg

"**T**his book offers a wide coverage of a unique multicultural, multimethod research endeavor on children's concepts of illnesses and their cure. In addition, it gives a reasonable introduction into doing research in practice with a team representing various professional backgrounds and cultures. The range of cultures studied is wide. The reader may well find his or her own, or at least one very similar, included. My guess is that this book is going to be the standard reference when dealing with children's illness conceptions. The chapter on the contents of medicine cabinets gives a vivid picture of the cultural determinants of diseases and their remedies. The last chapters of the book, directed to readers with varying interests–pediatrics, anthropology, health education, and/or policy forming–will offer reason enough for acquiring and reading the book."

Antti Uutela, PhD
Laboratory Director and Head,
Health Education,
National Public Health Institute,
Finland

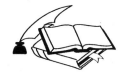

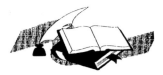

"There are known to be wide cultural variations in medicine use, in the status of children and in the relationship between families and the health care system. This book on children, medicines, and culture is a fascinating and rare example of productive cross-cultural work. The aims of the study on which it draws were to understand better cross-cultural variation in medicine use, to collect data relevant to planning health education for children, and to explore the use of different qualitative and quantitative research methods in carrying out an international study. Nine European countries and seven professional disciplines were involved. The multidisciplinary nature of the book's authors makes for a most unusual intermeshing of social and medical science perspectives. Different sections of the book explore contextual and structural factors that account for differences in medicine use; details of the local case studies; children's perceptions of illness and medicines; and concepts of illness, childhood, medication, and family life in different cultural settings. One of the most intriguing chapters reports on the contents of medicine cabinets in eight countries. Why do some families in Spain and Italy have more than 70 drugs in their household, and why are Finns the least home-medicated? What accounts for the variation in the proportion of over-the-counter medicines kept in different countries–from 36% in Athens to 74% in South Carolina? Other chapters suggest some underlying cultural differences here: parents and children perceive and define illness and normality differently; medical consultation rates vary; and there is a range of beliefs about the value of medicines such as antibiotics in treating childhood illness. *Children, Medicines, and Culture,* one of the most convincing demonstrations of medical anthropology's contribution in real

The Haworth Press, Inc.

Children, Medicines, and Culture

PHARMACEUTICAL PRODUCTS PRESS
Pharmaceutical Sciences
Mickey C. Smith, PhD
Executive Editor

New, Recent, and Forthcoming Titles:

Principles of Pharmaceutical Marketing edited by Mickey C. Smith

Pharmacy Ethics edited by Mickey C. Smith, Steven Strauss, John Baldwin, and Kelly T. Alberts

Drug-Related Problems in Geriatric Nursing Home Patients by James W. Cooper

Pharmacy and the U.S. Health Care System edited by Jack E. Fincham and Albert I. Wertheimer

Pharmaceutical Marketing: Strategy and Cases by Mickey C. Smith

International Pharmaceutical Services: The Drug Industry and Pharmacy Practice in Twenty-Three Major Countries of the World edited by Richard N. Spivey, Albert I. Wertheimer, and T. Donald Rucker

A Social History of the Minor Tranquilizers: The Quest for Small Comfort in the Age of Anxiety by Mickey C. Smith

Marketing Pharmaceutical Services: Patron Loyalty, Satisfaction, and Preferences edited by Harry A. Smith and Joel Coons

Nicotine Replacement: A Critical Evaluation edited by Ovide F. Pomerleau and Cynthia S. Pomerleau

Herbs of Choice: The Therapeutic Use of Phytomedicinals by Varro E. Tyler

Interpersonal Communication in Pharmaceutical Care by Helen Meldrum

Searching for Magic Bullets: Orphan Drugs, Consumer Activism, and Pharmaceutical Development by Lisa Ruby Basara and Michael Montagne

The Honest Herbal by Varro E. Tyler

Understanding the Pill: A Consumer's Guide to Oral Contraceptives by Greg Juhn

Pharmaceutical Chartbook, Second Edition edited by Abraham G. Hartzema and C. Daniel Mullins

The Handbook of Psychiatric Drug Therapy for Children and Adolescents by Karen A. Theesen

Children, Medicines, and Culture edited by Patricia J. Bush, Deanna J. Trakas, Emilio J. Sanz, Rolf L. Wirsing, Tuula Vaskilampi, and Alan Prout

Children, Medicines, and Culture

Patricia J. Bush, PhD
Deanna J. Trakas, PhD
Emilio J. Sanz, MD, PhD
Rolf L. Wirsing, PhD
Tuula Vaskilampi, PhD
Alan Prout, PhD
Editors

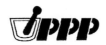

Pharmaceutical Products Press
An Imprint of the Haworth Press, Inc.
New York • London

Published by

Pharmaceutical Products Press, an imprint of The Haworth Press, Inc., 10 Alice Street, Binghamton, NY 13904-1580

The development, preparation, and publication of this work has been undertaken with great care. However, the publisher, employees, editors, and agents of The Haworth Press are not responsible for any errors contained herein or for consequences that may ensue from use of materials or information contained in this work. The opinions expressed by the author(s) are not necessarily those of The Haworth Press, Inc.

Library of Congress Cataloging-in-Publication Data

Children, medicines, and culture / Patricia J. Bush . . . [et al.], editors.
    p. cm.
    Includes bibliographical references and index.
    ISBN 1-56024-937-4 (alk. paper)
    1. Pediatric pharmacology–Cross-cultural studies. 2. Drug utilization–Social aspects–Cross-cultural studies. 3. Pharmacy–Social aspects–Cross-cultural studies. 4. Health attitudes–Cross-cultural studies. I. Bush, Patricia J.
RJ560.C46 1996
615.1′083–dc20
                                            95-17497
                                               CIP

CONTENTS

SECTION II: CROSS-CULTURAL REPORTS

SECTION IV: VIEWPOINTS

ABOUT THE EDITORS

Patricia J. Bush, MSc, PhD, is Professor Emerita, Department of Family Medicine, Georgetown University School of Medicine, Washington, DC. As a pharmacosociologist, she has long been interested in the medicine use process and especially the socialization of children into the use of medicines and abusable substances.

Deanna J. Trakas, PhD, is Director, Division of Medical Anthropology, Department of Social Pediatrics, Institute of Child Health, Athens, Greece. Dr. Trakas was the Project Leader for "The COMAC Childhood and Medicines Project," 1990-1993. Her anthropological research on medicine use in Athens, based on observations in neighborhood pharmacies and a review of home medicine cabinets, led to the suggestion from WHO/EURO to develop a comparative study in Europe.

Emilio J. Sanz, MD, PhD, is Associate Professor in Clinical Pharmacology, School of Medicine, University of La Laguna, Tenerife, Spain. He is the coordinator of the Regional Center for Drug Surveillance and Drug Information in the Canary Islands (Spain), and head of the group of "drug use in children" of the WHO-DURG (Drug Utilization Research Group).

Rolf L. Wirsing, PhD, MPH, is Professor of Anthropology and Medical Sociology at the Department of Social Work at the "Hochschule für Technik, Wirtschaft und Sozialwesen (FH)" in Gürlitz, Germany. As an anthropologist trained in the United States, he has cultivated a wide range of interests, ranging from methodology (e.g., comparative research) to medical anthropology (in particular pharmacoethnology and health behavior).

Tuula Vaskilampi, MA, PhD, is Docent in Medical Sociology in the Department of Community Health and General Practice, University of Kuopio, Finland. She performs studies in social sciences and community health.

Alan Prout, PhD, is currently Senior Lecturer in the Department of Sociology and Social Anthropology at Keele University, England, and was previously Senior Research Associate in Social and Political Sciences at Cambridge University. His interests are in the cultural performance of sickness, especially in relation to childhood and medical technology.

Contributors

Syed Rizwanuddin Ahmad, MBBS, MPH, is a researcher at Public Citizen Health Research Group, a consumer advocacy organization in Washington, DC, and is teaching at Georgetown University School of Medicine, Washington, DC. He received his medical degree from Dow Medical College, Karachi, Pakistan, and his public health degree from The Johns Hopkins School of Medicine and pharmacoepidemiology at the U.S. Food and Drug Administration. He is the recipient of the 1991 Olle Hansson Award, which gives recognition "to the work of outstanding Third World individuals in promoting the concept of rational use of drugs." His area of interest includes drug use in women and children.

Riitta Ahonen, MSc, PhD, a licensed pharmacist, is Senior Lecturer in Social and Administrative Pharmacy, University of Kuopio, Department of Social Pharmacy. Her training has emphasized social pharmacy, medical sociology, and research methodology in social science, pharmacology, and pharmacotherapy.

Anna B. Almarsdottir, PhD, served as Principal Investigator for the USA part of the COMAC Childhood and Medicines Project. She holds a pharmacy degree from the University of Iceland and worked in pharmacies and biotechnology research in her home country of Iceland before entering graduate school in the USA.

Pilar Aramburuzabala received a PhD at the School of Education of the Complutense University of Madrid (Spain) in 1995. She works for the New York City Board of Education as Educational Evaluator.

Chrysoula Botsis is Research Fellow in the AIDS unit of the University of Athens. Her research involves physicians' behavior toward patients with AIDS and children's health behavior. She served as the Greek National Coordinator for The COMAC Childhood and Medicines Project.

xiii

Giampaolo Canciani is a pediatrician specializing in Public Health. He is employed in the Emergency Medicine Department of the Trieste Pediatric Hospital where currently he is assisting in its data storage project.

Pia Haudrup Christensen has a postgraduate degree (Magisterkonferens) in anthropology from Copenhagen University. She is currently Research Fellow Associate at Brunel University in West London, England. Her ongoing doctoral research is on the cultural performance of childhood sickness in Denmark.

Concha Colomer, PhD, MD, is Professor in Health Promotion and Director of the WHO Collaborating Centre for Public Health Development, Instituto Valenciano de Estudios en Salud Publica (IVESP) Valencia (Spain), and Associate Lecturer in Public Health (University of Alicante). She is a member of the European Society for Social Pediatrics' Executive Board and of the European Training Consortium for Public Health.

Graham Dukes is a physician and lawyer. He spent eight years as head of WHO's Pharmaceuticals Programme for Europe. Since 1985, he has been Professor of Drug Policy Studies, University of Groningen, Netherlands, and he is also Director of Euro Health Group, the European arm of Management Sciences for Health, Boston.

Marcelino García, MD, received a PhD in 1995 in Clinical Pharmacology, Department of Pharmacology, School of Medicine, University of La Laguna, Tenerife, Canary Islands, Spain. Since 1992, he has been working at the Regional Centre for Drug Surveillance and Drug Information in the Canary Islands. Since 1990, he has been involved in the COMAC Childhood and Medicines Project and directed the study in Tenerife.

Trudie Gerrits studied Cultural Anthropology at the University of Amsterdam, and Education and Communication at the Agricultural University of Wageningen. At the moment she is Project Coordinator of the Medical Anthropology Unit of the University of Amsterdam. Prior to that she worked for five years at the Mozambican Ministry of Health.

Flora M. Haaijer-Ruskamp, PhD, received a masters degree in medical sociology at the University of Groningen, the Netherlands, in 1976. In 1984 she received a PhD in the Medical Faculty, University of Groningen, and since 1994 she has held a chair in that Faculty as Professor of Health Care in Particular Drug Utilization.

Outi Hallia, BA, is a student of cultural anthropology, currently working as a research assistant in the Department of Social Policy, University of Jyväskylä, Finland. She is preparing her master's thesis and is interested in cultural models of medication.

Anita P. Hardon, PhD, is a medical biologist. She has worked for both women's and health organizations and is currently Research Coordinator, Medical Anthropology Unit, University of Amsterdam. Her current research interests involve gender and reproductive health, and the use and provision of medicines in developing countries.

Abraham (Bram) G. Hartzema, PharmD, MSPH, PhD, holds the following positions at the University of North Carolina at Chapel Hill: Professor of Pharmacy Policy and Evaluative Sciences and Director of the Center for Pharmaceutical Outcomes Research at the School of Pharmacy; Clinical Professor of Health Policy and Administration at the School of Public Health; and Research Associate at the Cecil G. Sheps Center for Health Services Research.

Ronald J. Iannotti received his PhD in Developmental Psychology at the State University of New York at Buffalo. He has held teaching and research positions at Marietta College in Ohio, the National Institutes of Mental Health, and Georgetown University School of Medicine, and is currently at Miami University in Ohio.

Vida Jakovljevic has a PhD in Chemistry. She has been involved for many years in studies of drug utilization at the Department of Pharmacology, Toxicology, and Clinical Pharmacology, Faculty of Medicine, University of Novi Sad. Together with Professor Stanulovic, she initiated the use of DDDs and ATCs for comparative drug research. She has published more than 30 articles in this field.

Olli Kalpio, MA, is an ethnologist working as a researcher in the Department of Social Policy, University of Jyväskylä, Finland. He is preparing his doctoral thesis and his interests include children's explanations of illness and qualitative research methods and analysis.

Nila Kapor, PhD, is Professor of Human Development and Mental Health, University of Novi Sad, and Program Officer of UNICEF's Psychosocial Rehabilitation Program for Serbia and Montenegro. She has served as a consultant and advisor to the World Health Organization since 1973 and has participated in a number of cross-cultural investigations.

Aquilino Polaino-Lorente, PhD, MD, a psychiatrist, is Professor and Chair, Department of Psychopathology, School of Education, Complutense University of Madrid. He is interested in defining the role of the pedagogue in health education.

Patrizia Romito, a psychologist, has two doctorates, one in psychology and the other in mother and child health. Her research interests include the physical and mental health of mothers, social policies affecting motherhood, fatherhood, and families, and the doctor-patient relationship.

Ana Sabo is Associate Professor of Pharmacology, Department of Pharmacology, Toxicology, and Clinical Pharmacology, Faculty of Medicine, University of Novi Sad. Dr. Sabo's primary interests have been in pharmacoepidemiology. However, as a clinical pharmacologist, her interests have extended to patients' beliefs, attitudes, and compliance in taking medicines. She has more than 60 publications.

Milan Stanulovic, MD, MSc, DSc, is a Certified Pediatrician and a Certified Pharmacologist. He is Professor of Pharmacology at the Department of Pharmacology, Toxicology, and Clinical Pharmacology, Faculty of Medicine, University of Novi Sad. He initiated the discipline of pharmacoepidemiology not only in Novi Sad but throughout Yugoslavia. He is a member of national and international groups who are interested in drug utilization studies, and has had more than 30 WHO consultancies and more than 250 publications. Recently, he has become interested in sociocultural factors affecting medicine use.

Göran Tomson, MD, PhD, specialist in pediatrics and family medicine, is Associate Professor in International Health, Department of International Health and Social Medicine, Unit of International Health Care Research, Károlinska Institutet, Stockholm, Sweden. He is a member of The Károlinska International Research and Training

(KIRT) Committee and the Management Advisory Committee of the World Health Organization/Drug Action Programme (WHO/DAP), as well as several international networks.

Eleni Valassi-Adam, MD, Associate Professor of Pediatrics and Director of the Department of Social Pediatrics, Institute of Child Health, Athens, Greece, is the author of about 200 publications in scientific journals. Dr. Valassi-Adam is the editor of the *Archives of Hellenic Medicine*, the official journal fo the Athens Medical Society. She has edited two books on maternal and child health and has served as editor of *Paediatriki*, the official journal of the Hellenic Society of Pediatrics. Her interests also include health education and health promotion.

Sjaak van der Geest, PhD, a cultural anthropologist, is Professor at the Anthropological-Sociological Center, University of Amsterdam, the Netherlands. Currently he is investigating the social and cultural meaning of old age in Ghana.

Foreword

With almost every step that our understanding of medicine advances, we find ourselves, at a given moment, looking back over our shoulders in some wonderment as to why we did not fathom the matter earlier. Moving ahead is only exceptionally a question of new techniques and world-shattering new discoveries in the laboratory; in nine out of ten cases it is a matter of doing rather better with the means that are already available to us, and may have been so for a very long time. That is as true with respect to medicines and drugs as it is to the scalpel and the stethoscope. Goodness knows we have reason enough to acclaim the inventor; but there is also a risk that the invention will tempt us onto a new path before we have quite explored the promise of the old one. Thoughtfulness coupled with a dash of conservatism is not uncommonly the best way ahead.

My own involvement in matters of medicines and patients spans only some 35 years, and it is all too easy to attribute all the progress that we have made over that period to what people persist in calling the pharmacological revolution. But there also has been a quieter revolution going on, relating as much to the drugs that have always been with us as to the newcomers; it has been productive because it has put the individual patient, rather than the drug, firmly in the middle of the picture, which is where he or she obviously belongs. In the purest form of drug-centered thinking, the patient is almost an inconvenience; one proceeds from the test tube to the healthy rat, thence to the healthy dog, and thereafter to the healthy human volunteer. If a new drug shows its pharmacological effect in all these phases of study, one will then hasten to identify the most ideal patient population in which its merits can finally be confirmed. Ideal, that is, from the drug-centered point of view. The patients selected will be neither too old, too young, nor too ill; they will not smoke, drink, guzzle, or starve; they will not be pregnant, lactating, or black; they will take no other drug; and above all they will be passive and entirely compliant (which is to say meekly obedient), taking their medicines religiously with the requisite portion of water as the clock strikes seven, twelve, and five. They will have no expectations and no prejudices. They will be the clinical pharmacologist's angels, uncorrupted by the heterogeneity and noncompliance which rage in the bad world beyond.

That is no more than a caricature of the extreme drug-oriented approach to the medicine-patient interface, but all the elements in it are familiar. Too many medicines, for example, still come striding onto the market with the firm admonition that nothing is known as to their suitability for the young. Unless children appear to offer a particularly promising sales opportunity, the admonition may still be there five years later, with ethics offering a convenient excuse to carry out no systematic studies in those of tender age. And if, in due course, such investigations are finally set in train, they are likely to be limited to the bare questions of dosage, therapeutic effect, and safety. The young patient, like the adult patients before him, will still essentially be approached as a passive receptacle into which drugs are delivered to determine their pharmacological effects.

Children, happily, are not quite like that. They think for themselves; they know things; they have their fears and their anticipations; in the light of these things they may go their own way. What is more, they are surrounded by families who may have as great an effect on their well-being and their recovery as a pharmacy full of pills. Above all, they are as different from one another as the day is long. Even more so than in the adult, the effect of prescribing drug treatment to a child is therefore determined only in part by pharmacology and in very large measure by behavior and circumstances; it is as important to take account of the one as of the other in trying to understand and anticipate what treatment may achieve.

Again, one sometimes wonders why these aspects of drug treatment in children were not understood and looked into much earlier. My own pediatric teachers of a generation ago were indeed firm in their realization that "children are not merely small adults," but where medicines were concerned it did not lead them much further than algebraic formulas for calculating pediatric dosage and a number of rules about the hepatic breakdown and renal excretion of drugs in the very young. No further steps were perhaps possible so long as the doctor and the traditional dispensing pharmacist had a monopoly of authority on the scene. It was the arrival in the health field of what were still disparagingly called the "soft" sciences that, more than anything, cast a new light over things; much of what we are now learning is from the pen of the anthropologists, the sociologists, and the psychologists, and as much again has been contributed by a new and creative generation of doctors and pharmacists with wide open eyes.

An important step was the publication in 1992 of the proceedings of the COMAC Workshop on Medicines and Childhood, edited by Deanna Trakas of Athens and Emilio Sanz of Tenerife. It provided a monumental account of the reasons for a new approach to the field; it offered a reconsideration of what could be understood to constitute rational use of medicines in the young; it showed how drug utilization in children could reliably be measured, and above all what the determinants of utilization were likely to be. Based on work in eight countries it also provided a transcultural insight; finding out how Dutch children experienced illness proved as rewarding as discovering how children in Greece decide whether a medicine is "good" or "bad."

The present volume casts the net even more widely in regard to the countries involved and the questions that it seeks to answer. It presents the results of the COMAC study which the previous volume planned and recommended, as well as other studies and reviews. With so much material at hand, the reader is entitled to be told what he can expect of this book. To say that the facts that are now becoming known are fascinating or important (as many of them indeed are) is not enough. Much more essential is that they are now sufficient to provide anyone concerned with the use of drugs in children with a basis for working more effectively. That knowledge is not emerging in the form of universal rules, for there are some differences among countries and situations that may well persist.

The reader is, however, likely to find himself or herself noting numerous findings that are applicable to his or her own professional needs. If I am prescribing in Germany, what home remedies is the child also likely to be receiving? What does my young American patient already know about medicines from the media before I talk to him myself? How can I best ensure that a Greek child will indeed take what I am prescribing? These are the sorts of questions that the health practitioner will be asking: Researchers will ask others, but they too will find certain answers and some pointers as to where other answers may lie.

In recent years the World Bank has become as deeply involved as any other major international agency in issues of health (*Better Health in Africa* 1994; Dukes and Broun 1994; Investing in Health: The World Development Report 1993), for no nation can develop its fullest potential unless the available resources–including medicines– are used to the best advantage. One population group after another– the elderly, pregnant and lactating women, the indigent–have been the subject of studies to determine how medicines can best be used. Now, none too soon, it is the children's turn. The present volume deals very largely with medicines and children in the industrialized world, and one must hope that similar work will follow in countries at an earlier phase of development, for it is there that much of the world's future lies. In the 1960s, a child born in the developing world had only a 77 percent chance of surviving the first five years of life; some 30 years later, the chances of survival have increased to 89 percent *(Better Health in Africa* 1994). Income growth, schooling, and progress in science and medicine have all played their role, but if advance is to continue, all these things will have to be used to the very best advantage. That applies to the use of medicines in eliminating and curing disease in the young as much as it does to other advances in health care. Every credit is due to those who are making the effort to promote our understanding of how drugs can best be used in children, by children, and above all for children–everywhere.

Graham Dukes
Washington, DC

REFERENCES

Better Health in Africa. 1994. The World Bank, Washington, DC.

Dukes, G. and Broun, D. 1994. "Pharmaceutical policies." The World Bank, Washington, DC. (Discussion paper).

Investing in Health: The World Development Report. 1993. The World Bank, Washington, DC. ISBN 0-19-520890-0.

Trakas, D. J. and Sanz, E. J. (editors). 1992. *Studying Childhood and Medicine Use.* Athens, Greece: ZHTA Medical Publications.

Preface

The contributors to this book were members of a research group, some of whom began meeting for planning purposes in 1989.[1] A book, *Studying Childhood and Medicine Use: A Multidisciplinary Approach* (Trakas and Sanz 1992), was based on papers prepared for these early meetings. Subsequent meetings, held to facilitate the development of methods, instruments, and analysis plans, and to share results and plan reports, were funded through a European Economic Community (EEC) *Comité d'Action Concerté* (COM-AC) contract, COMAC/HSR MR4*-CT90-0319, awarded to The Institute on Child Health, Athens, Greece, with Deanna J. Trakas as the Project Leader. The official title of the Contract was "Medicine Use, Behaviour and Children's Perceptions of Medicines and Health Care." However, the working title used in this volume is "The COMAC Childhood and Medicines Project" and the researchers are referred to as the COMAC Research Group (CRG). The CRG consisted of a designated National Coordinator from each of nine European countries, members of their research teams, and consultants from the United States. Local research projects were funded by the university and research center affiliations of the National Coordinators and also by fellowships, grants, and stipends awarded by various agencies to individual research team members.

We believe this book, which presents the contributions of members of a research group, is unique in many ways. Few of the CRG's members knew each other or even each other's work or publications prior to meeting together. The CRG's members represented seven disciplines (health education, medical anthropology, medical sociology, pediatrics, pharmacoepidemiology, pharmacology, pharmacy) and came from ten countries (Denmark, England, Finland, Germany, Greece, Italy, Netherlands, Spain, United States, and Yugoslavia). The members represented both senior and junior level scientists. The process was previously unknown in health services research. Not unique were the attributes of all successful research

xxiii

team efforts: commitment to the project's goals, commitment to work together to succeed, respect for each other's contributions, and eventually, commitment to each other. As Deanna Trakas wrote in the Final Report to COMAC noting the concerted action objectives of the funding agency, "The entire project was, indeed, a concert, composed of different instruments and initially, different ways of playing them. Eventually, we learned to harmonize and began to produce a symphony–or at least not a cacophony–through the orchestrated efforts of first chairs and their willing accomplices in the ensemble."

"The COMAC Childhood and Medicines Project" was undertaken for several reasons. One was in response to the increased recognition that variations in medicine use among different populations have a social or cultural component. A second reason was to provide information that could be used for planning methods to educate children and their families about medicines. A third was to explore a combination of qualitative and quantitative methods for cross-cultural comparisons of medicine use.

The magnitude of differences in medicine use, even among the relatively similar Nordic countries, came as somewhat of a surprise to pharmacoepidemiologists in the 1970s following application of a new measurement tool, Defined Daily Doses (DDDs) (Nordic Council on Medicines 1979). DDDs permitted comparisons of the consumption of a particular chemical entity, thus overcoming problems attendant to using sales and production records to measure medicine use (Rabin and Bush 1974). For even a very high-specificity drug-condition pair, insulin and diabetes, the evidence indicated that differences in use of the medicine could not be accounted for by differences in the prevalence of the condition (Bergman 1979). Lacking differences in morbidity as more than a partial explanation, other candidates seemed likely to be: differences in structural factors relative to health care systems, differences in economic forces, differences in prescriber behavior, and differences in consumer behavior. While the first three candidates have received considerable research attention, consumer behavior other than purchasing has received little more than theoretical recognition. Thus, it appeared that a contribution could be made if it were possible to investigate and compare medicine use at the level of the family, and specifically to investigate and compare how cultural beliefs, attitudes, expectations, and behaviors regarding the use of medicines are transmitted to children within the context of their families.

The second impetus for "The COMAC Childhood and Medicines Project" arose from the observation, confirmed by research, that much medicine use among populations was "irrational" from a medical point of view (Sanz 1992). Health care providers and policymakers were often frustrated at the behavior of their populations in not doing what they were supposed to do–in not taking their medicines when they should (Wirsing and Sommerfeld 1992) and in taking products with no demonstrated evidence of efficacy. These concerns led to efforts to try to develop methods to educate consumers about rational medicine use. Such efforts were handicapped by lack of knowledge about how people learn about medicines and how people use medicines, although evidence began to accumulate that more medicine use was self-directed than resulted from contact with a health care provider (Kleinman 1980; Levin, Beske, and Fry 1988). Although it was obvious that medicine use was a frequent health behavior and that at some age children began to take some responsibility for medicine use, observations indicated that medicine use was rarely included as a topic in schoolchildren's health education curricula (Bush and Hardon 1990). If not learning about medicines in school, it seemed likely that children were socialized into medicine use within their families, with possibilities for some influence from their wider environments. Acquiring information about what families and children know and do appeared to have the potential for developing targeted medicine use education programs for future implementation.

Third, no methodology existed for comparing children's orientations toward medicines. Medical anthropologists had made significant contributions to our understanding of cultural orientations toward illness in general and the role of medicine use in particular in developing societies (Bledsoe and Goubaud 1985; Hardon 1987; Nichter 1980; van der Geest and Whyte 1989), and some efforts had been made to use qualitative methods in gathering information directly from American children in single-area studies (Bush and Davidson 1982; Korbin and Zahorik 1985). In 1987, anthropologists from Greece, Netherlands, and Sweden developed a common qualitative methodology to study children's health behavior, medicine use, and perceptions about them primarily through the mechanism of asking the children to make drawings of themselves when they were ill and to talk about their drawings (den Toom and Hardon 1992; Sachs 1992; Trakas 1992). From this effort, it became apparent that a common protocol held out promise for comparing medicine use information obtained from children and their families in different cultures. Although the protocol would reflect a multidisciplinary perspective, its focus on cultural aspects of medicine use meant that it would primarily reflect the methods of social anthropology but would incorporate quantitative methods where warranted.

The chapters in this book, which are based on "The COMAC Childhood and Medicines Project," are presented in four sections. Section One provides background and context. Its four chapters present more information about the Project, a discussion of traditional qualitative and quantitative methods in comparative research and how they relate to the methods used, a social-anthropological theoretical framework for studying medicine use in childhood, and contextual and structural factors that account in part for differences in medicine use among the different populations. Section Two consists of six chapters devoted to the results of comparisons among selected local studies. One chapter is devoted to comparisons of medicines kept in the households and one chapter to comparisons of how childhood fever is treated as reported by children and their primary caretakers. Presented in two chapters are comparisons of children's perceived benefits of medicines and comparisons of the decision makers involved in treating childhood illness among a U.S. community and two communities in Spain. Another chapter compares children's perceptions of illness and medicines as having pleasant and unpleasant aspects, and another reports children's concepts of dangers and side effects associated with use of medicines. The third section's six chapters are based on the special interests of four local teams of investigators, although these too are derived primarily from data acquired through use of the shared research methodology. They include issues in medicines and self-medication in families, understanding illness concepts of children from a developmental perspective, use of unconventional and conventional therapies, and parent-child agreement on perceptions and meanings of illness episodes and medicine use. The last section titled "Viewpoints" contains five chapters presenting the implications of the book from the perspectives of medical anthropologists and sociologists, health policymakers, health providers, health educators, and pharmacoepidemiologists.

The editors wish to acknowledge, with an abundance of gratitude, the support of COMAC and The Institute of Child Health, Athens, Greece, and the agencies who funded local studies. These were, in addition to the academic institutions associated with faculty and student investigators, in Denmark, Health Insurance Foundation Research Fund and The Danish Research Council for the Humanities; in Finland, The Academy of Finland; in Greece, Glaxo Pharmaceutical, Athens; in Spain, The General Directorate for Scientific and Technical Research, The Ministry of Education and Science; in the Netherlands, The Ministry of Welfare, Public Health and Culture; in the United States, The United States Pharmacopeial Convention, Inc., and The American-Scandinavian Foundation, Inc. Financial support facilitated not only this volume, but also two undergraduate dissertations, four master's theses, and six doctoral theses. The importance of funding new researchers in the area of children and medicines cannot be underestimated. As a result, there is an international group of young investigators who are very likely to carry on the work and to train others long after we editors have retired.

It has been said that a book's preface is a self-indulgent opportunity for the book's authors to acknowledge its shortcomings. We editors readily admit to shortcomings and we welcome your comments. However, we hope you will look beyond them to see this book as seminal, as a stimulus to the future. We will regard it as a success if it provokes discussion, criticism, and argument, but most of all, if it provokes an outpouring of research that is similarly international, collaborative, and multidisciplinary.

NOTES

1. The Planning Committee consisted of the following scientists (Note: Affiliations are those in effect when the Committee was meeting):

Amy Blue, PhD, Anthropologist, Department of Anthropology, Case Western Reserve, Cleveland, Ohio, USA

Patricia J. Bush, PhD, Pharmacosociologist, Professor and Director, Division of

Children's Health Promotion, Department of Family Medicine, Georgetown University School of Medicine, Washington, DC, USA

Maurice Cuthbert, MD, PhD, FIBiol, Senior Medical Officer, Research Management Department of Health, London, UK

Domingo A. Garcia-Villamisar, PhD, Psychologist, Assistant Professor, Faculty of Psychology, Central University of Barcelona, Tarragona, Spain

Flora M. Haaijer-Ruskamp, PhD, Pharmacosociologist, Professor, Department of Health Sciences and Pharmacology/Clinical Pharmacology, WHO Collaborating Center of Clinical Pharmacology and Drug Policy Science, University of Groningen, Netherlands

Anita Hardon, PhD, Medical Biologist, Anthropologist, Department of Cultural Anthropology, University of Amsterdam, Netherlands

Sussi Skov Jensen, PhD, Anthropologist, Institute of Anthropology, University of Copenhagen, Denmark

Berry Mayall, PhD, Sociologist, Thomas Coram Research Unit, London, UK

Dunja Moeller, PhD, Anthropologist, Institute of Ethnology, University of Hamburg, Germany

Marina Petronoti, MSc, Anthropologist, National Center for Social Research, Athens, Greece

Patrizia Romito, PhD, Psychologist, Istituto per l'Infanzia, Trieste, Italy

Emilio J. Sanz, MD, PhD, Clinical Pharmacologist, Reader, Pharmacology Department, Clinical Pharmacology, University of La Laguna, Tenerife, Spain

Johannes Sommerfeld, PhD, Anthropologist, Institute of Ethnology, University of Hamburg, Germany

Milan Stanulovic, MD, PhD, Clinical Pharmacologist, Professor of Pharmacology, Department of Pharmacology and Toxicology, University of Novi Sad, Yugoslavia

Vibeke Steffen, MA, Anthropologist, Institute of Cultural Anthropology, University of Copenhagen, Denmark

Mirjam den Toom, MA, Anthropologist, Department of Cultural Anthropology, University of Copenhagen, Denmark

Deanna J. Trakas, PhD, Anthropologist, Department of Social Pediatrics, Institute of Child Health, Athens, Greece

REFERENCES

Bledsoe, C. H. and Goubaud, M. F. 1985. "The reinterpretation of Western pharmaceuticals among the Mende of Sierra Leone." *Social Science and Medicine* 21(3):275-283.

Bergman, U. 1979. "International Comparisons of Drug Utilization: Use of Antidiabetic Drugs in Seven European Countries." *Studies in Drug Utilization—Methods and Applications,* edited by U. Bergman, A. Grimsson, A. H. W. Wahba and B. Westerholm. Copenhagen: World Health Organization Regional Office for Europe, pgs. 147-162.

Bush, P. J. and Davidson, F. R. 1982. "Medicines and 'drugs': What do children think?" *Health Education Quarterly* 9 (2&3):113-128.

Bush, P. J. and Hardon, A. P. 1990. "Toward rational medicine use: Is there a role for children?" *Social Science and Medicine* 31 (9):1043-1050.

den Toom, M. and Hardon, A. P. 1992. "Illness attitudes and perceptions of medicine in Dutch children." *Studying Childhood and Medicine Use,* edited by D. J. Trakas and E. J. Sanz. Athens, Greece: ZHTA Medical Publications, pgs. 93-104.

Hardon, A. P. 1987. "The use of modern pharmaceuticals in a Filipino village: Doctor's prescription and self-medication. *Social Science and Medicine* 25 (3):277-292.

Kleinman, A. 1980. *Patients and Healers in the Context of Culture: An Exploration of the Borderland between Anthropology and Psychiatry.* Berkeley: University of California Press.

Korbin, J. E. and Zahorik, P. 1985. "Childhood, health and illness: Beliefs and behaviors of urban American schoolchildren." *Medical Anthropology* (fall):337-353.

Levin, L. S., Beske, R., and Fry, J. 1988. *Self-Medication in Europe.* WHO Regional Office for Europe, Copenhagen.

Nichter, M. 1980. "The layperson's perception of medicine as perspective into the utilization of multiple therapy systems in the Indian context." *Social Science and Medicine* 14B (4):225-233.

Nordic Drug Council. 1979. *Nordic Statistics on Medicines 1975-1977. Part II. Nordic Drug Index with Classification and Defined Daily Doses.* NLM Publication No 3. Oslo.

Rabin, D. L. and Bush, P. J. 1974. "The use of medicines: Historical trends and international comparisons." *International Journal of Health Services* 4 (1):61-87.

Sachs, E. J. 1992. "Sweet medicine: The symbolic role of medicines in the socialization of illness behaviour (Sweden)." *Studying Childhood and Medicine Use,* edited by D. J. Trakas and E. J. Sanz. Athens: ZHTA Medical Publications, pgs. 143-152.

Sanz, E. J. 1992. "Hazards of medication in children." *Studying Childhood and Medicine Use,* edited by D. J. Trakas and E. J. Sanz. Athens, Greece: ZHTA Medical Publications, pgs. 93-104.

Trakas, D. J. 1992. "Heavy and light illnesses and medicines: Accounts from Greek children." *Studying Childhood and Medicine Use,* edited by D. J. Trakas and E. J. Sanz. Athens, Greece: ZHTA Medical Publications, pgs. 161-170.

Trakas, D. J. and Sanz, E. J. (editors). 1992. *Studying Childhood and Medicine Use.* Athens, Greece: ZHTA Medical Publications.

Van der Geest, S. and Whyte, S. R. (editors). 1989. *The Context of Medicines in Developing Countries: Studies in Pharmaceutical Anthropology.* Dordrecht/Boston/London: Kluwer Academic Publishers.

Wirsing, R. and Sommerfeld, J. 1992. "Compliance–a medical anthropological appraisal." *Studying Childhood and Medicine Use,* edited by D. J. Trakas and E. J. Sanz. Athens, Greece: ZHTA Medical Publications, pgs. 17-30.

SECTION I: INTRODUCTION

Chapter 1

The History of the COMAC Childhood and Medicines Project: A Reflection on Multidisciplinary Research

Deanna J. Trakas

The COMAC Childhood and Medicines Project[1] was completed in 1993 by a group of energetic and dedicated scientists who cooperated for more than three years in its planning and realization. This volume presents but a small portion of their energy which helped the Project grow beyond initial expectations. As the rationale, goals, and methodology are discussed elsewhere in this volume, this chapter addresses the Project's practical dimensions by recounting the multidisciplinary process by which the protocol was developed and implemented. It would be impossible to comprehend the Project outside of the context of its historical development and without recognizing the contribution of those scientists who helped form its foundations and who made it a reality.

THE PREHISTORY OF THE PROJECT

In 1981, a small study of medicine-use behavior in Greece was conducted through the Institute of Child Health, Athens. Systematic

1

observations of interactions in pharmacies were followed by home visits with the clientele where an inventory of medications in the home was made. The format was designed not only to record their numbers and types, but to prompt the informant to review health problems and the way in which they were handled (or not) through medications. Asking the informant to show the actual medications, preferably in their storage areas, provided a "solid" reference point from which to begin discussing the importance of medicines in the home. This technique, which had also been used independently in U.S. studies by Patricia J. Bush, was further refined during the COMAC Childhood and Medicines Project, producing the Medicine Cabinet Inventory (MCI; see Chapter 5), a central instrument for data collection.

Four years later, Graham Dukes, at that time Regional Officer of Pharmaceuticals, WHO/EURO, suggested that the anthropological perspective of the study be "renovated" and implemented on a cross-cultural basis in Europe. This indicated a recognition that there was room for comparative drug utilization studies in Europe to expand and to develop systematic methods of examining the behavioral dimension of "drug use," an on-the-ground (or "grassroots") investigation of psychosocial and sociocultural factors that are involved in "drug utilization."

The Regional Office of Pharmaceuticals promoted a meeting in 1987 to discuss the possibility of organizing a comparative study of the sociocultural differences related to medicine use in Europe. It was proposed that the study involve representatives from both northern and southern Europe since many of the differences in the pharmaceutical market had been observed to occur on this axis. Those present at the meeting discussed the rationale for an anthropological investigation of medicine use in Europe to complement the pharmacoepidemiological studies concerned with issues of prescription rates, sales rates, "compliance," and "rational drug use." Whereas these studies had demonstrated the considerable differences in medicine "use" among European countries, they usually did not provide explanations, or address the issue of people's actual behavior once away from the pharmacy or clinic. Anthropological investigations of medicine-use behavior on the other hand, had been confined to non-European countries and non-Western cultures, where the contradictions between the use of "traditional medicines" and modern pharmaceuticals is a pronounced interface which is attractive for its "exotic rather than its "rational" dimensions.

In response, a small intercountry study was conducted in Greece, Sweden, and the Netherlands, about children's perceptions of illness and medicines. Assuming that attitudes about medicines are developed, and possibly expressed, before adulthood, it was logical to focus on childhood as an important foundation in the evolution of adult medicine-use behavior. Children acted as the major participants in the study (rather than parents or pediatricians as had been the case in most previous studies of medicines and childhood). Following the suggestion of Lisbeth Sachs, Károlinska Institute, Stockholm, an anthropological interviewing technique was developed which began with children visually depicting their own illness experiences. The Drawing Interview became one of the cornerstones for data collection and analysis in the Project after scientists from additional disciplines had added to its design, direction, and methods of analysis.

The three-country study was presented at two meetings of the Drug Utilization Research Group (DURG EURO/WHO): the first at the Meeting on Medicine Use in Children, held in Novi Sad in 1988, and the second at the DURG Meeting in the Netherlands in 1989. In both meetings, the audience was composed primarily of pharmacologists, pharmacists, and physicians. The anthropological perspective may have raised some eyebrows, provoked some thoughtful frowns, but from the discussion that followed, there appeared to be a growing support for the participation of anthropologists in medicine-use studies conducted in Europe.

During the same time period, a brief proposal based on the three-country study was submitted to the Commission for Concerted Action Medical Research (COMAC). In response, the Commission extended an invitation for the composition of a Planning Committee which met in Brussels in March and June, 1989. A variety of scientific specialties was represented in the Committee and the sense of a multidisciplinary research effort was an integral part of the Project from the very beginning. However, the challenge of creating a multidisciplinary project was evident during the planning meetings. At least two "factions" developed at the first meeting: the "hard" scientists (e.g., clinical pharmacologists) and "soft" ones (e.g., anthropologists). Phrases such as "rational drug use" and "compliance" fell hard on the ears of the anthropologists; those having conducted studies using these concepts were dismayed when attempts were made to demystify this terminology; the lack of anthropological interest in "sample size" and "dummy tables" was received without enthusiasm by the clinical pharmacologists and physicians.

The organization and functioning of COMAC was explained to the Planning Committee by Andre E. Baert, its Director. As constituted in 1990, COMAC was composed of six research divisions: Aging, Life-Style Diseases, AIDS, Cancer, Pharmaceuticals, and Health Services Research (HSR). The Project was assigned to the HSR Division. COMAC provided financial support for the *coordination* of the Project (e.g., meetings of National Coordinators and representatives of local research teams, exchange of data, exchange of personnel and other costs of coordination. One of the goals of COMAC was to foster cooperative research within the European Community, following the guidelines of "concerted action," i.e., a concert– an orchestrated ensemble–wherein each musician performs under the direction of a conductor, i.e., the Project Leader. In order to make the metaphor a reality, clearly a common language needed to be developed; a language that would facilitate a true discourse among scientists from so many diverse specialties, and, indeed, cultures.

Members of the Planning Committee were invited by the Project Leader to give an overview of the issues in medicine use and childhood from the prism of their specialties. The clinical pharmacologists presented findings about adverse drug reactions in children and the use of antibiotics, vitamins, and appetite stimulants; the sociologists placed consumer behavior in the context of various models; the psychologists raised the issue of developmental levels and defining "the healthy child;" the anthropologists discussed the differences between the "folk," the "popular," and the biomedical health systems.

COORDINATION MEETINGS

The Protocol was approved by COMAC in December, 1990, and the first Coordination Meeting was held in Athens in April, 1991. Some local teams sent new members and new teams joined the effort. Despite the new synthesis of the group, the spirit of the earlier planning meetings was rekindled, and the protocol, a document which now needed to be put into practice, was rediscovered. The planning meetings were characterized by a distinct lack of hierarchy wherein all members worked together in a spirit of equality, each sharing ideas from their areas of expertise with the others and taking on pieces of the task at hand consistent with their areas of expertise. Decisions were reached through a process of consensus, rather than arbitration. This method of working together was to continue throughout all the coordination meetings and workshops of the Project.

Pilot studies were conducted in the summer of 1991 followed by a second coordination meeting for their evaluation in Rhodes, Greece, in the autumn. Most of the local research teams began data collection for the main study by January, 1992. By this time, ten teams in nine countries were represented in the Project, the synthesis of most local research teams had been solidified, and several had obtained economic support for their local studies. In cases where local funds were not obtained, data collection and analysis were conducted by volunteer field researchers who viewed their field work as a learning experience and an opportunity to attend coordination workshops. This was enhanced by their attendance at Coordination Workshops.

Some teams were quite extensive: they included field researchers, consultants, and auxiliary scientific, technical, and administrative personnel. Other local research efforts were realized primarily by one field researcher, scientifically supervised by the National Coordinator, and, in one case, the coordinator was also the sole researcher. If the terms "local team" and "National Coordinator" seem to be exaggerations given the small size of some teams, it should be emphasized that the responsibilities of National Coordinators in all countries were not confined to directing a large team of researchers, but also involved locating funding sources and securing administrative "team members" from university and research affiliations.

During 1992-1993, three additional Coordination Workshops were held in Athens and Tenerife, Spain, to encourage the "continual analysis" of local data and to facilitate the exchange of data. Unlike many intercountry epidemiological and statistical studies, the qualitative data gathered in this Project required continual review in order to formulate comparative categories that could be used across local studies (e.g., "cross-culturally"). A major part of one meeting was devoted to developing these categories and resulted in a consensus report which served as the guideline for the preparation of country reports in the form of interpretative essays. A "computer meeting" was arranged for standardizing a code book for handling the quantitative data with the purpose of developing future comparative publications. The final workshop was arranged for drafting the Final Project Report to COMAC (Trakas 1993). Excerpts from local study reports were compiled in a document for review by the team members. The participants also worked to pull together theoretical threads, lines of discussion, and interpretations. Thus, the Final Report was truly a group effort, and held onto the spirit of concerted action to the end.

Comparative subprojects had been performed and the meetings provided the opportunity for their presentation in plenary sessions and working groups. Some local teams, by the nature of their composition, had implemented methods beyond those stated in the project-level protocol. Some added quantitative methods such as measures of children's autonomy, knowledge of medicines, developmental levels, and locus of control. Others concentrated on the collection of information through the use of qualitative methods, such as participant observation, the use of adult health diaries (parental or school nurses), and in-depth interviews with parents. This enriched the quality of the Project which had designated a modest number of instruments precisely to allow for local research teams to, not only conform to their use, but to add to them; indeed some members of the Project used both Project level instruments and additional ones in order to develop Master's Theses and Doctoral Dissertations. This is perhaps one of the most exciting dimensions of the concerted action which involved scientists at various levels of their careers ranging from experts in the field to those completely new to it.

REFLECTIONS ON THE MULTIDISCIPLINARY RESEARCH EXPERIENCE

While pleas and plans for multidisciplinary research are often heard, its implementation often falls short of original goals. It is an effort that "looks good on paper" but has challenges that must be identified and met. The COMAC Childhood and Medicines Project had the additional dimension of being multicentered, with local teams formed in various configurations in terms of disciplines involved.

Some national teams were multidisciplinary and multicentered; others were homogeneous, drawing their members from the same scientific discipline as the coordinator. Both types have their value in a concerted action, multidisciplinary project. At the local level, coordinators with multidisciplinary and multicentered teams faced challenges similar to those of the Project Leader; for example, to develop a basis for a "balance" between the scientific disciplines represented, to maintain communication links between centers, and to draw together the multidimensional data into a cohesive end-product. Coordinators of homogeneous teams had the security of working entirely within their "own territory" at the local level, developing strong perspectives. Their challenge arose when presenting discipline-specific methods of analysis and interpretations of data at coordinating workshops. Still other local teams worked with a "binary" approach; e.g., one physician and one behavioral scientist, or one pharmacosociologist and one medical anthropologist. This helped to balance the team so that it could manage the demands of, for example, classifying medicines by pharmacological properties as well as describing and interpreting their "meaning" to the consumer. These various combinations certainly led to the fluidity of exchanging and explaining different types of data among members of the group.

As the end of the contract drew closer, it was realized that the Project and the support of COMAC had allowed the members of the group to move and to be moved. The movement was actually visual in plenary sessions where participants began by sitting strategically in clusters, either by scientific background or by country. Slowly, our static positions would shift; first by shifting *in* our chairs, then by shifting chairs, then by changing seats altogether. Working groups were formed spontaneously during coffee breaks and meals to focus on exchanging specific information, refining data collection instruments, or analyzing the esoteric meaning of results. The energy and conclusions were then shared with the entire team. We found that we had became quite mobile, not only in moving to different seats during plenary sessions, but in being able to move out of our own scientific backgrounds to respect and embrace each other's perspectives.

NOTE

1. The coordination for the COMAC Childhood and Medicines Project, Contract MR4*-CT90-0319, was administered through the Institute of Child Health, Athens, Greece. The official title of the Contract was "Medicine Use, Behaviour and Children's Perceptions of Medicines and Health Care."

REFERENCE

Trakas, D. J. (editor). 1993. *Medicine Use, Behaviour, and Children's Perceptions of Medicines and Care Services.* Final Report to COMAC/HSR. Child Health Institute, Athens, Greece. (unpublished).

Chapter 2

Cross-Cultural Comparative Research: A Discourse on Using Qualitative and Quantitative Methodologies

Rolf L. Wirsing
Deanna J. Trakas

The methodological approach of the COMAC Childhood and Medicines Project[1] was inspired primarily by anthropological and sociological concepts. The goal was to discover another kind of "truth" other than that provided by pharmacoepidemiological data, to obtain a deeper picture of what people, especially children, do with and think about medicines. Thus, we began with a methodological frame which included ethnographic interviews followed by content analysis, and to some degree also participant observation. These qualitative techniques are well known to experienced anthropologists.

However, because some of our cooperating teams from several nations also included scientists trained in quantitative techniques and hypothesis testing, we discovered that we also needed to learn from each other about the value of using both qualitative and quantitative methods of data collection. We often found ourselves in debates about the merits of qualitative versus quantitative research, each "camp" faced with the difficulties of using either one or the other approach. These debates were exacerbated when we wanted to reach a consensus on how to do cross-cultural comparisons. We now believe that all of the participants who were part of our concerted action benefitted from these discussions and successfully resolved most of the difficulties.

This chapter presents the methodology of the COMAC Childhood and Medicines Project to familiarize the reader with the methodological issues. In the first part, those methodological issues are addressed that continually presented themselves during the course of designing and carrying out our multidisciplinary, multimethod, and multicultural study. The second part of the chapter summarizes the research questions and the specific instruments and approaches actually used.

But now we turn to an examination of the deeper methodological questions that arise when qualitative and quantitative research methodologies are used in cross-cultural comparative research.

METHODOLOGICAL ISSUES

Comparative Research in General

Importance in Anthropology

Most anthropologists probably would agree that their discipline has always been a comparative one. This is not to mean that comparisons are exclusive to anthropology or to any other discipline but that comparisons are an inherent aspect of human thinking. Lay persons, as well as scientists, make comparisons and the only difference between their respective endeavors is that the latter observe certain methodological rules to help them proceed in a more systematic fashion.

Methodological Rules

Scientific comparisons are made by examining specific qualities or patterns of complex research units, such as individuals or cultures. This allows for the comparison of, e.g., apples and oranges or, perhaps, the Kung Bushmen of the Kalahari desert with factory workers in post-industrialized societies. Apples and oranges are "members" of the general category fruits and can be compared according to specific qualities such as color, weight, size, nutritive value, etc. African Bushmen and U.S. factory workers are members of different cultures and can be examined according to such cultural patterns as marriage customs, residence rules after marriage, division of labor, and organization of time.

In order to make comparisons there must be a defined standard that operationalizes the conditions under which two elements should be considered equal or unequal with respect to the quality/ pattern being observed. Setting standards of equality is more common in, but not exclusive to, the natural/positive sciences than in interpretative ones such as anthropology. There exist universally agreed-upon standards for many one-dimensional qualities important in natural sciences (e.g., weight, length, or time) but there are practically none for many qualities, patterns, and complex configurations that interest anthropologists. Minimal standards for the cross-cultural classification, comparison, and theorizing of a variety of simple cultural patterns, such as kinship structures (Murdock 1949) or concepts of disease causation (Clements 1932; Foster 1976; Murdock 1980) have sometimes been reached in earlier cross-cultural studies. However, there are practically no agreed-upon standards for establishing equality or differences among complex cultural configurations such as highly elaborated ideational systems. But even if established or recommended classifications are available and used, no anthropologist engaged in cross-cultural comparisons can ever be certain if such preconceived categories will prove theoretically useful for his or her particular research question. Anthropologists doing fieldwork have usually ignored such categories or standards and have attempted to discover those concepts and categories that are grounded in data or seemed useful for the understanding of what happened in the field.

The Need for a Theoretical Goal

All (good) scientists recognize that the process of making comparisons is not an end in itself; it is done with a theoretical goal in mind. Thus, to discover that two cultures are similar or dissimilar regarding concepts of disease causation may be interesting, and even contribute to our knowledge, but the discovery remains at the descriptive level. An anthropologist (or any other scientist for that matter) should never stop at this point but should proceed with the next level, i.e., the question of why any two cultures differ or are similar with respect to a quality/pattern.

The answer to this question usually arrives in the form of a general statement, a working hypothesis, that is grounded in the data. Such a general statement will be proposed by the anthropologist on the basis of his or her extensive knowledge of the cultures compared and by taking into account the theoretical discussions in the existing literature. The ultimate goal of comparison is thus to generate new theoretical insights or to support existing theories that make understandable or effectively explain what has been observed and classified.

Regional Comparative Studies as Cooperative Field Studies in Anthropology

Early Cross-Cultural Studies

Comparisons across cultures with the aim of theory testing have a long history in anthropology. The first study of this type was done about 100 years ago and is ascribed to Tylor (1889). It was based on the codification and quantitative analysis of published ethnographic sources from an unknown number of cultures (more than 100) from all around the world. But with the emergence of a culture-relativistic and an anti-theoretical stance under Boas (1896), cross-cultural studies, as they became to be called, soon fell into oblivion. They become popular again with Murdock's (1949) *Social Structure*. Their golden age was in the 1960s and 1970s (see also Wirsing 1975). Now the number of published worldwide cross-cultural studies that are performed in the library is dwindling. They have become slowly replaced by regional comparative studies performed in the field. Since our concerted action was primarily a regional comparative study, focusing on regionally close European societies, some of its major methodological characteristics and problems are outlined in this chapter.

Regional Comparative Studies

Regional comparative studies are coordinated field studies done by cooperating anthropologists within at least two regionally close cultures. Well-designed studies of this type are still rare (for examples of current and presumably well-designed regional comparative studies see Kramer 1980; Munroe and Munroe 1986; and Johnson and Johnson 1987, all of which are cited in Johnson 1991). The reason for this scarcity is the traditional individualism of anthropological researchers and their image of the brave, lone researcher enduring hardships in exotic, even dangerous settings (Johnson 1991, p. 15).

Methodological characteristics. Regional comparative studies are always carried out with a theoretical problem in mind. The problem is in the form of one or more research questions that ask about the antecedents or consequences of particular customs or beliefs that are known to vary between cultures. The issue of the selection of cultures has, however, been given little thought in actual field research. Ideally, the cultures selected should both maximize the cross-cultural variation of the phenomena under investigation and minimize within-culture variation. But, with few exceptions, sampling among viable societies–as in our project–has been opportunistic, relying on the availability of funding, the voluntary (or, occasionally supported) participation of professional colleagues in the selected societies, and other factors not driven by design. The selection and comparison of only two cultures is by far the most common in anthropology (Johnson 1991, p. 13), but there are already a few regional comparisons with more than ten cultures (see also Munroe and Munroe 1991, p. 155).

Modern comparative field studies–such as ours–employ a variety of data collection procedures ranging from qualitative to quantitative and from standardized to unstandardized methods. But to ensure comparability between units (i.e., cultures) and subunits (e.g., individuals), it is advisable that anthropologists use uniform, preset, and standardized techniques in addition. To these belong standardized observations and the formal interviewing of informants as individual respondents. We might add that our study exclusively relied on a set of uniform instruments that we had agreed upon in various cooperative meetings (see below).

Problems of comparative studies. Regional comparative studies are not without problems. A particular problem frequently raised by cultural relativists is the cultural equivalence of central theoretical concepts (e.g., our concept of "medicine") and the standardized measures (i.e., our set of interview questions) employed by all of the research teams. No simple translation of the questions from, e.g., an English original into, e.g., German, Spanish, and Finnish, however well done, will guarantee that Germans, Spaniards, and Finns understand them in the same way as was intended. Cultural nonequivalence endangers the validity of relevant concepts and questions and leads to errors of interpretation. While there are ways to diminish this problem (e.g., by a simple wording of questions and back translation procedures (see Brislin, Lonner, and Thorndike 1973, p. 32) we more heavily relied on the use of more than one question or measure for each dimension under investigation and on the use of triangulation. Triangulation of results by means of multiple methods of data gathering that also include standard ethnographic enquiry also ensures that such errors of interpretation can be kept at a minimum (see also below).

Another problem relates to the limited scope of generalizations in regional studies that use only two societies. Many anthropologists, after they notice interesting differences between two cultural units feel tempted to decide that the differences must be correlated with some other differences. At this point, almost any anthropologist could think of a theoretical rationale to explain this "correlation" (see Johnson 1991, p. 13).

Problems of interpretation are also apt to arise if one compares large complex nations rather than relatively homogeneous cultures. In complex nations, such as the United States or European cultures, the respective subunits–such as cities, families, and individuals–are likely to vary greatly with respect to the phenomenon under investigation. If the variation in our national sample of subunits does not reflect the true variation in the nation (as might easily happen if we only study a small number of families from one or two locations in each nation), differences between nations based on the modal or typical values of such samples are difficult to explain. For instance, the American research team noticed that there were huge differences between the family medicine-cabinet inventories stemming from Washington DC and those coming from Chapel Hill, North Carolina. Since the U.S. team thus tapped only part of the true within-nation variation, it can never be certain whether the true (but unmeasured) variation within the U.S. is larger or smaller than the (observed) between-nation variation, such as between the U.S. and Germany. The actual observed difference between the American samples raises the additional questions, "Which one of the two American locations–if any–should be considered typical for the American nation?" and "What do the observed differences between the inventories of either Chapel Hill or Washington and those of one selected German city, such as Hamburg, mean?"

Qualitative Research

Characteristics and Advantages of Qualitative Research

Qualitative research that dwells on words rather than numbers has always been the dominant approach of certain social sciences, notably of anthropology and history, but is also used in sociology and psychology. The interpretations and generalizations deriving from qualitative data are presented in written prose supplemented by supporting data, such as simple statements of fact from a variety of sources, a story told in the words of the researcher or informant, or a citation that uses the original words of a research subject.

Its obvious strengths are twofold. It provides rich descriptive data and it helps to understand selected cultural phenomena of *one* group or society under investigation.

Descriptive data, "emic" concepts, and different levels of investigation. Qualitative data aid in making descriptive generalizations about human thinking and behavior that are typical for one group, one culture or one society. The richness of its data derives from the fact that generalizations are supported from many sources of data collected by different methods at different levels of investigation. Anthropologists are likely to rely heavily on data generated by qualitative and unstructured participant observation in "natural" contexts and by informal questioning of informants as cultural reporters. These procedures are ideal for eliciting cultural constructs as "emic" concepts and for richly describing processes within social situations.

Qualitative researchers (in contrast to quantitative researchers) pay much attention to the specific language used in a situation in order to understand a specific behavior or cultural domain. By listening carefully to the way people discuss a phenomenon and to what words they use and what conceptual and moral distinctions they make, the researcher can learn the situation-specific "emic"[2] concepts and points of views relevant to the members of the culture under investigation.

Anthropologists doing qualitative field research focus on different levels of investigation. Levels of investigation can be individuals, aggregates of individuals (e.g., households), or frequently occurring social situations. They constitute the level at which data is collected. The concept of "level" indicates that there is a hierarchy of types of levels, and that data collected at a lower, e.g., individual level can be aggregated to make statements about a next higher level, for instance the family or household level. It also means that data can be collected at each level without necessarily resorting to data at its lower level. Anthropologists, for instance, talk with individuals, collect data on households from documents, household heads or informants, and observe the participants and interactions within frequently occurring social situations.

Understanding cultural phenomena. Qualitative research is more than mere description. It is also done with the goal of "understanding" selected cultural phenomena. However, unlike in quantitative positivistic research, events are not "explained" in deductive fashion by appeal to preconceived universal laws but by pointing out empirically observed regularities and relationships that fit an emerging theory. Qualitative anthropological research also achieves an "understanding" of cultural phenomena by, e.g., preserving the chronological flow that leads up to the phenomena in question and by analyzing the social, cultural, and historical context and structures in which these processes and phenomena usually occur. Additional understanding is also achieved by not ignoring the cognitions, meanings, and values, i.e., the "emic" point of view, which the research subjects associate with the phenomena in question. This approach is especially appropriate for the understanding of seemingly unique cultural complexes and ideational institutions that are marked by historical and cultural embeddedness, by cognitive and symbolic elaborations, moral complexity, and by a limited geographical distribution.

The "understanding" we thus achieve does not yield the "objective truth" but perhaps a glimpse into the complexities of human thought and action. It sustains the discussion about morally important issues, refines the debate about them, and provides food for further thought (Buchanan 1992, p. 131ff).

Answers to Critics

Critics with a different conception of what "real" science ought to be "about" typically operate from a scientistic or positivistic tradition that has idealized investigative models borrowed from the natural sciences. They start with preconceived theories and concepts from which they deduce hypotheses to be tested. They then stress a strict division between researcher and data collector in order to reduce personal bias and favor the manipulation of the research settings. Finally, they insist on the replicability of findings, and value exactness and precision by means of quantification.

Testing theories or creating new hypotheses? Let us address each point in turn. First, the idea that science should attempt to test (or "falsify") existing theories. While nobody denies that testing preconceived theories is an important goal of science, approaches are also needed that are suited to the generation of new theories solidly grounded in data. The latter is an ideal domain for qualitative research. Its pool of rich data is a useful source for new theoretical insights, not just a testing ground for preconceived theories. Qualitative research may thus lead to unexpected findings, to new concepts and hypotheses that go beyond initial preconceptions (Miles and Huberman 1984, p. 5). For instance, while doing research in Germany, it became apparent that nearly all of the parents we talked to had some disdain for antibiotics and often a clear preference for therapies and medicines which are unconventional by scientific medical standards. We also noticed that those parents that had acted on their preferences tended to be those with more education. These unexpected observations made us think of a variety of hypotheses that might explain this phenomenon. Could it be that these parents had a deeper immersion into the German ideology of naturalism, wished more autonomy from the dominance of medical experts, and had the financial means to pay for having more choices? (see also Chapter 4 in this book).

Researcher-centered biases. Second, one frequently hears the objection that qualitative research is too intuitive, personal, and

individualistic, and that it lets the biases and values of the researcher influence data collection, analysis, and interpretation. There is no
doubt that qualitative research is researcher- and author-centered in
the sense that the researcher is both the research tool and the inter-
preter of the data. But this need not be a disadvantage. The personal
involvement of the researcher with research subjects creates the
very conditions under which meaningful and complex data can be
collected, while too much distance would result in an unfriendly
detachment and might interfere with discourse. Similarly, instead of
treating personal involvement merely as a source of bias, we can
exploit it. How people react to the presence of the researcher may
be as informative as how they respond to other social situations
(Hammersley and Atkinson 1989, p. 15).

A self-conscious researcher is not just a data recording machine
but an active part of the setting under investigation. Under these
conditions the researcher is well advised to constantly reflect on his
or her own role, motives, values, and behaviors and not be deceived
by too simple answers to his or her questions. This attitude is not just
the traditional skepticism or internal criticism that wants to penetrate
through the mist of deception, misunderstanding, and bias to get at
the real truth, but is introspection coupled with intellectual curiosity
in the search for additional angles, categories, or interpretative para-
digms. Such an attitude has been called "disciplined subjectivity"
(Erickson 1973, in Borman, Le Compte, and Goetz 1986).

Another way to guard against too much subjectivity is to either
work in teams, both inside and outside the field, and to seek the
commentary and critique from other researchers, colleagues, or even
from the research subjects themselves (Borman, Le Compte, and
Goetz 1986, p. 44). Observations of social situations in which the
scientist actively participated might also be supplemented by other
observations of similar situations in which the researcher had a less
conspicuous role.

Reliability. Third, questions of reliability have to be addressed
differently, because qualitative studies cannot and do not want to
control or manipulate the setting or phenomenon under study. It
therefore should come as no surprise if studies of the same or similar
settings done by different researchers may yield different results.

One solution, if there is any, must lie in explicitly stating what questions are under investigation, what data sources were used and in delineating clearly those strategic moves that were still under the control of the researcher. While researchers in the field are not always free to behave in ways that elicit data relevant to their research, they always have some strategic choices open to them, such as what social situations and local sites should be entered and when, how actively they should participate and what should be their focus of attention. And if it is at all feasible, they should describe or define the social, cultural, and historical context of their interactions and the social actors present or alluded to.

Another solution to the question of reliability may be in the use of methods of triangulation. Triangulation "means that each piece of information gained or each conclusion reached must be considered tentative or idiosyncratic until it has been corroborated by information collected by other means or from other sources" (Denzin 1978, in Borman, Le Compte, and Goetz 1986). Triangulation can be accomplished among different researchers working in a team by openly discussing their respective data and inferences or between different methods of data collection by examining data relating to the same phenomenon from participant observation, interviewing, and documents. Triangulation, however, is no golden way to absolute "truth." Cultural "truth" is always situation- and context-dependent. Ridding data of such contexts (even if we only mean by this the cleaning of our data from the "artifacts" produced by different settings or approaches) is equivalent to ignoring valuable information (see Silverman 1989, p. 226). But if we can live with this critique, the observation that different kinds of data lead to the same general conclusions makes us more confident in those conclusions (Hammersley and Atkinson 1989, p. 199). We, for instance, supplemented our insights gained from qualitative interviews (e.g., about medicine use) with data won in a more systematic fashion (e.g., from the medicine cabinet report). We checked our knowledge about, e.g., our own health system by consulting corresponding publications, and we validated what children said with the accounts of their parents.

Questions of precision. Fourth, qualitative studies are accused of lacking exactness and precision because their observations are not

measurable or not recorded in quantified amounts that can be analyzed statistically (Borman, Le Compte, and Goetz 1986, p. 51).
But exactness by means of numbers only makes sense if we are
dealing with units that can be measured with respect to dimensions
for which we have a standard of measurement. This is rarely the
case in qualitative research that investigates unique and multidimensional events, context-dependent patterns of thought, and units
on different levels of analysis. Furthermore, for most of the important dimensions that interest the qualitative researcher, there may
not exist a meaningful and agreed upon way to measure or classify
it. We are then better advised to stick to meaningful words rather
than to assign numbers to selected qualities according to a research-
er-invented rule. And finally, exactness and precision by means of
numbers are not always necessary to prove a point. Words, carefully
chosen, a concrete incidence well summarized, a story skillfully
told full of meaningful metaphors, can prove far more convincing to
a reader than pages of numbers (Miles and Huberman 1984, p. 15).

Quantitative Research

Quantitative research is usually what the lay public thinks about
when they hear the word "research." But quantitative research is
not only research employing numbers. Scientists link it with logical
positivism, with experimental and survey research, with measurement and statistical analysis. While some anthropologists would not
want to dirty their hands with any techniques of quantification, we
agree with Silverman (1989, p. 223) that it may sometimes be very
useful to use certain quantitative measures, however crude they
may be.

Use of Quantitative Measures in a Qualitative Comparative Study

For us quantitative research simply meant structured interviews,
the systematic assignment of numbers to answers, and statistical
analyses using computer software packages. We used such methods
because they proved convenient for the quick collection of information on simple and theoretically unproblematic questions whose
answers lend themselves easily to numbers. They were an effortless

way to systematically learn about the health history of each sampled child, to collect information on the socioeconomic status of the participating parents or to determine the kind and number of medicines stored in the house. But unlike scientists allied with positivism, we had no intention of testing or "falsifying" preconceived theories or of doing fanciful statistical analyses. What we did, however, was to reduce our data by computing univariate and bivariate distributions and to sometimes attempt to "verify" our inductively arrived at hunches and hypotheses.

Quantification thus was used for nothing else but the systematic assignment of numbers to the answers of structured questions according to a set rule. The numbers we used were mostly of the nominal type and symbolized nothing more than a limited, often dichotomized set of exhaustive and mutually exclusive categories, such as the number 0 to a "yes" and 1 to a "no" answer to each question of the health history which inquired about the past incidence of certain childhood diseases. Sometimes our numbers were of the ordinal type, which meant that numbers assigned to the qualities could be ordered from high to low. An example would be the classification of family heads into an ordered set of a limited number of social strata on the basis of their years of education and/or income. Sometimes our numbers had the meaning of a single count, such as the number of children in the house or the number of medicines stored in the home.

Some of us who were more closely allied with positivistic logic tried to quantify complex behavioral patterns. While many of us shied away from this endeavor, some teams developed "scales" for the purpose of measuring complex theoretical concepts that cannot easily be observed or ascertained with a single indicator or question. Each of these resulting scales, such as the "autonomy scale" for children, consisted of a number of questions whose answers were quantified and combined into a numerical index. In order to develop this scale, qualitative techniques with children and mothers were used first by an anthropologist to derive a preliminary list of what things children might do on their own relative to medicines. To be a scale this list had to demonstrate tests of internal reliability and each item had to have at least face validity. Two of the items in the original version inquired into buying over-the-counter medicines and picking up prescriptions independently. Each commercial establishment where medicines were sold within a half-mile radius of the study children's schools was visited to confirm that children, the age of those in the study, bought medicines and picked up prescriptions, most often, however, as directed by a parent. The resulting scale had to correlate with other behaviors in a sensible way. For instance, older children and children taking medicines regularly for chronic illness, such as asthma, should score higher on the scale than younger children or children rarely taking medicines. Furthermore, among those who scored high on the scale, the medicines had to be in a location such that children were physically able to access them (Iannotti and Bush 1992). The construction of the autonomy scale can serve as an impressive example where qualitative research generates, enlightens, and informs quantitative research. It can thus more easily evade one of the most frequently heard critiques leveled against quantitative research, i.e., the frequent lack of isomorphism between measures and reality (Krenz and Sax 1986, p. 58).

METHODOLOGY OF THE COMAC CHILDHOOD AND MEDICINES PROJECT

Research Questions

Our project was inspired by our conviction that there was a need for a cross-cultural study of medicine use in Europe that used anthropological rather than pharmacoepidemiological methods. We began with the formulation of research questions that were to aid us in the discovery rather than the testing of hypotheses. These questions included the following:

1. Under what circumstances are medicines given to children? Who takes the responsibility to medicate? When is medication stopped and who decides?
2. What is the level or "type" of children's and parent's knowledge about medicines in regard to their efficacy, dosage, characteristics, use, form, and source?

3. What are the symbolic meanings attached to children's medicines in various European cultures; e.g., differences in medical ideology and perceptions of medicines, cultural codes of regarding appropriate health and illness behavior?
4. Are there differences in children's models for staying healthy and where do medicines enter as part of this strategy?
5. What do children/parents believe about medicines and their action within the body, how they work, and association with the treatment of specific bodily parts or symptoms?
6. Who are the brokers in children's health? Do they differ according to cultural setting?

Research Design

We wanted to promote a research design weighted in the direction of, but not necessarily restricted to, qualitative and anthropological methodology. The members of the Planning Committee could see early on that this was not going to be an easy task, given its multidisciplinary and multicultural composition.

We were aware that the collection of qualitative data is a labor-intensive operation, that may last for months if not years. This reason and the wish to generate rather than test theory may explain why qualitative researchers have only studied a limited number of cases without worrying too much about representativeness. Its labor-intensive style makes it focus on only those cases that seem theoretically fruitful.

One selection strategy we could have followed is "theoretical sampling" (Glaser and Strauss 1970). This kind of sampling views selection and interpretation as an ongoing process that is geared by the considerations of an emerging theory rather than by representativeness. It is a strategy that selects each new case according to theoretical considerations arising during the continual review and analysis of the cases already selected. Selection of new cases would stop the moment we were confident that our hypotheses need no further revisions and that new cases add no new information.

Unfortunately, the conflicts inherent between the needs of qualitative and comparative research forced us into long discussions of how many children should be sampled and how. Even though qualitative anthropologists are not usually concerned about issues of representativeness and of studying large numbers of subjects, we were swayed by the logic of comparative anthropologists and scientists who stressed that we are not dealing with homogeneous cultures but pluralistic societies where a great variation of responses can be expected. We settled on the "reasonable" number of 100 healthy children, 50 each in two age groups, and their families for each local study. We hoped to gain their parent's informed consent and the children's participation from two schools located in "middle class" urban or suburban neighborhoods. The latter was decided on to control for variation due to social status. The children should be six to seven and ten to eleven years old. The two age-groups were chosen in order to tap children at different stages of their mental development and to compare them with respect to their perception and autonomy of medicine use.

In the final product, study populations ranged from 19 to 215 children per country (see Table 2.1). A major impediment to our first goal of 100 children was related to gaining permission from school authorities (national departments of education, school boards, etc.) to conduct the initial stage of the research in schools.

TABLE 2.1. Number of Children Participating

Location	Boys	Girls	Total
Vanløse, Denmark	14	17	31
Keele, England	19	14	33
Jyväskylä, Finland	26	25	51
Hamburg, Germany	14	12	26
Athens, Greece	47	41	88
Trieste, Italy	29	36	65
Amsterdam/Groningen			
Netherlands	10	9	19
Madrid, Spain	62	38	100
Tenerife, Spain	63	52	115
Chapel Hill, USA	51	52	103
Novi Sad, Yugoslavia	75	75	150

In some countries, the school system was already burdened by several research projects being conducted in schools. Thus, other avenues of reaching the study population were implemented (e.g., interviewing children in summer camps and a follow-up with their parents, networking through contacts with parents).

Methods of Data Collection

Data collection instruments used in concerted action projects are expected to be uniform for each local study. We had this goal in mind when designing the following instruments for the COMAC Project:

1. Ethnographic Interviews with Children ("Drawing Interview")
2. Socioeconomic and Health History Questionnaire for Parents
3. Fever Interview for Parents
4. Fever Interview for Children
5. Home Medicine Cabinet Inventory

The way they were used is presented in following chapters. Here we simply want to give our readers a description of the instruments.

Ethnographic interviews with children were conducted in all local studies in the project. In all but one study, the interviews took place after each child had completed (or tried to complete) a drawing of him/herself (or another person) during an illness episode. The drawing was used as an aid to help the children recall their episode, not as a diagnostic or therapeutic tool. After completion of the drawing, the child was asked to describe what was happening in the picture.

The interviews were unstructured, but focused on a variety of themes regarding the last remembered illness episode:

- what it feels like to be sick,
- what the concrete symptoms were,
- why a person comes to feel this way,
- who is with the sick child,
- quantitative and qualitative information about medicines,
- conceptions of what medicines do to the body,
- how one becomes well again, including alternative therapies,

• information about the process of becoming sick and getting better.

By using this technique, the children were allowed to report their episode (or that of someone else, even a fictitious figure) in their own words. Interviewers were trained not to prompt the children by using leading questions. If the designated thematic topics listed in the following paragraphs had not been spontaneously discussed by the child by the end of their narrative, they were asked specific questions about them.

During visits to the children's homes, information was collected about the family's socioeconomic characteristics and health history to gain a fuller picture of the familial contexts of the children in local studies. In some studies, these data were collected by highly structured questionnaires (i.e., socioeconomic data and health history), in others by ethnographic interviewing techniques.

The Fever Interview for Parents and the Fever Interview for Children, developed by the COMAC Project members, were made available to all National Coordinators who decided as to their use in their local study. This was designed to supplement the children's interview narratives and other parent's responses to questions about family health history, treatment of illness in general, and use of medicines. Each interview protocol consists of a standard set of closed and open questions. Where implemented, it was used during home visits, where parents and children were interviewed separately. Some local teams preferred to use parts of it in semistructured interviewing techniques.

The Home Medicine Cabinet Inventory was designed to prompt parents to actually show the interviewer where medicines were stored in the home–or at least to present the medicines to the interviewer. The explicit goal was to record each and every medicine in the home. The Inventory requested:

• the characteristics of each medicine (e.g., brand name, package, date of expiration, place of storage).
• the method of purchase (OTC, Rx) or how acquired (e.g., relative, friend, etc.).
• the reason it was used/being used and by whom.

- other comments (e.g., effectiveness, lack of use, adverse reactions).

Other techniques and instruments, both qualitative (adult journals to record illness episodes in children, participant observation in schools) and quantitative (autonomy scales, developmental measures) were used by some local teams.

ANALYSIS OF DATA

We also struggled with problems during qualitative data analysis. We soon encountered that data analysis is a laborious task that starts the moment the first case is selected and that takes months or years to complete after the last case had been interviewed and its answers transcribed. After all, we had to read, reread, analyze and subject to data reduction hundreds of pages of text in order to draw conclusions. While we have clear conventions for the data reduction of quantitative data in the form of predefined categories, codes, and numbers, there are only few agreed-upon canons or shared ground rules for drawing conclusions from qualitative data. So we were often left to our own logic and procedures.

In short, ethnographic (or unstructured) interviews were analyzed by long and tedious content analyses. These included the Drawing Interview with the children, interviews with parents, and, where used, adult journals of children's illness episodes. The qualitative Drawing Interview data were used both in local study and cross-cultural interpretative essays.

Those national teams that had many questions in common and had asked them in standardized ways coordinated their efforts and produced a common code book. This code book defined the rules which cooperating teams then used in the assignment of codes (i.e., numbers) to the answers of the set of shared instruments and quantifiable questions. These included the answers to the Fever Interview for Parents, the Fever Interview for Adults, and the Home Medicine Cabinet Inventory. The code book enabled each team to produce a data matrix of quantitative data that could be exchanged and used for quantitative cross-cultural comparisons. These approaches are represented in the contributions to this book.

CONCLUSION

What do we want to leave the reader with? Our conclusion–or rather closure–to this chapter is to give our reader the incentive to read each comparative chapter and each interpretative essay of local study results. This is the only way that the pros and cons of qualitative vs. quantitative research can be "resolved" in our reader's minds. Readers may also view the remainder of the book as a challenge to cherished ideas about what is "science," explanation and proof or understanding and meaning (or both?). If that is not the goal, readers are asked to read selected chapters; in most of them will be found qualitative and quantitative approaches intermixed. Is not that the beauty of the multimethod approach?

NOTES

1. The COMAC Childhood and Medicines Project was funded through a European Economic Community (EEC) *Comité d'Action Concerté* (COMAC) contract, COMAC/HSR MR4*-CT90-0319, awarded to The Institute on Child Health, Athens, Greece, with Deanna J. Trakas as the Project Leader. The official title of the Contract was "Medicine Use, Behaviour, and Children's Perceptions of Medicines and Health Care."

2. "Emic" derives from the word "phonemic" and refers to the culture-specific concepts and conceptual distinctions that make a difference to the insiders of a group. "Emic" is usually contrasted with "etic" (which derives from "phonetic") to refer to the language, concepts, and point of view of an observer or cultural outsider.

REFERENCES

Boas, F. 1896. "The limitations of the comparative method of anthropology." *Science* 4: 901-908.

Borman, K. M., LeCompte, M. D., and Goetz, J. P. 1986. "Ethnographic and qualitative research design and why it doesn't work." *American Behavioral Scientist 30* (1): 42-57.

Brislin, R. W., Lonner, W. J., and Thorndike, R. M. 1973. *Cross-cultural Research Methods.* New York: Wiley & Sons.

Buchanan, D. R. 1992. "An uneasy alliance: Combining qualitative and quantitative research methods." *Health Education Quarterly 19* (1): 117-135.

Clements, F. E. 1932. "Primitive concepts of disease." *University of California Publications in American Archaeology and Ethnology 32*: 185-252.

Foster, G. M. 1976. "Disease etiologies in nonwestern medical systems." *American Anthropologist 78*: 733-782.

Glaser, B. G. and Strauss, A. L. 1970. *The Discovery of Grounded Theory. Strategies for Qualitative Research.* Chicago: Aldine.

Hammersley, M. and Atkinson, P. 1989. *Ethnography. Principles in Practice.* London: Routledge.

Iannotti, R. J. and Bush, P. J. 1992. "The development of autonomy in children's health behavior." *Emotion, Cognition, Health, and Development in Children and Adolescents*, edited by E. J. Sussman, L. V. Feagans and, W. Ray. Englewood Cliffs, NJ: Erlbaum, pgs. 53-74.

Johnson, A. 1991. "Regional comparative field research." *Behavior Science Research 25* (1-4): 3-22.

Krenz, C. and Sax, G. 1986. "What quantitative research is and why it doesn't work." *American Behavior Scientist 30* (1): 58-69.

Miles, M. B. and Huberman, A. M. 1984. *Qualitative Data Analysis. A Sourcebook of New Methods.* London: Sage.

Munroe, R. L. and Munroe, R. H. 1991. "Comparative field studies: Methodological issues and future possibilities." *Behavior Science Research 25* (1-4): 155-177.

Murdock, G. P. 1949. *Social Structure.* New York: Macmillan.

Murdock, G. P. 1980. *Theories of Illness: A World Survey.* Pittsburgh: University of Pittsburgh Press.

Silverman D. 1989. "Six rules of qualitative research: A post-romantic argument." *Symbolic Interaction 12* (2): 215-230.

Taylor, E. B. 1889. On a method of investigating the development of institutions applied to the laws of marriage and descent. *Journal of the Anthropological Institute of Great Britain and Ireland 18:* 245-272.

Wirsing, R. 1975. "Probleme des interkulturellen Vergleichs in der Ethnologie." *Sociologus 25* (2): 97-126.

Chapter 3

Hierarchies, Boundaries, and Symbols: Medicine Use and the Cultural Performance of Childhood Sickness

Alan Prout
Pia Christensen

The studies carried out as part of the COMAC Childhood and Medicines Project had their starting point in the observation that differences among countries in pharmaceutical prescription, sale, and use cannot be fully explained by differences in their disease patterns or in the structure and regulation of their pharmaceutical markets. It was suggested that there may be a "cultural" component in medicine use. The COMAC protocol[1] proposed a cross-cultural study of the social and cultural factors that might influence pharmaceutical use for childhood illness.[2] The basic notion was that local studies may be able to show cultural patterns in the meanings associated with medicine use and that these patterns, learned in childhood, may be used to explain variations in pharmaceutical use enacted in adult life.

This chapter is the result of some social anthropological reflection on the various local studies and the material they have produced. We do not discuss the data but rather aim to draw out some theoretical insights which may be of value in thinking about the reports in this volume as well as in planning future studies.[3]

We have organized our discussion around two themes. The first asks the following question: What do children's accounts tell us about sickness as a cultural event? Our initial discussion of this question concerns the social position of children and how it mediates their cultural experience. We then look at sickness as a broad cultural event, arguing that therapies play an important symbolic role in marking the boundaries between health and sickness and various graduations of sickness. This leads to a discussion of how pharmaceuticals, as a specialized form of therapy, communicate messages about hierarchy, authority, and power.

The second theme follows on from this by suggesting how we might conceptualize differences in the social environments within which health and sickness practices take place (and within which medicine use is embedded). Once again, we draw upon the concepts of hierarchy and boundary, suggesting that different configurations of these are important in forming the social structural settings within which cultural differences arise.

THE SOCIAL POSITION OF CHILDREN

A growing field of the anthropology and sociology of childhood suggests that childhood can be seen as a social and cultural construction and that children can be understood as social actors with their own perspectives on the social world (e.g., Prout and James 1990). Children can be seen as engaged in social interaction, confronting the world, making sense of it and attempting to change it. Rather than assuming that they are formed rather than forming social life, we should look for the points at which children act and the methods or strategies they employ. Conventionally, adults have been viewed as being in charge of and having responsibility for children, and this emphasis has tended to obscure children's own role and contribution. These views not only dominate popular perceptions of childhood illness but likewise have proved influential in most research studies of this area (for a discussion, see Prout 1992 and Christensen 1994). These constitute children as not only particularly vulnerable (in general and to illness) but also to be the passive recipient of adult care.

Our approach challenges traditional assumptions in studies of childhood illness, drawing on more recent notions of childhood as a social construction and children as social actors. This position is specified further by the application of a well-known anthropological model of health care systems. In this structural analysis three basic sectors are distinguished: a popular, a folk, and a professional sector (Kleinman 1980). The professional sector consists of the institutionalized diagnostic care and treatment in Western societies (European and North American) based in natural science medicine or biomedicine. The folk sector includes both what has been called complementary medicine or alternative medicine (such as homeopathy), and traditional healing systems (such as herbalism). The popular sector consists of the domestic and household-based lay management of health and illness. Studies have shown that approximately 70 to 90 percent of all treatment to be carried out is in the popular sector in both Western and non-Western societies. Although perhaps too rigid in the distinctions it draws, the strength of this model is that the influence and importance of each of the sectors can be put on an equal footing. It provides a framework for exploring the nature of social relations and the social positions of patients and healers within different clinical realities (Whyte 1992).

Children in Europe and North America do not have any formal professional status in health care. Therefore we may see children as being "doubly constrained": first in relation to the social structures of professional knowledge, control, and power; and second in their relationships with adults. From this point of view, seen within the formal hierarchies of the health care system, children appear as dependent. However, if we look more closely at the informal aspect of these relations, we might see how children are able to negotiate and possibly alter their social positions and relationships. From this perspective children are as such no longer seen as passive recipients in the health care system, but rather as active participants in structures and processes.

Recent studies of family health have stressed the importance of recognizing that the traditional emphasis on women as the main health care providers conceals some of the interactive character of family health care which necessarily needs to include the perspective of both men and children (e.g., Prout 1988; Backett 1990). These two studies, as well as those of Christensen (1993) and James (1993), have revealed that children develop their own ideas and strategies of (inter)actions in relation to health and illness in social contexts such as those at school and in the family. Some of these studies have pointed to the active role of children in everyday social negotiations with parents or professionals. A study of school sickness absence in England, for example, showed that children, without having any formal power in decision making, could, through informal action, persistently claim illness or feign symptoms (Prout 1988). Through operating in the sphere of "vulnerability" (that is, potential rather than actual harm), children were able to negotiate the complex process of a sickness absence decision. Another study (Christensen 1993) showed Danish children engaged with adults (at home, school, and after-school centers) in similar initial negotiations about the classification of a child's complaints or the meaning of undefined sensations. These negotiations would then go on to include others about care and treatment.

It is useful to focus on children as social actors in the popular sector of the health care system, i.e., on children's experiences and agency around health and illness in households (or equivalent settings) in which they are brought up. This does not, however, exclude examining children's role in the professional sector. While it is easy to assume that children are passive recipients in settings such as the clinic where the work of Strong (1979) and Davis (1982) has shown that children become muted actors, it is more difficult to avoid noticing the active participation of children in the structures and processes of their home. Nevertheless, studies such as those by Bluebond-Langner (1979) have shown even terminally ill children in hospitals to be actively engaged in complex social interaction and a struggle to comprehend their situation. Further understanding of their specific contributions will inform our understanding of the health care system as a whole, acknowledging the complex relations between children and social institutions and of the formal and informal hierarchies that influence children's lives (Nader 1980).

SICKNESS AS CULTURAL PERFORMANCE

A particular focus of this chapter is on what children experience and learn through their participation in the cultural performance of sickness. Frankenberg (1980, 1986) and Young (1982) have pointed out that being sick is always located within a wider social and cultural context. "Sickness" (used as an analytically precise term distinct from "disease" and "illness") can be viewed as a process concept through which different worrisome biological or behavioral signs and changes get a socially recognizable meaning which constitutes them as "symptoms." The result then constitutes the person's sickness in a given culture. This approach implies a focus on how disease (biological pathologies and abnormalities) and illness (personal sensations and experiences) are socialized and the means by which social relations create, form, and distribute sickness. Relating this notion of sickness as an interpretive process to the study of childhood illness implies a focus on the ways in which illness is enculturated and conceptualized by children.

In many of the studies reported in this book, children's accounts showed that their illness experience is not only about different bodily sensations and their significance, nor is it solely focused on receiving and responding to different treatments and cures. Children emphasized the social processes of illness. This suggests that children are engaged in a much larger project: illness episodes are broad cultural events through which children comprehend the social relations and structures of their world.[4]

We suggest, therefore, that illness episodes are best understood as broad cultural events through which children experience the structure of their world and the social relations within it. During illness they learn, *inter alia*, fundamental aspects of the social processes that occur between children and adults in their specific social and cultural context. These include child-adult hierarchies, relations of power, and the distribution of knowledge.

Illness episodes (including common events such as minor accidents) may be seen as repetitive performances in which children and adults experience, substantiate, and confirm the social roles and relationships of everyday life. An example of such analysis is found in Frankenberg's (1985) study of northern Italian children. This was based on over 200 essays entitled "What happens in your house when someone gets ill?" collected from 11- to 13-year-old children. Frankenberg's interpretation concerned the cultural performance of sickness in the Italian village as taking on the cultural form and content of the local Catholic and Communist "*festas.*" Events such as these may be significant in this process because they can be distinguished by their dramatic form from the ongoing flow of actions and speech which always surrounds us (Hastrup 1988). The meaning of sickness was, therefore, understood as part of a much larger social and cultural context.

Childhood Sickness as a Cultural Event

An overall finding of the studies was that, in general, children did not spontaneously refer to or mention the role of pharmaceuticals in illness and its treatment. This is not to say they did not recognize the role of medicine (both as a professional activity and therapeutic substance) but rather that they did not dwell on this aspect and were not particularly concerned with therapeutic effect, efficacy, or side effects. They stressed that becoming and being ill, and being treated and becoming well, is a process that involves both intense care and concern from their household members and relative isolation from their nonhousehold age mates. Children saw the nonpharmaceutical therapeutic actions of their caretakers as the most important aspect of their recovery. For example, in the English study, 18 (of 35) children described taking medicine. Only three children thought that medicines "get you better."

Nevertheless, that a pharmaceutical was "used" in relation to illness acted for children as a symbol of being sick, that is, as an event related to, but different from, other significant events. Children were engaged in classifying and categorizing pharmaceuticals in relation to other sorts of consumables. They described form, color, size, and taste in the same way as they would discuss food, sweets, and drinks and were involved in understanding how these classifications overlapped and differed. Children provided vivid descriptions of how to take a medicine in order to avoid its unpleasant taste or how to get access to (more) medicine that tasted good. For example, in the Danish study a ten-year-old Danish boy described his success in getting access to medicine. His younger brother had had a cold and was given some cough medicine. His older brother recognized that it was a very tasty medicine and imitated a cough in order to have some. He explained that he was not sure that he had actually convinced his mother that he was ill but she had nevertheless allowed him some of the medicine every day together with his younger sibling.

Another general quality of the data was that accounts from both children and adults showed children as more or less dependent on and under the control of adults. In many situations (including medicine taking) children did not have great scope for independent action, so while children are social actors, they are social actors of a particular kind. This means that we cannot read off cultural aspects of sickness from children's accounts in any simple way. Children's social position as relatively dependent and controlled always mediates their experience. In the second half of this chapter we discuss how different social environments structure the degree to which children are given independent action. For the moment, however, we simply note that given their position, dependency and control are likely to figure in any understanding of how children experience and learn from illness as a broad cultural event.

Danish and English children described therapy as integral to social relationships and interactions. In their descriptions, therapies were inseparable from the therapist (that is anyone providing care, –mother, general practitioner, or teacher). By describing different therapeutic actions, children explained the roles, statuses, and positions of specific persons involved in an illness episode. Children in both age groups mapped out the quest for pharmaceuticals in this way. They described, for example, how the doctor was consulted to prescribe medicine, the pharmacy where they subsequently bought it, and the persons involved in the transactions. They also spoke about where pharmaceuticals were kept in the house and who and how they were used by family members. They sometimes denoted specific actions to characterize particular persons. Six- to seven-year-old children, for example, described doctors simply stating that: "The doctor prescribes medicine."

Another example comes from a seven-year-old Danish girl. She explained that: "When I am ill, my mother always puts a cloth with cold water on my forehead." This is also an example of how the general notion of "being ill" was marked and distinguished by the specificity of a therapy.

Overall, then, children emphasized the experience of illness as a social process. Being ill was expressed through describing the social roles, (inter)actions and social positioning of the persons involved, and by pointing to specific characteristics such as alterations of the household and work setting. Bodily sensations, emotional distress, or contexts of becoming ill were given only secondary attention in recounting the illness episode. This is not to say that children's accounts did not include explicitly or implicitly some notion of the "natural" course of illness but the primary concerns of children's accounts were the social aspects of an illness, especially changes to everyday life. Diffuse bodily sensations were embedded in, give significance to, and take meaning from, the wider social processes.

Therapy as a Symbolic Boundary Marker

Children's references to therapy played a particular part in their accounts of sickness as a cultural event. Children spoke about a wide range of therapies, not only medicine taking but many other actions as well, as part of the social interaction between themselves and immediate family members, relatives, doctors, and other health care workers. The children pictured therapy as a significant symbol of these processes, especially the way in which different therapeutic actions mark the crossing of boundaries in the process of becoming, being, and recovering from illness.

The application of a therapy, or the move to a different one, marked the passage from one stage of becoming or being ill to another; it was one of the practices that distinguished one phase from another. One such feature in the European context in the classification of illness was for many children symbolized in "temperature taking." A general observation from all of the studies was that children in both age groups explained that, in terms of somatic experience, they were the first person to know that they were ill or not feeling well. Nevertheless the children also drew attention to the fact that to be socially and culturally classified as ill "the thermometer" often played a decisive symbolic role. For example, in the Danish study, a ten-year-old girl said: "I felt ill, then my father took my temperature and he said, 'Yes you are ill.'" In confirming her own prior understanding, temperature taking may not only mark the boundary from "health" to "illness" but may also become the symbol of recovery. As another ten-year-old Danish girl concluded in an essay:

I yawned and got out of bed. I took a glass of water because I was thirsty. Mummy shouted to me that I should go back to bed, but I said I feel well now. Mummy looked at me and said: "We must take your temperature." It showed 37.2°C. Mummy exclaimed: "But, you are well. Run out and play with the others, but wrap up well."

Prout (1986) addressed similar observations in his study in an English primary school. In the school the secretary held a central and powerful position in children's illness episodes. She used a thermometer to record whether a child had fever. On this basis she then made a final judgement of whether a child was "actually ill" and hence unable to conduct his/her school work. This procedure was conducted (more or less) detached from the complaints or symptoms the child forwarded to her. More than establishing a reliable diagnosis, her own action initiated other actions and powerfully delegated the child to an altered position in the school.

These examples show how, what is at one level an instrumental action–taking the temperature–was given symbolic meaning by both children and adults. It was an action which signified the possibility of transition from one state to another, thus marking and facilitating subsequent steps and stages of the sickness performance for children and adults.

An essay written by a ten-year-old Danish boy is full of such boundaries, transitions and their markers:

One morning I feel ill. I call my mummy and I say. I have tummy ache, mummy. Yes I'm on my way. Mummy I have a tummy ache. My mother went to my bed and touches my forehead. What a warm forehead you have. We walked down into the lounge. My mother brings the duvet. And my dad has left for work a long time ago. My mother takes my fever (temperature); it is very high. My mother calls the doctor. Ten minutes later the doctor arrives. He says that I have got a fever. The doctor leaves again and my mum says you must have some medicine. I get sick; my mother runs to get a cloth. When she has wiped up she said that she would go to the pharmacy. She would be back home in ten minutes. I got tea and medicine and we read some books, then we made some drawings. Then it was lunch time. Dad came home and discovered that I was ill. The time went past. At one o'clock my dad and I talked together and watched a cartoon. I got medicine, I slept a bit. It was evening. I watched a children's programme and got soup. I was going to sleep now. . . . The next morning I was well again. I was happy and also my dad and my mum. The end.

The symbolic meaning of therapeutic actions does not, however, have a fixed relationship to transition through stages and across boundaries. Like all symbolic boundary markers, the symbols of sickness provide a specific form or structure but not a fixed meaning. Symbolic communication requires acts of interpretation and, therefore, different people will attach their own specific meaning to a symbol. Both adults and children may agree about the structure of therapy and both parties may see it as a symbolic boundary marker in sickness but it may not bear the same meaning for each of them. Indeterminacy is thus inherent in symbolic relationships. So while adult's and children's understanding of the symbols of sickness may gradually come into closer alignment through experience, interaction, and negotiation, this process will never be complete.

Pharmaceuticals and the Communication of Hierarchy

Because they are substances, pharmaceuticals present a concrete possibility for self-care and often serve to specify and classify symptoms (Van der Geest and Whyte 1989). We suggest that in relation to children our understanding of the role of pharmaceuticals must be broadened and seen as part of the way therapeutic actions communicate meaning about power and hierarchy. This process can be observed in the ways in which access to medicines is enacted and controlled. In the Danish study, for example, painkillers such as Panodil®[5] were named by children as "adult pills," sometimes with them adding comments such as ". . . you know, prohibited for children under 12 (years old)." However in everyday experience, children found that tablets restricted to adults may in fact be divided and provided in a smaller dose. This shows that pharmaceuticals can express complex and ambiguous messages: adults and children are classified as different and unequal; at the same time access is implicitly negotiable for children. By dispensing the tablet into smaller pieces the once "prohibited" becomes accessible.

Access to medicines and being able to use them without consulting others (especially biomedical practitioners) has been suggested as being one of the "charms" of pharmaceuticals (van der Geest and Whyte 1989). Unlike most other therapies which involve others in undertaking the treatment, using a pharmaceutical makes it possible not only to act within the private domain but also to engage in different exchanges within families, households, and other like social settings. This indirectly contributes to the process by which the power and hierarchical status of medicine is redistributed from the doctor and pharmacy to the level of family and peers. It thus has the possibility of affecting power relations such as that shown above where for children the use of a pharmaceutical "strictly for adults" marks the achievement of a (possibly) new status—a person who can negotiate the hierarchy of power relationships within the household.

Implicit in this view of pharmaceuticals is the notion that they might express some of the hierarchies of health care. This could happen at several different levels. On a macro social level pharmaceutical use is embedded in both specific market structures and state regulations and legislation. At an intermediate level it is sometimes subject to gatekeeping when, for example, a prescription from a doctor is necessary for access to a wanted pharmaceutical. This may also happen when a medicine is purchased over the pharmacy counter. Some medicines cannot be dispensed without the authority of a medical practitioner, which clearly places the pharmacist as subordinate to the authority of medicine. When a medicine can be obtained over the counter (OTC), the lay consumer may be subordinated to the recommendations of the pharmacist—once again creating a hierarchy. Finally on the family level the relations of power and knowledge emerge between child and adult, this time with the adults in the gatekeeping position of control.

In reviewing the data from the various countries, it is clear that all the studies showed strong biomedical dominance. Running through the interviews with both children and adults was an implicit acknowledgement of biomedicine as the authoritative source of knowledge, understanding, and action on child health. This is not to say that some parents did not have doubts about or criticisms of biomedicine or were not prepared to use alternatives to it; biomedical dominance is contested. Nevertheless, when it came to their children's health, parents were reluctant to take risks or experiment with alternative forms of therapy. While parents felt that they were competent to treat most of their children's minor ailments, they often implied that their competence had limits. It stood hierarchically lower than that of biomedicine and they were ultimately dependent on the professional skills of biomedicine. Related professions such as nursing and pharmacy were also placed in this hierarchy—as lower than biomedicine and drawing their legitimacy from it. In the Dutch study (Gerrits, Haaijer-Ruskamp, and Hardon 1995), for example, biomedical dominance and hierarchy were quite explicit. Dutch parents (most often mothers) were shown to judge whether they should treat children's illness according to how serious they thought it was. Although there was variation in what counted as seriousness, common and moderately severe illnesses were thought of as treatable at home but when they were seen as serious, or becoming serious, a medical doctor was consulted. In this case the doctor: ". . . takes over the decision-making process on medicine use and other therapies." (Gerrits, Haaijer-Ruskamp, and Hardon 1993, p. 2) Another example, this time from the Finnish study (Vaskilampi et al. 1993), makes a similar point: pharmaceuticals were ranked by adult respondents in their power according to whether they were available OTC or by prescription from a doctor only; OTC medicines that were recently prescription-only status were ranked in an intermediate position.

Children's interviews were full of references to restrictions and regulations concerning pharmaceuticals. For example, many children of all ages understood that the doctor prescribes medicine and that an adult in the household (usually their mother) distributes it to the child. Children pointed to their own role as one of cooperating in taking medicine. For example: "My mother pours the medicine and I take it."

In general children seemed to comply and cooperate in having a specific treatment, even though they might stress the unpleasant taste of a pharmaceutical and that they took it with food to make it easier to swallow. They also usually accepted that to be ill implied restrictions of their behavior.

However, both children and parents described episodes when competition for control also entered their relationship. Children sometimes challenged the control, decision-making power, and responsibility of adults during the process of illness and recovery. Children's objections may be understood as their attempt to keep control or regain power of their body–thus asserting their claim on a higher position in the hierarchies of health care. This is also shown in their rejection of unwanted, unintelligible, or unpleasant interference in their body, e.g., several children explained that they did not like to have their temperature taken rectally. Their rejection might take a more diffuse expressive form. A seven-year-old Danish girl said: "I don't like to have my temperature taken; I scream."

A more purposeful form was illustrated when children rejected a suggested treatment and insisted on another–for example, when children objected to home remedies such as resting or having specific food suggested by the parent. Children also objected to the use of pharmaceuticals, as a story told by a six-year-old Danish girl illustrates. On the previous day the girl had experienced a headache and her mother therefore offered her a "headache pill." The girl explained how she refused to take the tablet stating, "Because I don't want to." Instead she had insisted on helping her mother clean some chairs and proclaimed proudly, ". . . and then it made the headache disappear."

MAPPING CULTURAL DIVERSITY

In the first section we have suggested that therapies acted as symbolic markers of changes and graduations of health, illness, and healing. Therapy was for children embedded in social relations and interactions and thus served to define the status and position of persons involved in an illness episode. Accordingly the performance and communication of hierarchy was implicit in therapeutic acts. This allowed us to suggest that from the perspective of the child, pharmaceuticals act as powerful symbols of children's position within the broader social structures of society.

Childhood Illness in Diverse Cultural Contexts

So far we have focused on the meaning of therapy from the perspective of the individual child. The following section suggests a theoretical framework for understanding pharmaceutical use in different cultural contexts. In our discussion the family or household will form the unit of analysis. The relevance of this unit of analysis is a consequence of our focus on pharmaceutical use (and childhood illness more generally) from the perspective of children and their parents. Through it we acknowledge the family/household to be at the core of the popular health care sector. At the same time we develop a set of concepts relating to hierarchy and boundary that might be used to differentiate different sorts of of social and cultural context in further work on childhood health and illness.

We noted above that the dominance of a biomedical perspective on illness and therapy is hardly surprising. Biomedical dominance is well established in the countries of Europe and the USA. There are some differences between them but they all fit this overall pattern. In addition, the samples with whom the data were produced for the various COMAC studies were deliberately "middle class"— those groups whom the social anthropologist Mary Douglas would define as part of the "core community" (Douglas 1992). As Douglas suggests, the members of this group are exactly those who would be expected to support the claims of biomedicine to status, specialized professional skill, and expert knowledge.

In order to see diversity in medicine use we may have to look at a wider range of households. In the rest of this chapter we will develop some theoretical speculations about how differences might be considered and identified empirically. Our approach is to suggest a map of cultural possibilities by using some anthropological concepts to imagine a series of social environments within which therapy, including medicine use, is embedded.

Our starting point is the so-called "grid and group" approach introduced and developed by Mary Douglas (see, for example, 1992). This is a framework for analyzing cultural settings. The essence of the notion can be stated quite simply: the terms "grid" and "group," which from this point we will refer to by the more intuitively obvious terms of "hierarchy" and "boundary" signify two dimensions then when put together can with some justice be claimed to capture a great deal about the many different social environments within which individuals relate to each other.

The first dimension is *hierarchy* (what Douglas calls grid). It refers to the different degrees to which social groups are structured. Cultures can be placed on a continuum. At one end it is highly structured; individuals have little scope for negotiating their courses of action with others and are caught in a tight grid of ascribed behavior. At the other end of the continuum social environments are only loosely structured; behavior is open to individual preference and is highly negotiable with others in the social field.

The second dimension we call *boundary* (Douglas refers to this as group). It speaks of the different degrees to which the boundaries between a social group and other social groups are open or closed. In closed boundary environments membership is highly regulated, members are strongly consocial and, while it may be made difficult to leave the group, serious breaches of its rules may lead to complete expulsion. In contrast, open boundary groups are loosely constituted, the barriers to membership are not great, and members do not spend a great deal of time together.

These dimensions are combined to create a fourfold typology of social environments:

1. those with relatively open boundaries and a relatively weak hierarchy;
2. those with relatively open boundaries but a strong hierarchy;
3. those with relatively closed boundaries but a strong hierarchy;
4. those with relatively closed boundaries but a weak hierarchy.

There is now extensive literature refining the conceptual dimensions of this framework and clarifying methodological procedures in its use. It has been shown how different social environments shape and constrain individual behavior (in that environment) and how the environments are linked to characteristic sets of beliefs and have been used as theoretical tools in the ethnographic analysis of a wide variety of social settings (see, for example, Douglas 1982, 1987, 1992). These include topics with a direct health relevance. (See, for example, Douglas's [1992] analyses of "cultures of risk" in relation to the AIDS virus.)

The four positions shown above are, of course, extremes and any number of intermediate combinations might be found. Nevertheless, the theory generates four (ideal) types of social environment. The content of these environments is not given in the framework and is empirical; it can (and has) been used to compare many different groups. Essentially the framework is a useful guide to empirical study–suggesting questions to ask about the characteristics of social environments that shape and constrain individual beliefs and actions. It helps to move us beyond the vague notion of "culture" toward the detailed comparison of some abstract dimensions that can be translated into meaningful features of social situations.

Hierarchy and Boundary in Household Health Care

We suggest that this theoretical framework might help to throw light on our previous discussion. One possibility is to think of sickness as a cultural performance which is shaped (but not rigidly determined) by the social environment of which it is a part. Hierarchy and boundary combinations might play an important role in this. By way of illustrative speculation, we offer the following map (Table 3.1) of hierarchy and boundary differences as they apply to the different environments within which family/household (that is popular sector) health care takes place.

We have restricted our discussion to family/household health largely for reasons of convenience and clarity of presentation. In many respects, however, this is bound to be misleading. Households are embedded in wider social structures and cultures. In recent times medical social anthropologists and sociologists have been concerned with demonstrating the complex connections between economy, social structure, local culture, and health beliefs and practices (Scheper-Hughes 1987; Currer and Stacey 1984). It is also clear that all families and households have more or less permeable boundaries (Bernardes 1985, 1986) with other social institutions and networks. One direction for future studies of childhood and medicine use should be to look at households in these wider terms.[6]

What we have called *consumerist* households are characterized by medical pluralism. No one system of therapy would be dominant; individuals would be relatively free to choose which forms of

TABLE 3.1. Hierarchy, Boundary, and Household Health Care

B *Isolated* Strong hierarchy Open boundary	C *Conventionalist* Strong hierarchy Closed boundary
A *Consumerist* Weak hierarchy Open boundary	D *Dissenting* Weak hierarchy Open boundary

therapy they preferred. The choice of experimental and innovative therapies of all types would be encouraged to the extent that fads and fashions in health care (including preventive health) would tend to come and go quickly. Individuals might actively seek out new approaches and set new trends. Health action would be flexible, mobile, and practices might be borrowed from the conventionalist, dissenting and even the idiosyncratic spaces in an *ad hoc* manner. For example, in cases of acute life-threatening illnesses, there may be a sudden shift to the conventionalist space and a reliance on orthodox medicine. On the other hand, if conventional therapies prove ineffective (as is often the case with chronic illness), there may be a shift to the dissenting space and the use of alternative therapies.

In these households the emphasis would be on the (relative) autonomy of the child to decide when they are ill and what the appropriate therapy might be. Except at the extreme corner the degree of choice given to a child would not be the same as that accorded to adults, but compared to children in conventionalist households we would expect it to be relatively high. Most likely it would be marked by a relatively high degree of negotiation between adult and child about whether they are "really" ill, what the costs and benefits of staying home sick might be, what the appropriate therapy might be, and what their preference is. Choice of therapy and negotiation around sickness would be one of the ways children in these settings learn that their life is under their own control.

Conventionalist households have (relatively) strong hierarchy and closed boundaries. Here medical pluralism is weaker than the previous type. In Western societies biomedicine is the most prestigious and a series of controls would be in place to limit access to alternative modes. There would be sanctions of those who strayed outside the dominant forms of healing. Illness would be seen as a consequence of behavior that breached the rules of health promulgated by the health professions, although contact with outsiders or groups seen as deviant might also be seen as dangerous. The boundary between health and sickness would be strong and entry into sickness would be regulated by accredited specialists. The type of therapy used would be strongly symbolic of taking the proper course of action in the face of sickness.

In conventionalist households there would be stress on strict adherence to officially recommended preventive and therapeutic actions. Children would have little chance to negotiate their status as well or sick and little choice about the form of therapy used. A strong distinction would be drawn between home remedies and biomedical ones, and children would be made aware of the importance of specialist knowledge and professional qualifications. Health rules will be strong and might include not associating with polluting things and people. Many of the COMAC studies showed this sort of pattern, although rarely in an extreme form and often with a tendency toward a mild form of consumerism. It would be useful to explore further when and how children and their caregivers break from conventionalist approaches and use more strongly consumerist and/or radical strategies. Families in which a child develops a chronic condition may, for example, make such a shift.

Idiosyncratic households (with a strong hierarchy but weak boundaries) are by definition rare. The notion might be applied to households dominated by isolated individuals who develop strong and rigid but (in comparison to the wider context) bizarre and unusual notions of health, illness, and therapy–people who might be pejoratively labelled as "health nuts." Here the boundaries between illness and health are strong but the range of social life which is thought of as sick is very large. Only idiosyncratic preventive and curative actions will return a person to the (narrow) range of health. An example from England illustrates the point. For a number of years, passersby in Oxford Street, London, were accosted by a man bearing a billboard and a selection of pamphlets giving advice about the health benefits of a low-protein diet. His pamphlets suggested that almost all personal ill health and most social problems are caused by a high-protein diet and could be simply cured by the changes he advocates. His ideas were strongly held and quite impervious to the objections raised with him during the multitude of conversations he must have had over the years. When he died in early 1994, the news was reported on national television; he had become well known–a fondly remembered eccentric who was completely unsuccessful in recruiting adherents to his views.

Children would be unfortunate indeed to find themselves in an idiosyncratic environment. They would find little scope for negotiating about sickness or therapy because this would be governed by the strong and rigid ideas of their caretaker–for example that ill health is caused by a high-protein diet. At the same time, the notions governing health action would appear bizarre by the standards of other groups which the child participated in. Such households are presumably rare.

Finally we turn to the *dissenting* households. These can be thought of as linked to organized enclaves of opposition to the conventionalist view. Radical critiques would be made of the conventional modes of therapy (especially biomedicine) which would be viewed with suspicion and the authority of its practitioners would not be accepted. The world of conventional therapy might be seen as inimical to health, even acting conspiratorially to undermine the well-being of people. Like the idiosyncratic environment, dissenters would develop a preference for local remedies and charismatic therapists. In this case, however, oppositional or unusual views would have been successful in enrolling adherents, producing a powerful belief underpinned by a somewhat sect-like social organization. The tendency would be for the boundary between health and sickness to be relatively weak because of ever-present threats from the conventional world. On the other hand, specific practices advocated by the dissenting groups would be symbolically powerful in prevention and cure. Possible examples include self-help groups for chronic illnesses who sometimes develop strong adherence to nonconventional therapies. Extreme examples might include Christian Scientists who see sin as the cause of illness and prayer as the therapy and who reject biomedical treatment. Here therapy is seen as highly symbolic; prayer in the face of sickness signifies belonging to the group acceptance, but using conventional therapy is taken as a rejection of the group teaching.

In this final type of setting children would have a degree of freedom to negotiate illness and therapy for two reasons: first, the emphasis in such households would be on children choosing to become "real" believers in whatever the dissenting view might be; second, children's voices might be heard as part of the general position of mistrusting authority and listening to those marginalized by the system. Chronically ill children taking part in self-help group activities may be in such a position—with a self-help group championing their objections to conventional therapy. In more extreme cases (such as Christian Scientists) these negotiations would take place in a context of strong group pressure toward the acceptance of the beliefs of the dissenting minority. As children grew up they would be expected to make a personal commitment to belief and failure to do so would result in expulsion from the group. Clearly there is much scope for studies of health and illness practices of marginal groups.

CONCLUSION

The COMAC Children and Medicines Project was an opportunity to think about how social anthropology (and akin disciplines such as medical sociology) might develop a deeper understanding of the cultural context of medicine taking. The reflections in this chapter suggest that pharmaceutical use can be understood as a practice embedded in a social and cultural context. Therefore, if medicine use is to be understood, it must be studied in and as part of the situation as a whole. Our suggestion is that medicine-taking is embedded in therapy-giving, which in turn is embedded in the cultural performance of sickness. This approach requires that sickness is seen as a broad cultural event that draws on and reproduces wider features of the social environment. Every social environment will have its own set of meanings and there is no substitute for detailed ethnographic enquiry into these. Nevertheless, we have suggested that differences in the way boundaries and hierarchies are constructed deserve particular attention. Future studies need to diversify the contexts within which medicine use (whether in childhood or adulthood) is studied so that comparative material might be used as a means developing, modifying, and refining the ideas we have sketched here.

NOTES

1. The COMAC Childhood and Medicines Project was funded through a European Economic Community (EEC) *Comité d'Action Concerté* (COMAC) contract, COMAC/HSR MR4*-CT90-0319, awarded to The Institute on Child Health, Athens, Greece, with Deanna J. Trakas as the Project Leader. The official title of the Contract was "Medicine Use, Behaviour and Children's Perceptions of Medicines and Health Care." In Denmark, additional support was received from the Health Insurance Foundation Research Fund and The Danish Research Council for the Humanities.

2. "Illness" is used here in a general sense, including the subjective experience of disease. Conversely "sickness" is an analytical concept. We address a more specific definition of these concepts later in the chapter.

3. This chapter proposes some theoretical ideas based on children's understandings of illness and therapy (including pharmaceuticals) in different European cultural contexts. The distinctiveness of these understandings in relation to gender, age, and other aspects of social status will be analyzed in later publications. Here children's age and gender are used in a descriptive sense.

4. The distinctiveness of an illness episode (or e.g., minor accident) in everyday life may be illustrated using the example of a game of football in school. The game is rolling over the field, children are engaged in shouts and actions, running and kicking the ball. However, as soon as a child stumbles and falls on the ground, the match will stop. The game is interrupted by the whistle or shout of an adult or initiated by the children themselves. The previous flow of the game and noise is contrasted by the almost rigid roles and actions performed by adult and child. The adult inspects, organizes, and provides help. The other children often take a more passive role as spectators or they may run off to seek further adult assistance. For a further discussion see Christensen (1995).

5. Panodil® is a brand name of paracetamol (a painkiller) encountered in the Danish study. Panodil® can be obtained in two forms as over-the-counter medi-

cine in a pharmacy, one more generally used form although intended for adults, and one of a weaker strength/form intended especially for children.

6. Particular social and cultural settings and their embeddedness in wider social structures raise a number of difficult theoretical issues which are beyond the scope of this chapter. James and Prout (1995) discuss these at length, arguing that one problem with Douglas's approach is that it treats patterns of hierarchy and boundary as stable (at least in the long run). They suggest that on the contrary the patterns should be seen as mixed and in flux. Any given family or household is likely to display all the patterns to one degree or another (although perhaps tending toward one). Hierarchy and boundary patterns might be thought of as a set of partial connections recursive between different "levels." Furthermore, it might be preferable to theorize the patterned combinations as a grammar of strategic action rather than stable social environments. Most health work in the family, for example, is embedded in the flow of sometimes contradictory demands on family members and appears more as a set of contingent trade-offs among these demands rather than a fixed and consistent set of beliefs or attitudes.

REFERENCES

Armstrong, D. 1983. *Political Anatomy of the Body: Medical Knowledge in Britain in the Twentieth Century.* Cambridge: Cambridge University Press.

Backett, K. 1990. "Studying Health in Families." *Readings in Medical Sociology* edited by S. Cunningham-Burley and N. P. McKeganey. London: Routledge and Kegan Paul, pgs. 67-84.

Bernardes, J. 1985. "Do We Really Know What 'The Family' Is?" *Family and Economy in Modern Society* edited by P. Close and R. Collins. London: Macmillan.

Bernardes, J. 1986. "Multidimensional development pathways: A proposal to facilitate the conceptualization of family diversity." *Sociological Review,* 34: 590-607.

Bluebond-Langner, M. 1979. *The Private Worlds of Dying Children.* Princeton: Princeton University Press.

Christensen, P. H. 1993. "The social construction of help among Danish children: The intentional act and actual content." *Sociology of Health and Illness,* 15(4): 488-502.

Christensen, P. H. 1994. "Vulnerable bodies: Cultural meanings of child, body, and illness." Presented meeting Royal Anthropological Institute. Pauling Center for Human Sciences, Oxford.

Christensen, P. H. 1995. "The Danish participation in the COMAC Medicines and Childhood Project." *Childhood and Medicine Use in Cross-Cultural Perspective: A European Concerted Action* edited by D. J. Trakas and E. Sanz. Luxembourg: Office for Official Publications of the European Community, (EURO Report), pgs. (in press).

Currer, C. and Stacey, M. 1986. *Concepts of Health Illness and Disease.* New York/Oxford: BERG.

Davis, A. 1982. *Children in Clinics*. London: Tavistock.

Douglas, M. 1973. *Natural Symbols*. Harmondsworth: Penguin.

Douglas, M. (editor) 1982. *Essays in the Sociology of Perception*. London: Routledge and Kegan Paul.

Douglas, M. 1987. *How Institutions Think*. London: Routledge and Kegan Paul.

Douglas, M. 1992. *Risk and Blame: Essays in Cultural Theory*. London: Routledge and Kegan Paul.

Frankenberg, R. 1980. "Medical Anthropology and development: A theoretical perspective." *Social Science and Medicine* 14B: 197-207.

Frankenberg, R. 1985. "Malattia come festa: Sickness as celebration and socialization: Children's accounts of sickness episodes in a Tuscan community." Paper presented Annual Meeting American Anthropological Association, Washington.

Frankenberg, R. 1986. "Sickness as cultural performance: Drama, trajectory and pilgrimage. Root metaphors in the making social of disease." *International Journal of Health Services* 16(4): 603-626.

Gerrits, T., Haaijer-Ruskamp, F. and Hardon, A. 1994. "The perceptions and attitudes of Dutch children and their mothers about illness and the use of medicines." *Childhood and Medicine Use in Cross-Cultural Perspective: A European Concerted Action* edited by D. J. Trakas and E. Sanz. Luxembourg: Office for Official Publications of the European Community, (EURO Report), pgs. 123-128.

Hastrup, K. 1988. "Kultur som analytisk begreb." *Kulturbegrebets: Kulturhistorie* edited by H. Hauge and H. Horstbøll. Kulturstudier 1. Aarhus: Universitetsforlag, pgs. 120-139.

James, A. 1993. *Childhood Identities. Self and Social Relationships in the Experience of the Child*. Edinburgh: Edinburgh University Press.

James, A. and Prout, A. 1995. "Hierarchy, Boundary and Agency: Toward a Theoretical Perspective on Childhood." *Sociological Studies of Childhood* edited by A. M. Ambert. London: JAI Press.

Jenks, C. 1982. *The Sociology of Childhood: Essential Readings*. London: Batsford.

Kleinman, A. 1980. *Patients and Healers in the Context of Culture: An Exploration of the Borderland Between Anthropology, Medicine, and Psychiatry*. Berkeley, CA: Berkeley University Press.

Nader, L. 1980. "The Vertical Slice: Hierarchies and Children." *Hierarchy and Society* edited by G. M. Britain and R. Cohen. Philadelphia: Ishi.

Prout, A. 1986. "'Wet children' and 'little actresses': Getting sick in primary school." *Sociology of Health and Illness* 8(2): 111-137.

Prout, A. 1988. "Off school sick: Mothers' accounts of school sickness absence." *Sociological Review* 36: 765-790.

Prout, A. 1992. "Children and childhood in the sociology of medicine." *Studying Childhood and Medicine Use* edited by D. J. Trakas and E. J. Sanz. Athens, Greece: ZHTA Medical Publications, pgs. 123-139.

Prout, A. and James, A. 1990. "A New Paradigm for the Sociology of Child-hood..?" *Constructing and Reconstructing Childhood: Contemporary Issues in the Sociological Study of Childhood* edited by A. James and A. Prout. London: Falmer Press, pgs. 7-34.

Scheper-Hughes, N. (editor). 1987. *Child Survival: Anthropological Perspectives on the Treatment and Maltreatment of Children*. Dordrecht: D Reidel.

Strong, P. M. 1979. *The Ceremonial Order of the Clinic*. London: Routledge and Kegan Paul.

van der Geest, S. and Whyte, S. R. 1989. "The charm of medicines: Metaphors and metonyms." *Medical Anthropology Quarterly* 34: 345-366.

Vaskilampi, T., Kalpio, O., Ahonen, R., and Hallia, O. 1995. "Finnish study on medicine use, health behavior, and perceptions of medicines and health care." *Childhood and Medicine Use in Cross-Cultural Perspective: A European Concerted Action* edited by D. J. Trakas and E. Sanz. Luxembourg: Office for Official Publications of the European Community, (EURO Report), pgs. 191-220.

Whyte, S. R. 1992. "Pharmaceuticals as folk medicine: Transformations in the social relations of health care in Uganda." *Culture, Medicine and Psychiatry* 16:163-186.

Young, A. 1982. "The anthropologies of illness and sickness." *Annual Review of Anthropology* 11: 257-285.

Chapter 4

Acquiring Medicines in Europe and the USA

Flora M. Haaijer-Ruskamp

The act of acquiring medicines is performed within different circumstances depending on where one lives. These differences determine to a considerable extent the use of medicines. Medicine use varies greatly among countries, as is widely recognized. A variety of medical traditions has led to different views about medicines and their use, which is also reflected in policy regarding pharmaceuticals even in countries with comparable socioeconomic backgrounds. Take, for example differences in overall drug use, as measured by volume and expenditure (Table 4.1).

Table 4.1 presents a general picture, but similar variations appear when more detailed information is examined. For example, psychotropic drug use in 1986 was in Denmark 120 DDD/1000 (Defined Daily Doses/1000) inhabitants/day, in Finland 76, and in the Netherlands 33 (Bakker 1989).

Prescribing "rationality," i.e., prescribing consistent with pharmacological knowledge and opinion, requires attention to more than volume and expenditure. Comparing the 50 most frequently sold medicines in France, Germany, Italy, and the UK it was recently noted that in France and Italy 50 percent of the expenditure was for medicines of proven effectiveness, 70 percent in Germany, and 95 percent in the UK. At the same time 20 percent of the expenditure in France and Italy and 12 percent in Germany were spent on medicines of dubious value (Garattini and Garattini 1993). These four countries have only seven products in their top 50 in common: ranitidine, omeprazol, nifedipine, enalapril, captopril, simvastatine and acyclovir, underlining the diversity of medicine use patterns.

TABLE 4.1. Percentage of Diagnoses Ending in Medication and Pharmaceutical Expenditure per Person Including Hospitals (wholesale prices in U.S. $,1992)

Country	Diagnosis with Medication (%)	Pharmaceutical Expenditure (U.S. $)
Finland[1]	51	109[3]
Germany[2]	70	184
Italy[2]	95	166
Netherlands[2]	56	101
Spain[2]	79	126
UK[2]	74	88
USA[2]	67	152

[1]Riihimäki S: Särkylääkeiden käytön ongelmia sekä lääkkeiden määräämi- nen terveyskeskuksessa. Master's Thesis. University of Kuopio, Depart- ment of Social Pharmacy, Finland 1989.
[2]IMS, as quoted in Nefarma: farma feiten 1994.

To understand how such variations can occur, it is important to take a close look at the context of medicine use. In recent decades many contextual factors have been identified as being relevant. They include characteristics of the society, of patients, of physician practices, and of the prescribing physicians themselves. The most important factors identified are given in Table 4.2.

The focus in the remaining chapters in this book is on the family as a source of variation in medicine use. The focus in this chapter is on how people may acquire their medicines in the different coun- tries concerned in view of the organization of health care and phar- maceutical policy. The issues addressed are the availability, both physical and financial, of medicines for different segments of the population and the quality of the available medicines. For the pre- scribing physician and the consumer, the structure of health care and drug policy determine the available options. One cannot, however, isolate the health care system completely from the other

TABLE 4.2. Factors Influencing Medicine Use

Level	Relevant Factors	Policy/Instruments
I population	Regulation, financing and availability of medicines and health care, power of the pharmaceutical industry, culture, tradition, beliefs regarding health and illness	Legal instruments, requirements of drug registration, health insurance and reimbursement systems for drugs
II practice	Urbanization; proportion of elderly and female patients, lower economic class patients; practice size, single-handed practices, health centers	Organization of health care/structure of health care
III physician	Age, gender, attitudes and working style (e.g., tendency of physicians to act instead of to 'wait and see,' disease vs. patient orientation, perceived patient demand), training and education, use of information sources, doctor-patient interaction	Physician education, information available to physicians
IV patient	Age, gender, social economic class, social circumstances, expectations and demands, compliance	Patient education, reimbursement system

Source: Cialdella et al. 1991; Dukes 1985; Haaijer-Ruskamp and Hemminki 1993.

relevant factors. In looking at the health care systems within the countries involved in The COMAC Childhood and Medicines Project,[1] other contextual factors are first examined, beginning with differences in medical opinion.

FACTORS ACCOUNTING FOR DIFFERENCES IN MEDICINE USE

Differences in Medical Opinion

In general, little is known regarding the effect of medical opinion as reflected in different prescribing patterns for different diseases. Most international comparisons look at patterns of medicine use without the context of the indication. The scant data that exist which take the indication into account point to a substantial effect. For example, a comparison of the treatment of sinusitis, tonsillitis, and otitis media between the Netherlands and Sweden, showed that in Sweden antibiotics were used much more often than in the Netherlands. In Sweden the antibiotic of choice was the small spectrum phenoxymethylpenicillin, while in the Netherlands the antibiotic of choice was usually a broad spectrum. In the case of otitis media, these differences could be explained by differences in the national medical literature and local trials (Haaijer-Ruskamp 1992). More recently, *The Lancet* noted a possible underuse of morphine and morphine derivatives in Europe in the treatment of pain of terminal cancer patients, in particular in the southern European countries (Thomsen et al. 1993; Zenz and Willweber-Strumpf 1993; Zylics 1993). It appears that in southern and eastern European countries, terminal cancer is still often kept secret from the patient, rendering the prescribing of morphine rather difficult. In some southern European countries (for example Italy), prescribing of morphine requires extensive bureaucratic procedures going back to legal measures before World War II that were originally meant to stop illegal morphine trade in a time when the value of morphine for terminal cancer patients was not appreciated.

Although, undoubtedly, more such examples of differing medical opinion can be found, it is safe to assume they will lessen in the near future. Medical knowledge is increasingly becoming international with a rapid exchange of information between scientists. In important diseases, international consensus meetings are held on treatment, such as in the case of asthma (International Guidelines for the Treatment of Asthma 1992). Large international databases are set up to facilitate meta-analysis–for example by the Cochrane Centre at Oxford–and thus promote consensus in medical opinion.

Availability of Medicines

In addition to differences in medical opinion underlying the variation in drug use patterns, many "nonmedical" factors are influential. One such is the registration policy in the different countries, which determines the number of drugs on the market (Table 4.3).

The variation in the number of drugs on the market when looking at the individual preparations is much more than if only the active substances are taken into account reflecting differences in approval policies. One reason, for example, for the relatively high number of medicines on the German market has been the tolerance for com-

TABLE 4.3. Number of Medicines on the Market, All Preparations and Active Ingredients

Country	Different Preparations	Active Ingredients
Denmark[1]	3,789	902
Finland[1]	3,700	1,000
Germany[1]	23,431	2,900
Greece[1]	4,888	812
Italy[1]	9,029	1,545
Netherlands[1]	8,195	1,600
Spain[1]	10,817	1,897
USA[2]	9,079	1,260

[1] Muller and Dessing (1994).
[2] Johnson, K. (1994).

bination products, in contrast to other countries. With increasing internationalization, such differences will probably disappear in the long run. In the European Union, efforts to harmonize approval procedures date back to the beginning of the 1980s with the Committee for Proprietary Medicinal Products (CPMP) playing a key role as coordinator. Multi-state approval procedures, making registration possible based on the registration in at least two other member states, have simplified approval at the national level. Since 1987, national registration authorities are obliged to consult the CPMP for "high-tech" preparations, for example those based on biotechnology, in a so-called concertation procedure. The aim is to judge highly innovative products as uniformly as possible. From January, 1995, the harmonizing role of "Europe" will be intensified when the new European Medicines Evaluation Agency (EMEA) starts its work in London. The close cooperation within Europe has eased collaboration with the USA and Japan. Registration authorities of the three power blocks now confer on a regular basis.

The data in Table 4.2 refer to medicines as defined by law; so-called alternative medicines are excluded, although in some countries, notably German speaking, these comprise an important part of the market. Other countries seem to be catching up; countries with a low turnover for homeopathic products show high growth rates (Figure 4.1).

Health Insurance and Medicines

The medicines available on the market are of course essential in shaping patterns of medicine use. As essential, if not more, is the extent that medicines are affordable; a situation that is influenced by drug pricing and reimbursement policies. Traditionally, health insurance in Europe has been dominated by the principle of solidarity, while in the USA the accent has been on self-help. Solidarity means the acceptance of the responsibility that all who are in need have access to medical care. The principle of solidarity implies the direct involvement of public health authorities, as is the case in most European countries. The impact of the different principles governing health care insurance in the USA and Europe is well illustrated by the percentage of public expenditure (Table 4.4).

FIGURE 4.1. Growth in Turnover of Homeopathic Products in Europe

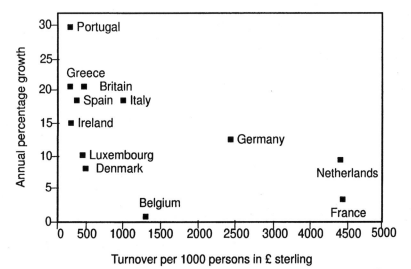

Source: Leufkens, Haaijer-Ruskamp, and Baker 1993.

Faced with continuously rising costs, the natural response of European countries has been to intervene directly with a number of cost-containment measures. Pharmaceutical expenditure figures strongly in these policies, because access to and use of drugs is supposed to be more amenable to regulation than other health care provisions (Lovatt 1992). Moreover, the increase in pharmaceutical expenditure has been significantly larger than the total health expenditure in a number of countries, such as the Netherlands, Italy, and the USA. The USA has been faced with more than only a steep increase in pharmaceutical expenditure. Here, health care in general has become so costly that a large proportion of the population cannot make use of it. An overview of the reimbursement situation in Europe is given in Table 4.5, including direct price control and measures intended to promote rational prescribing. In all these countries, virtually the total population is covered by insurance plans. Health insurance legislation and regulation are enacted at the national level, although in some countries regional states or prov-

TABLE 4.4. Public Expenditure as Percentage of Total Health Expenditure (1989) and Percentage of Public Expenditure of Total Pharmaceutical Expenditure (1987)

Country	Public Health Expenditure (% of total)	Public Pharmaceutical Expenditure (% of total)
Denmark	84%	45%
Germany	72%	70%
Greece	89%	21% (1986)
Italy	79%	66%
Netherlands	73%	67%
Spain	78%	59% (1983)
UK	87%	79%
USA	42%	11%

Source: Redwood 1992.

inces are independent to a considerable degree in matters other than the reimbursement of medicines.

In all countries reimbursement of drugs is limited to prescribed drugs; self-medication is not covered. Southern European countries seem to rely mainly on a combination of control of drug prices and a positive list plus copayment. Prices in these countries are also low in comparison to the others. Copayment is usually related to the therapeutic value of drugs (as described and defined in the positive lists) as well as the medical need for groups of patients. In Italy, for example, recent legislation has been enacted that identifies a limited number of "essential" medicines that are 100 percent reimbursed after a 5000 lire payment; however, children, elderly and pregnant women are exempt from this fixed amount. The category of "therapeutically valuable" medicines are reimbursed for 50 percent, and the remainder are represented by a list of nonreimbursable drugs. In the UK, a fixed amount is charged from which many patient groups

TABLE 4.5. Reimbursement of Pharmaceuticals in Europe

	DE	YU	D	GR	I	NL	E	UK
PRICE RELATED								
Individual product prices controlled				Yes	Yes		Yes	
Company profits controlled								Yes
Promotion of generics	Yes		Yes			Yes		X
REIMBURSEMENT								
Positive list	Yes	Yes		Yes	Yes		Yes	
Negative list	Yes		Yes			Yes	Yes	Yes
Copayment[1]	25-50%	0-50%		25%	0-100%		60%	£4.75
Reference prices	Yes		Yes			Yes		
Budget for prescribers			Yes					Yes

DE: Denmark; YU: Former Yugoslavia; D: Germany; GR: Greece; I: Italy; NL: Netherlands; E: Spain; UK: United Kingdom.
[1]Percentages represent the charge to the patient.
Sources: Report on the Measures taken by Member States for the implementation of Directive 89/105/EEC, March 1994; Rutten and van Hout 1994.

(including elderly, children, pregnant women) are exempt. Interesting new developments include the introduction of reference pricing and indicative budgets for prescribers. A reference price system implies that a patient is reimbursed up to the limit determined for the cluster of drugs to which the prescribed drug belongs. If the price for the prescribed drug is above this limit, the patient has to pay the difference out of pocket. Drugs are clustered in terms of pharmacologic or therapeutic equivalence. In fact, in reference pricing, the patient is used in order to put pressure on prescribers to prescribe the cheaper products. At the same time it is an indirect way of controlling prices; a pharmaceutical company will lower drug prices to remain below the reimbursement limit in order to safeguard the use of its products. Another way to keep prices down is to encourage the use of generic preparations; when the patent of a brand name is ended, generic products come on the market, usually at a much lower price than the original. In some European countries, as in some states in the USA, the pharmacist is entitled to substitute generics for brand-name products. The use of generics is not common in all countries. In Greece, Italy, and Spain, it is very limited or nonexistent, whereas in Denmark, Germany, the Netherlands, and the UK, it is increasing rapidly. In 1992, generics represented 29 percent of the medicines prescribed in Germany, 43 percent of those in the UK, 70 percent of those in Denmark, and in the Netherlands 24 percent of the medicines prescribed (Joossens 1994). Health insurance has traditionally not been so much a part of the national policy, as it is considered to be the responsibility of the individual. In 1992 a further increase was forecasted in Germany (18 percent), the UK (18 percent), and the Netherlands (34 percent) (IMS 1992).

Budgets for prescribers have been introduced in the UK and Germany. In Germany, in particular, where, in a measure introduced in 1993, sanctions were included for not keeping to the budget, the effect has been enormous. A decrease in prescribing occurred mainly in drug groups presumably prescribed for a wider range of indications than medically and pharmacologically indicated, such as lipid-lowering drugs (-42.8 percent), vascular drugs (-34.2 percent), blood circulation products (-26.5 percent), vitamins (-25.4 percent), minerals (-22.6 percent) (Arzneimittelbrief 1993). The decrease was so strong that overall spending fell short of the budget in 1993. As mentioned before, the situation relative to drug reimbursement in the USA is completely different from Europe. Only the unemployed and very poor are insured in Medicaid and the elderly in Medicare. For the rest, health insurance is usually related to the job situation, being one of the secondary employment benefits. However, in case of change of jobs or unemployment, health insurance benefits may be lost. Moreover, acceptance within a health insurance plan is not obligatory. Coverage can be excluded for certain preexisting diseases or pregnancy, or premiums can be raised greatly. Employers are not obliged to get health insurance for their employees. About 49 percent of small companies do not provide health insurance coverage, whereas large companies have tried to cut back on expenditure by limiting coverage. An increasing number of middle income people, in particular, have lost coverage; 37 million people are not insured, 22 million are estimated to be underinsured (Van Kemenade 1994). This, in combination with the high percentage the USA spends on health care (more than 12 percent of GDP in 1993) has made the need for health care reform clear. In September, 1993, the Clinton Plan for health care reform was made public (Greenberg 1993). In the USA system of private enterprise, no uniformity exists regarding drug reimbursement. In any case, reimbursement for medicines in some form is not assumed as it is in most European countries. Many insurance plans (and even capitated prepaid plans) do not cover medicines at all. Medicare, health insurance for the elderly, does not cover medicines for ambulatory patients in any state. Medicaid, public health care for the poor, covers drugs but varies among the states in providing coverage. If insurance plans cover drugs, they seldom cover 100 percent of the expenditure. Many of the reimbursement schemes are used as in Europe, in particular positive and negative lists, deductibles, copayments, and encouragement of the use of generics. Price control of individual products obviously does not fit the American system. In the Clinton Plan, reimbursement for drugs for everybody was included with a choice between a copayment of $5 per prescription or 20 percent per prescription after a deductible of $250 was met—with a maximum copayment of $1000 annually. Quantity limits and prescribing frequency were not mentioned in the plan.

Although it is unlikely that nationwide coverage of drugs will in fact be implemented, it does indicate that the USA is considering moving to more solidarity in its health insurance plans. Ambulatory Medicare patients are the most likely next group to be covered for prescription drugs but even these are highly likely to have a deductible and/or copayments.

Availability of Care

For patients the availability of accessible care is an important factor when deciding to seek professional care or rely on self-care. For the use of medicines, outpatient care is the most relevant. In Europe it is mainly provided by general practitioners and primary care health centers, and in the USA mainly by private physicians and outpatient clinics. In general, it is estimated that 80 to 90 percent of the costs for medicines are generated in outpatient care. Two professions dominate the field: general practitioners (GPs) and pharmacists. In countries with a high number of GPs, competition for patients is strong. It is to be expected that in such situations giving in to patient demand is more attractive then "saying no." Such processes are strongest in systems where the remuneration system is one of fee-for-service. Not giving in to patient demand in such systems may lose patients. It is therefore to be expected that in a country such as Germany, GPs will be more sensitive to patient demand than a country such as the UK where GPs do not have to compete for patients and their income is relatively little determined by the amount of services provided (Table 4.6).

General Practice is well developed in the European countries; the number of GPs is large enough to make them easily available and in most cases their care in the public system is free of charge. The position of GP is particularly strong in countries where it has a gatekeeper role for access to hospital care. Greece is the exception in the general European picture. Contrary to the other countries, in Greece primary care is poorly developed; the system relies heavily on secondary care provided in outpatient clinics and public and private hospitals. The government has tried to develop a network of health centers, but only 180 of the 400 have been realized, mainly in rural areas. Many people use private services for which considerable payments are made.

TABLE 4.6. General Practice and Pharmacists

| Country | General Practitioners | | | | | Pharmacists |
	GPs	Persons/GP	Gate Keeper	Remuneration	Patient Cost	Inhabitants/ Pharmacist
DE	3,300	1,600	yes	mixed system	95% free[1]	4,644[2]
YU	3,800	2,000	no	salary	free	4,600
D	29,000	2,000	no	fee for service	93% free	3,950
GR	850[3]	1,900	no	capitation/salary	free (public)	1,124[4]
I	67,000		yes	capitation/salary	copayment	3,700
NL	6,500	2,350	yes	mixed system	60% free	10,570/2.6 50[5]
E	40,000	2,500	yes	capitation/salary	free	2,207
UK	30,000	1,800	yes	mixed system	free	5,020
USA	74,715	3,480	sometimes	mixed system	0-100% free	2,155

DE: Denmark; YU: former Yugoslavia; D: Germany; GR: Greece; I: Italy; NL: Netherlands; E: Spain; UK: United Kingdom.
1 95% of the patients.
2 Sources: Statistik Denmark 1994; Holme Hansen, Claesson, and Frokjet, 1994.
3 The GP is almost unknown in Greece; other physicians working in outpatient centers may have different payment schemes; in the USA, GP includes family practitioners (FP).
4 Greece National Pharmacist Association.
5 Second figure represents the number of inhabitants per pharmacist drugstore owner.
Sources: Grol et al. 1993; Boerma, De Jong, and Mulder 1993; Croix Verte 1990; Rajaniemi 1992; Weiner 1994.

The number of inhabitants per pharmacy varies greatly. In Spain, a pharmacist seems to be nearby for most patients, while in the UK this is less clearly the case. The Netherlands have a complicated system of distribution for pharmaceuticals, relying on pharmacists as well as dispensing GPs and drugstore owners for packaged self-medication preparations. The number of 10,570 inhabitants per pharmacy is therefore inflated.

Self-Medication

Most physical complaints are dealt with at home without any professional help; the extent varies with the accessibility of professional care. Where access to professional care is poor, self-medication tends to be used as a substitute for prescribed drugs (Leibowitz 1989). A market research study investigated the response to health complaints in the USA–a country with unequal access–and the Netherlands; 59 percent of the respondents chose self-medication in the USA and 31 percent in the Netherlands. For similar complaints, 15 percent in the USA chose to go to the physician and 25 percent to do nothing, in comparison to respectively 26 percent and 43 percent in the Netherlands (Van Rossum 1993). However, accessibility of professional care is not the only reason for choosing self-medication. Data from another marketing research effort (Secodip 1991) show that respondents in the UK–with a health care system similar to that of the Netherlands–responded to the same question with 55 percent choosing self-medication, 26 percent choosing to visit the doctor, and 17 percent choosing to do nothing. People in both the USA and the UK seem from these data more prone to use self-medication than the Dutch. In the UK people seem, however, to use professional care more readily than in the USA; they were much less likely to indicate they would do nothing. These data should be interpreted with care, however, since nothing is known regarding their representativeness. They do however indicate a trend that is consistent with other data–the Dutch are low users of medicines and the use of professional care is related to its accessibility.

Table 4.7 shows that the Dutch are relatively low spenders on self-medication, as they are low spenders for total pharmaceutical consumption (Table 4.1). Germany is a high consumer of medicines, including self-medication in particular (Table 4.1). Greece is

TABLE 4.7. Self-Medication Expenditure per Person (in Guilders, Retail Price) and Percentage of Expenditure for Self-Medication of Total Pharmaceutical Expenditure (1993)

Country	Self-Medication Expenditure/Person	Percent Expenditure for Self-medication
Germany	106	16
Italy	42	10
Netherlands	29	8
Spain	37	12
UK	51	13
USA	70	28

Source: IMS 1994.

exceptional regarding the legal status of self-medication in that self-medication drugs do not exist officially with the exception of aspirin and paracetamol.

Health authorities in many countries consider a switch to more self-medication as a possible way to contain public pharmaceutical expenditure; switching from prescription-only status to self-medication status is one way of stimulating this trend. The analgesic ibuprofen was one of the first drugs to be switched to self-medication status and is now a self-medication drug except in Greece. Other frequently prescribed drugs such as H2 antagonists for peptic ulcers, other nonsteroidal inflammatories (NSAIDs), and hydrocortisone are in many countries in the process of being switched to self-medication status. In the UK, 14 such switches took place since 1993; the most recent one concerned cimetidine and famotidine, both H2 blockers.

Advertising of Medicines

Prescribers and consumers alike all over the world are bombarded with information and advertising about medicines. Advertising and other promotional activities of the pharmaceutical industry are considered to be one of the most important influences on actual medicine use. In particular, in a time of growing self-medication, advertising directly to the public is getting more and more important (Chetley 1993). All industrialized countries recognize the influence of advertising and have set up legal standards concerning the promotion of medical products in order to regulate the contents of the advertisements. In the European countries, advertising directly to the public is limited to self-medication products, while in the USA this is also allowed for prescription-only medicines. On the international level, two important guidelines have been published. In 1992 the European Communities published the Directive on the Advertising of Medicinal Products, while already in 1988 the WHO published its Ethical Criteria for Medicinal Drug Promotion. The importance and relevance of the latter standard was reinforced in a new resolution of the World Health Assembly of the WHO in 1994 asking the countries of the world to pay new attention to the problem of advertising with unsubstantiated claims. At present, it is not clear to what extent the countries involved in the COMAC Childhood and Medicines Project actually differ in the amount of advertising to which their populations are subjected. It is safe to assume that in all countries, such advertising occurs widely, and that in all countries the information is biased.

In a recent International Organization of Consumers Unions (IOCU) study (Kaldeway et al. 1994), 183 advertisements to the public from 11 countries were analyzed in regard to their adherence to the EU and WHO standards. The study included advertisements from Denmark, Finland, Germany, the Netherlands, the UK, and the USA. Direct comparison among countries was not legitimate; the advertisements differed too much in terms of content and numbers. However, overall there appeared to be little compliance with the international standards. Only three advertisements complied completely with the international standards. In particular, information about contraindications, side effects, and warnings was lacking.

Marketing pharmaceuticals to the public is not limited to advertising in magazines. The pharmaceutical industry has, partly in reaction to the stricter regulations from the authorities, developed many other ways to reach the public. Direct advertising on television and radio happens regularly and there are more indirect ways. In some popular TV series, for example, attention is given to the positive aspects of medicines, and this is paid for by the pharmaceutical industry (Chetley and Mintzes 1992). A recent trend, in the USA as well as in Europe, features "information campaigns," preferably with famous people acting as informers, which concern a specific disease but not a specific single product, in order to prevent problems with the authorities. The information campaigns on TV provide toll-free numbers people can call to get information about the disease. Also there are multiple choice tests published in magazines and journals, and articles about some disease in magazines ending with the offer of a booklet for people who want to have more information, etc. These campaigns are intended to increase general patient demand; they suggest to the public "maybe you're sick." The health authorities appear to have little to counter these new tactics. The press, however, does give attention to this phenomenon. *The New York Times* (April 10, 1994), described success of this tactic in getting people to the doctor with complaints suggested in the promotional activities, but who had no apparent medical need (as quoted in *Nederlands Tijdschrift voor Geneeskunde* 1994).

CONCLUSION

The acquisition of medicine is subject to a number of regulations that differ for every country. To a certain extent, these regulations shape actual patterns of medicine use. In this chapter, the context is given for the countries involved in The COMAC Childhood and Medicines Project, based on data available from different sources. Although the data are not complete for every country, they do give an overall impression, of diversity.

On the one hand, there is a clear tendency toward internationalization. The pharmaceutical industry operates at a global level; health authorities in the different countries meet each other more and look at each other's solutions for the problems they encounter in their own countries. In the European Union a number of recent directives strengthens rationalization of pharmaceutical policies. At present, most European directives are concerned with technocratic aspects. The national health authorities are still largely in control.

More important for convergence of pharmaceutical policies than direct intervention in policies at the European level may be the increased collaboration and exchange of information it has brought about, not only among European countries but also between Europe and the USA. All countries are faced with the problem of the rapid increase in costs for medicines. The nature of the problems differ— some countries face high levels of use of low-cost medicines, whereas others have low levels of use of expensive medicines. In the future one may expect prices to converge; in high-price countries there is strong pressure to have lower prices, whereas in low-price countries the need to value innovation will lead to higher prices in the long term (Redwood 1992). On the other hand, regarding reimbursement systems, convergence is not as clear. The northern European countries are directing their measures primarily at the demand side, i.e., the prescriber, with negative lists and reference pricing, while the southern European countries and the USA are primarily oriented toward the supply side with systems of positive lists and patient charges. However, even here one can see signs of further convergence. France has now also turned toward prescribers by establishing prescribing guidelines, and Denmark has a positive list and copayments. Moreover, the USA may be ready to introduce more elements of solidarity in its system, whereas in Europe more self-help elements are being introduced with more responsibility and more financial contributions by the patients. The recent European directive regarding labeling, patient information, and promotional activities of the industry should increase the possibility of uniformity of drug information. Besides these bureaucratic measures, the increased interchange of information in professional journals as well as in the mass media provides a climate favorable for further internationalization of knowledge and beliefs. Professional medical organizations, as well as patient and consumer organizations operate frequently at an international level which regulates information to their own members. Medical tourism, where groups of patients seek care in another country when the desired care is not provided in their own, happens regularly and may even be entitled to reimbursement (Hughes 1992). All these trends toward internationalization do not imply that medicine-use patterns will be the same in the near future.

In a recent study in Belgium, medicine use by adolescents for a headache appeared to be higher in the Flemish-speaking community than in the French-speaking community, despite an identical health care structure (Joossens 1993). Findings such as these emphasize that even in similar contexts, medicine use may still differ because of different interpretations, attitudes, and beliefs. This issue is the central theme of the studies reported in this book.

NOTE

1. The COMAC Childhood and Medicines Project was funded through a European Economic Community (EEC) *Comité d'Action Concerté* (COMAC) contract, COMAC/HSR MR4*-CT90-0319, awarded to The Institute on Child Health, Athens, Greece, with Deanna J. Trakas as the Project Leader. The official title of the Contract was "Medicine Use, Behaviour and Children's Perceptions of Medicines and Health Care." In the Netherlands, the study was also supported by The Ministry of Welfare, Public Health, and Culture and the Northern Centre of Health Care Research, University of Groningen.

REFERENCES

Arzneimittelbrief, 1993. Wo haben die Kassen Ärtzte gespart? *Der Arzneimittelbrief,* 62-63.

Bakker A. 1989. "Vergelijking met het buitenland; is Nederland anders?" *Pharmaceutisch Weekblad* 124:950-955.

Boerma, W. G. W., De Jong, F. A. J. M, and Mulder, P. H. 1993. *Health Care in Europe.* Dutch College of General Practitioners/Netherlands Institute of Primary Health Care, Utrecht.

Chetley, A. 1993. *Problem drugs.* Health International (HAI Europe), Amsterdam.

Chetley, A. and Mintzes, B. (eds). 1992. *Promoting health or pushing drugs.* Health Action International (HAI Europe), Amsterdam.

Cialdella, P., Figon, G., Haugh, M. C., and Boissel, J. P. 1991. "Prescription intentions in relation to therapeutic information: A study of 117 French general practitioners." *Social Science and Medicine,* 33:1263–1274.

Croix Verte, 1990. As quoted in *Zelfzorg* 1993 (Sept): pg. 6. *Denmarks Statistik* 1994, Copenhagen.

Dukes, M. N. G. 1985. *The Effects of Drug Regulation.* Lancaster, MTP Press.

European Communities. 1992 Council Directive on the Advertising of Medicinal Products. 92/28/EEC. March 31.

Garattini, S. and Garattini, L. 1993. "Pharmaceutical prescriptions in four European countries." *The Lancet* 342:1192-1193.

Greenberg, D. 1993. "The Clintons present their health plan." *The Lancet* 342: 797-798.

Grol, R., Wensing, M., Jacobs, A., and Baker, A. 1993. *Quality Assurance in General Practice; the State of the Art in Europe.* Dutch College of General Practitioners/European Working Party on Quality in Family Practice, (EQuiP) Utrecht.

Haaijer-Ruskamp, F. M. 1992. "Geneesmiddelengebruik in Europa." *Pharmaceutisch. Weekblad,* 127: 1291-1297.

Haaijer-Ruskamp, F. M. and Hemminki, E. 1993. "The Social Aspects of Drug Use." *Drug Utilization Studies–Methods and Uses* edited by M. N. G. Dukes. WHO Regional Publications, European Series 45: 97-124.

Holme Hansen, E., Claesson, C., and Frokjet, B. 1994. *Apoteksfarmaceuternes funktiones i de Nordisk Landr.* Copenhagen 1994.

Hughes, C. 1992. "European law, medicine and the social charter." *British Medical Journal,* 304: 701.

IMS (Institute for Medical Statistics). 1992. Strategic forecast study.

IMS (Institute for Medical Statistics). 1994. As quoted in *Zelfzorg* 6:(June) supplement.

International Consensus Report on Diagnosis and Treatment of Asthma. 1992. Bethesda, MD: National Institutes of Health.

Johnson, K. 1994. (Personal communication).

Joossens, L. 1994 (April). *De Evolutie Van de Verkoop Van Generieke Geneesmiddelen in de Europese Unie.* Hearing of the Committee for Public Health and Environment, Chamber of Representatives, Brussels.

Joossens, L. 1993. *Geneesmiddelen.* Onderzoek–en informatiecentrum van de verbruikersunie, Brussels.

Kaldeway, H., Wieringa, N. F., and Herxheimer, A. 1994. *A Searching Look at Advertisements.* Scienceshop for Medicines, University of Groningen and International Organization of Consumers Unions.

Leibowitz, A. 1989. "Substitution between prescribed and over-the-counter medications." *Medical Care,* 27: 85-94.

Leufkens, H. G. M., Haaijer-Ruskamp, F. M., and Bakker, A. 1993. *De toekomst van het geneesmiddel in de Gezondheidszorg.* Bohn Stafleu Van Loghum, Houten/Zaventem.

Lovatt, B. 1992. "The role of health economics in marketing new pharmaceuticals worldwide." *Journal of Research in Pharmaceutical Marketing,* 4: 19.

Muller, N. F. and Dessing, R. P. (eds) 1994: European Drug Index. Amsterdam Medical Press, Alkmaar.

Nederlands Tijdschrift voor Genees unde. 1994; 138:1042.

Nefarma. 1994. Farma feiten (Pharmaceutical facts).

Rajaniemi, S. 1992. Reimbursement of medicine expenses out of social insurance funds in the Nordic countries and EC member states. Kansaneläkelaitoksen julkaisuja M:84, Helsinki.

Thomsen, O. O., Wulff, H. R., Martin, A., and Singer, P. A. 1993. "What do gastroenterologists tell cancer patients?" *Lancet,* 341: 473-476.

Redwood, H. 1992. *The Dynamics of Drug Pricing and Reimbursement in the European Community.* Oldswicks Press, Felixstowe.

Report on the Measures Taken by Member States for the Implementation of Directive 89/105/EEC. 1994 (March). Brussels.

Rutten, F. F. H. and Hout, B. A. 1994 (April). *Economic Evaluation and Reimbursement of Drugs; Current Policies and Future Trends.* 8th Conference on Pharmaceutical Medicine, Rome.

Secodip. 1991. As quoted in *Zelfzorg* 1993; 5 Sept pg. 9.

Van Kemenade, Y. W. 1994. "Het plan-Clinton." *Medisch Contact,* 49: 829-832.

Van Rossum, Z. T. 1993. Based on data from NDMA as quoted in *Zelfzorg* 5: 11-12.

Weiner, J. P. 1994. "Forecasting the effects of health reform on US physician workforce requirements." *Journal American Medical Association* 272(3): 222-230.

World Health Organization. 1988. Ethical Criteria for Medicinal Drug Promotion. WHO Geneva.

Zenz, M. and Willweber-Strumpf, A. 1993. "Opiophobia and cancer pain in Europe." *Lancet,* 341: 1075-1076.

Zylics, Z. 1993. "Opiophobia and cancer pain." *Lancet,* 341: 1473-1474.

SECTION II:
CROSS-CULTURAL REPORTS

Chapter 5

Medicines at Home: The Contents of Medicine Cabinets in Eight Countries

Emilio J. Sanz
Patricia J. Bush
Marcelino García

with Riitta Ahonen, Anna B. Almarsdottir,
Pilar Aramburuzabala, Chrysoula Botsis,
Giampaolo Canciani, Trudie Gerrits, Vida Jakovljevic,
Ana Sabo, Milan Stanulovic, and Rolf L. Wirsing

Research dating back to the 1970s confirmed suspicions that the majority of illness symptoms are either ignored or self-treated (Knapp and Knapp 1972; Bush and Rabin 1976). It is not until symptoms persist, worsen, or interfere with activities of daily living that most people bring them to the attention of the formal health care system. These observations stimulated concerns with the quality of self-care, its extent and nature, and concerns about the care provided by parents to children. Central to these concerns was the role played by medicines and how and why they are used differently by people who are in similar states of health.

In addition to morbidity, medicine use has been studied relative to demographic factors (e.g., age, gender, family size), economic and convenience factors (e.g., family income, health insurance; physical distance from a physician or a pharmacy), and factors related to the medicine itself (e.g., cost, prescribed or nonprescribed). Most of these investigations have relied on clinic or pharmacy records to obtain data (Bergman and Griffiths 1986; Sanz and Boada 1988; Sanz, Bergman, and Dahlstrom 1989; Serradel, Bjornson, and Hartzema 1991). Some investigations have involved home interviews (Bush and Rabin 1976, 1977; Cunningham-Burley and Irvine 1987; Gagnon, Salber, and Greene 1978; Jackson et al. 1982; Maiman, Becker and Katlic 1985; Rabin and Bush 1975; Segal 1990; Van den Brandt et al. 1991). One cross-national study performed in 12 areas of seven countries involved home interviews about medicine use in association with morbidity and use of health care services (Kohn and White 1976).

Considering the prevalence of self-care and the expected relationship between medicine availability and medicine use, it is surprising that household medicine inventories have not been performed with greater frequency. Exceptions are studies by Knapp and Knapp (1972) in a mid-western U.S. city; by Helling et al. (1987) of persons 65 years and older in the United States; by Chrischilles et al. (1992) in four United States areas; by Puche et al. (1982) who recorded the household medicines in Granada, Spain; by Trakas in 1981 who observed interactions in pharmacies in Athens, Greece, and then made home visits to the clientele where inventories of medications were made; and by Bush (Bush and Almarsdottir 1993; Moore, Bush, and Iannotti 1991a; 1991b) who twice inventoried the medicines in the homes of African Americans in Washington, DC, with the second inventory following the first by a year on average. In these studies, medicines in the home were seen and recorded, but in both the Chrischilles and Helling studies, reports only were made about the medicines taken in the two weeks prior to the interview. In the Puche study, reports were made of the medicines in 1,548 households to determine the type and quantity, source of acquisition, and storage location. Risks were noted relative to self-administration and accessibility to children less than five years old.

Comparing the results of the household medicine inventories of the Knapp study with the Bush study suggests that, within the same country, there may be considerable differences between different populations in the numbers of medicines kept in the home, but also similarities relative to characteristics such as the kinds of medicines found most frequently and household storage locations. In the Knapp study of 278 Ohio households, each with one child under 21 years, the average household had 4.8 persons and 22.5 medicines (5.3 prescribed and 17.2 nonprescribed), or an average of 4.7 medicines per household member. In the Bush study in 196 Washington, DC households, each with two children under ten years, the average household had 5.3 persons and 7.3 medicines (2.5 prescribed and 4.8 nonprescribed), or an average of 1.4 per household member.

An issue in The COMAC Childhood and Medicines Project was to investigate differences and similarities among the study locations with respect to the number of medicines, kinds of medicines, storage location, and use of medicines. This information, which is the subject of this chapter, is a first step toward explaining children's perceptions about medicines and expectations regarding their use.

METHODOLOGY

All of the medicines were inventoried in 400 homes in nine different locations in eight countries in the framework of The COMAC Childhood and Medicines Project.[1] A basic instrument, the Medicine Cabinet Inventory (MCI), was used in the following participating study locations: Amsterdam/Groningen, the Netherlands; Athens, Greece; Chapel Hill, United States; Hamburg, Germany; Jyväskylä, Finland; Madrid, Spain; Tenerife, Spain; Trieste, Italy; and Novi Sad, Yugoslavia. The MCI was adapted from the one used previously in Washington, DC (Bush and Almarsdottir 1993; Moore, Bush, and Iannotti 1991a, 1991b). Additional information was gathered by some research teams in addition to that required by the common MCI.

The home of each child participating in the study was visited to collect the data. The selection of the children and their families is described in Chapter 2.

Except in Jyväskylä, during the home visit the interviewer asked the parents to show all the medicines kept in the household. In some locations, the inventory began with three questions: What medicines are used and stored at home? Which are the most commonly used? Which are considered indispensable? The reactions of the parents ranged from spontaneously volunteering to take the interviewer to storage locations to simply beginning to name the medicines without showing them to the interviewer. In the latter case, the interviewer then asked the parents to show the medicines.

In Jyväskylä, an inventory of household medicines was taken via a structured form (modified MCI) left at each home following the interview of the children's parents. The parents returned the form by mail. Forty forms were returned from the 46 households where forms were left. Two of these forms indicated that there were no medicines in the household.

For each medicine, a complete record was made including the name, therapeutic category, prescription versus over-the-counter (OTC) status, dose form, days since acquired, for whom acquired, place acquired, days since last used, for whom last used, place kept, purpose of last use, expiration status, future use intention, and for whom intended. Each research team administering the MCI used the same variables and codes. Therapeutic categories were not defined by a standard pharmacological classification, but by one developed for the study. However, the teams in Madrid and Tenerife also used the names of the medicines to classify them by ATC codes (WHO 1993).

The analysis of the appropriate use of drugs by families in Madrid and Tenerife was performed as follows. Two different variables were assigned to each drug found in the MCI: (1) the official pharmacological classification of the drug (ATC codes), and (2) the study code reflecting the parent's opinion of the drug's purpose. However, this information was not available for 1,310 (51 percent) of the 2,587 medicines found in the Madrid and Tenerife households. The last use (or the intended use) was considered erroneous when the respondent's opinion of the drug's purpose was in serious disagreement with the pharmacologic (ATC) classification or when the indicated use was potentially dangerous, e.g., antibiotics or analgesics for vitamins, antiepileptics for analgesics, antacids for antidepressants or oral contraceptives, analgesics for tranquilizers.

In Chapel Hill, Madrid, and Tenerife, both the children and their primary caretakers were administered health locus of control scales. The concept of locus of control means that individuals have beliefs along a continuum that varies from a conviction that one can significantly affect (or is responsible for) the state of one's health (internal) to the conviction that one is helpless, that the state of one's health is largely out of the individual's control (external). The health locus of control scale used for the children was the nine-item Children's Health Locus of Control (CHLC) Scale shortened and adapted by Bush, Parcel, and Davidson (1982) from a longer version developed by Parcel and Meyer (1978). The CHLC requires dichotomous (yes/no) responses. The stability of the factor structure of the nine-item version has been shown (O'Brien, Bush, and Parcel 1989). The Multidimensional Health Locus of Control (MHLC) Scale consisting of 18 items measured on a six-point Likert Scale (Wallston, Wallston, and DeVellis 1978) was administered to the adults.

RESULTS

The MCI was administered in almost all of the households of the children included in the study in each location (Table 5.1). The number of households participating varied from 14 or 15 in Amsterdam/Groningen, Hamburg, and Novi Sad to 99 in Madrid, depending on the sample obtained for the general study. Where the study was more qualitatively oriented as in Amsterdam/Groningen and Hamburg, the number of families tended to be small. A total of 400 families with a total of 1,511 members was surveyed. Each family had at least one primary caretaker (usually a parent) and one child either about seven or about ten years old. Surprisingly, the average size of the families was very similar (four members) in most of these different locations with only Madrid and Hamburg having slightly smaller families of three members on average, and Jyväskylä having slightly larger families of five members on average.

A total of 6,554 medicines was found in the 394 households studied (Table 5.1). The average number of medicines per person varied from two in Jyväskylä to seven in Chapel Hill. There were threefold differences in the average number of drugs per household among the eight locations. Whereas in Jyväskylä there was an average of eight medicines per household, in Chapel Hill this value was 24 and in Novi Sad 23. The average number of medicines per household in the rest of the European locations was around the

TABLE 5.1. Description of the Samples

Variables	Location*									
	AmGr	At	CH	Ha	Jy	Ma	NS	Te	Tr	Total
Number:										
Households	15	32	59	15	40	99	14	85	35	394
Persons	67	130	215	52	197	325	56	331	138	1511
Medicines	203	353	1401	200	320	1793	323	1440	521	6554
Mean:										
Persons/household	4	4	4	3	5	3	4	4	4	4
Medicines/person	3	3	7	4	2	6	6	4	4	4
Medicines/household	14	11	24	13	8	18	23	18	15	17

*AmGr: Amsterdam & Groningen (NL), At: Athens (GR), CH: Chapel Hill (USA), Ha: Hamburg (D), Jy: Jyväskylä (SF), Ma: Madrid (E), NS: Novi Sad (Y), Te: Tenerife (E), Tr: Trieste (I).

mean of the total sample, ranging from 11 (Athens) to 18 (Madrid and Tenerife). Very few families (one or two) in each location stated that they did not have any medicines at all. At the other extreme, a few families in Spain and Italy showed more than 70 drugs stored in their households.

Another cultural difference appears to be reflected in the percentage of over-the-counter (OTC) drugs (Table 5.2). About 40 percent of all medicines in the homes were OTCs except in Amsterdam/Groningen (51 percent), Chapel Hill (74 percent) and Jyväskylä (51 percent) where the percentage of OTCs exceeded the percentage of prescription (Rx) drugs.

The number of drugs per household member varied among the different age groups (Table 5.3). The average number of drugs stored for multiple children and/or adults was small. In all of the locations except Jyväskylä and the two locations in Spain, medicines for females 15 to 64 years were most frequent.

The most common categories of drugs are shown in Table 5.4. Medicines in three therapeutic categories (topical, cough/cold, analgesic/antipyretic/nonsteroidal antiinflammatory drugs [NSAID]), were found most frequently in four locations, (Athens, Chapel Hill, Hamburg, and Trieste) accounting for more than half of the medicines. In all of the remaining locations, two of these three therapeutic categories ranked among the top three. Also ranking among the top three in Amsterdam/Groningen (11 percent) were homeopathic remedies, in Jyväskylä (14 percent) were eye/nose/ear medicines, and in Madrid (11 percent) and Tenerife (10 percent) were antiinfectives. Hamburg (8 percent) was the location with the second highest proportion of homeopathic remedies. In addition to homeopathic remedies, Amsterdam/Groningen (12 percent) and Hamburg (10 percent) accounted for the highest rates of medicines in the vitamin/mineral category. The digestive category was highest in Madrid (11 percent), Tenerife (11 percent), and Hamburg (10 percent). The pattern of drugs in Novi Sad households was quite different from the other locations, with the highest proportion of antibiotics (24 percent) and a relatively high proportion of cardiovascular and digestive medicines (7 percent). The low rates of oral contraceptives in all the locations suggest that this category was underreported.

TABLE 5.2. Over-the-Counter (OTC) vs. Prescription (Rx) Medicines*

| | Location* | | | | | | | |
Variables	AmGr	AT	CH	Ha	Jy	Ma	Te
Percentage:**							
Rx	48	55	26	57	38	61	51
OTC	51	36	74	43	51	36	38
Don't know	1	9	0	0	11	3	11
Average Number:							
Rx/household	7	6	6	7	3	11	9
OTC/household	7	4	18	6	5	6	7
Don't know	0	1	0	0	0	1	2

* No data available from Tr and NS.
** Percentages based on the total numbers from each location.

TABLE 5.3. Average Number of Medicines/Household by Gender and Age

Persons	Location[1]							
	AmGr	At	CH	Ha	Jy	Ma	Te	Tr
Female <3 yr	2	3	2	-	0	3[2]	4	0
Male <3 yr	-	0	-	-	2	0	5	0
Female 3-14 yr	1	1	3	4	1	5	2	3
Male 3-14 yr	1	1	4	4	1	6	3	3
Female 15-64 yr	4	3	6	4	1	3	4	4
Male 15-64 yr	3	2	4	2	1	3	3	2
Female >64 yr	0	0	4	0	-	4	-	0
Male >64 yr	0	0	-	0	-	1	-	1
Multiple children	0	1	1	0	0	0	1	0
Multiple adults	1	2	0	0	0	0	0	0
Adults and children	1	0	1	0	0	0	0	1
Unknown	0	0	0	1	0	1	0	0

[1] No data available from NS.
[2] Data omitted on one child with 22 medicines.

85

TABLE 5.4. Percentage of Medicines by Therapeutic Category[1]

Category	Location								
	AmGr	AT	CH	Ha	Jy	Ma	NS	Te	Tr
Analgesic/antipyretic	17	33	21	19	24	22	21	25	24
Topical	23	13	16	19	19	9	8	8	14
Cough/cold	8	12	20	17	9	16	4	20	13
Vitamin/mineral	12	7	7	10	9	4	4	6	4
Gastrointestinal	5	7	8	10	7	11	7	11	8
Eye/nose/ear	3	4	7	5	14	3	3	3	7
Antiinfective	1	8	5	3	0	11	24	10	7
Homeopathic	11	0	4	8	0	0	0	0	1
Antihistamine	1	6	5	0	5	3	3	2	3
Antiasthmatic	2	3	2	4	4	1	4	4	1
Psychotropic	3	2	3	1	3	3	4	2	1
Cardiovascular	1	4	1	4	0	2	7	4	2
Oral contraceptive	2	0	0	0	0	1	0	0	0
Other	13	1	5	0	6	14	11	3	16

[1] analgesic/antipyretic includes non-steroidal antiinflammatory (NSAID); cough/cold includes decongestants, sore throat medicines, antitussives/expectorants, combinations; gastrointestinal includes antacids, antidiarrheals, laxatives, and other stomach medicines; psychotropic includes antidepressants, antipsychotics, tranquilizers, sedatives, and hypnotics; cardiovascular includes antihypertensives, diuretics, and heart medicines.

Many kinds of dosage forms were found in the homes, the most frequent being solid oral preparations such as capsules and tablets (Table 5.5). The second most frequent were liquid oral forms and the third were the topical preparations. In only Amsterdam/Groningen were there more topical than liquid oral dosage forms. In Novi Sad, the proportion of drugs in the tablet/capsule dosage form, 88 percent, was about twice that found in the other locations.

In all locations, the pharmacy was the most frequent source for acquiring the medicines, even if they were OTC (Table 5.6). The amount of drugs purchased in other stores, e.g., supermarkets, was only significant in Amsterdam/Gronigen (45 percent) and Chapel Hill (14 percent), locations in which OTC drugs accounted for a majority of the MCI composition. Rarely were medicines acquired from friends or relatives; the location with the highest rate was Hamburg at 5 percent.

The most common place for keeping medicines was the kitchen (both in the refrigerator and elsewhere) or the bathroom (Table 5.7). There were differences in storage from one location to another. Almost half of the drugs in Madrid were stored in a room other than the kitchen or the bathroom, whereas in Jyväskylä almost three-fourths were kept in the kitchen. More than half of the families kept their medicines in only one place in the household; this trend is consistent everywhere but in Novi Sad, where drugs were frequently stored in two or more places. Rarely were any of the medicines locked up or in a place inaccessible to children.

A substantial proportion of the drugs stored in the homes had expired and many (10 to 30 percent) had not been used for more than a year (Table 5.8). In fact, of the total medicines in Madrid and Tenerife, the respondents stated that a third of them probably would not be used in the future.

In the two Spanish locations, it was possible to perform a combined analysis of the respondent's perception of the medicine's indication (purpose of the last or intended use) in relation to its ATC pharmacological classification. The proportion of erroneous indications reported by the respondents for each therapeutic category of drugs is reported in Table 5.9. Ten percent of the medicines were considered to have erroneous indications. The analgesic/antipyretic/ NSAID category and cough/cold remedies were the most frequent

TABLE 5.5. Percentage of Total Medicines by Dosage Form

Dose Form	Location								
	AmGr	At	CH	Ha	Jy	Ma	NS	Te	Tr
Capsule/tablet	46	41	49	38	46	39	88	36	34
Inhaler/spray	5	1	5	7	3	3	1	4	3
Injection	0	1	0	0	0	0	0	3	0
Liquid (oral)	15	36	28	22	16	19	1	26	29
Suppository	2	1	1	5	2	6	1	6	3
Eye/ear/nose/throat drops/lozenges	1	0	1	0	15	0	0	0	2
Topical	31	5	15	17	14	14	8	12	22
Other	1	14	1	12	7	19	1	13	7
Total percent[1]	100	100	100	100	100	100	100	100	100

[1] Not all columns add to 100 due to rounding errors.

TABLE 5.6. Percentage of Total Medicines by Place Acquired

Place Acquired	Location[1]								
	AmGr	At	CH	Ha	Jy	Ma	Te	Tr	
Pharmacy	51	91	69	87	88	96	84	96	
Clinic/hospital/MD	1	1	8	0	7	3	0	2	
Other store	45	0	14	1	2	0	0	0	
Friends/relatives	0	3	0	5	1	0	2	0	
Don't know	3	6	8	7	2	0	14	2	
Total[2]	100	100	100	100	100	100	100	100	

[1] No data available from NS.
[2] Not all columns add to 100 due to rounding errors.

TABLE 5.7. Percentage of Total Medicines by Place Kept and Number of Places Kept

Variable	Location[1]							
	AmGr	At	CH	Jy	Ma	NS	Te	Tr
Place Kept:								
Bathroom	1	16	39	6	26	0	9	58
Bedroom	17	7	5	1	9	7	11	3
Kitchen—fridge	1	14	1	16	6	0	1	1
Kitchen—other place	33	36	35	72	18	64	44	24
Other place/room	31	27	16	5	42	29	27	13
Other	18	0	5	0	0	0	8	3
Total percent[2]	100	100	100	100	100	100	100	100
N Places Kept:								
One only	ND	ND	56	51	61	43	75	86
Two only			32	40	26	57[3]	24	11
Three or more			12	9	13		1	3
Total percent	100	100	100	100	100	100	100	100

[1] No data available from Ha; ND: No Data.
[2] Not all columns add to 100 due to rounding errors.
[3] Two or more places.

TABLE 5.8. Percentage of Medicines Expired and Time Since Acquired

Variables	Location[1]						
	AmGr	At	CH	Ha	Ma	Te	Tr
Percent expired:	12	17	29	ND	13	13	10
Time since acquired:							
0-1 month	11	18	10	7	ND	21	13
>1-6 months	28	29	24	37	34	17	27
>6-12 months	18	17	21	24	16	5	20
>12 months	33	6	31	29	17	7	18
Don't know	10	30	14	3	33	50	22
Total percent	100	100	100	100	100	100	100

ND: No data
* No data available from Jy; in NS, 7 percent of medicines expired and no data available on time since required.

TABLE 5.9. Medicine Use and Intended Medicine Use Indication Errors in Madrid and Tenerife

Variables	Drug Category										
	H	P	AB	AH	V	D	Ast	An	C	Total	(%)
Total N meds	23	79	354	66	179	375	84	791	636	2587	
N information[1]	11	36	151	28	84	158	59	413	337	1277	
N errors[2]	4	8	32	5	13	21	6	23	19	131	
Percent errors	36	22	21	18	15	13	10	6	6	10	
Indication error category:											
Analgesics	1	3	23	2	9	8	5	-	-	51	(39)
Antibiotics	1	-	-	2	3	4	1	9	15	35	(27)
Digestive	-	-	2	-	-	-	-	6	2	10	(8)
Cough/Cold	2	1	3	-	-	4	-	-	-	10	(8)
Vitamins	-	-	3	-	-	-	-	3	1	7	(5)
Psychotropics	-	-	-	-	1	1	-	4	-	6	(5)
Antihistamines	-	1	1	-	-	3	-	-	-	5	(4)
Cardiovascular	-	2	-	1	-	-	-	1	1	5	(4)
Eye/nose/ear	-	1	-	-	-	-	-	1	-	1	(1)
Contraceptives	-	-	-	-	-	1	-	-	-	1	(1)
Total[3]										131	(100)

H: Hormones, P: Psychotropics, AB: Antibiotics, AH: Antihistamines, V: Vitamins, D: Digestive, Ast: Antiasthmatics, An: Analgesics, C: Cough/Cold.
[1] Number of medicines with information available about the indication for the last use or intended use.
[2] Number of medicines used for, or intended to use for, an erroneous indication.
[3] Does not add to 100 due to rounding errors.

drugs kept at home, and most of them appeared to be used in a manner consistent with recommendations. When not, they were most often mistaken for antibiotics or vitamins. More than a fifth of antibiotics were misclassified; they were described as analgesics or "cold" remedies most frequently.

In three locations, Chapel Hill, Madrid, and Tenerife, some of the psychosocial variables from other instruments were analyzed together with MCI variables. Because the study was not designed to investigate differences in medicine use among different socioeconomic status (SES) subpopulations, the samples were selected purposefully from middle-class strata. Therefore, as expected, there was no significant relationship between SES and the number of household medicines.

The percentage of children who said that the household medicines were accessible to them was 60 percent or higher for the youngest age group in the three locations and ranged from 71 to 85 percent for the ten-year-olds (Table 5.10). The actual accessibility of medicines to children could be even higher because some children may have responded according to what they believed they were "supposed" to say.

In Jyväskylä, data from a Health Inventory (HI), an instrument inquiring into the chronic disease status of family members, was related to the number of medicines present (Table 5.11). To analyze the possible influence of the presence of a chronically ill person in the family on the number of drugs in the MCI, the HI was used to indicate the presence or absence of a chronically ill person, and the average number of medicines per household was divided into three intervals, each encompassing one-third of the drug distribution (< 6, 6-9, > 9) (Table 5.11). In those 17 households where there was a chronically ill person, the number of medicines kept was much higher than in the 28 households in which no member had a chronic illness. A similar trend was observed in Madrid and Tenerife.

In Madrid and Tenerife, the number of medicines per household was compared with the health locus of control scale data of parents and children. There was no correlation between the Children's Health Locus of Control (CHLC) scale and the number of medicines at home. However, the locus of control scale of the parents (MHLC) was positively correlated with the number of medicines in

TABLE 5.10. Percentage of Children Stating that Medicines Are Accessible

	Location		
Age	Ma	Te	CH
7 years	65	60	85
10 years	81	71	85

TABLE 5.11. Relationship between Medicines and a Household Member with a Chronic Illness (Jyväskylä)

	Illness State	
N Medicines	No Chronic	Chronic
< 6	12	0
6-9	12	6
>9	4	11

Chi square 15.50, p< 0.0001.

Madrid households (Table 5.12). Moreover, the more internal the MHLC scale scores of the parents, the more medicines stored at home and the more they consisted of OTC drugs compared with Rx drugs. These data suggest that an internal health locus of control may represent the feelings of some parents that medicines are a personal tool they can choose and use to preserve or achieve health independent of professional care.

DISCUSSION

In this study, the amount of information gathered in the nine different locations varied somewhat from one to another as did the number of families studied in each location. Instruments similar to the MCI have been used in studies performed in cross-sectional and longitudinal studies in a single location, but this is the first time (to

TABLE 5.12. Spearman Correlations between Parental Multidimensional Health Locus of Control (MHLC) Scale and Household Medicines in Madrid and Tenerife

	Location		
Variables	Ma	Te	All
N total medicines	0.28**	0.08	0.24**
% Rx/household	−0.27**	−0.04	−0.13*
% OTC/household	0.30**	−0.02	0.17*
% medicines intend to use/household	−0.15	−0.15	−0.03

Rx: prescription only; OTC: Over the counter.
 * $p \leq 0.05$; ** $p \leq 0.01$.

our knowledge) that a medicine inventory has been implemented on a cross-cultural basis. While the MCI is time-consuming when the number of medicines is many, if used correctly, it provides an indication to the extent of the household's pharmacomedicalization, dependence of families upon medicines, and erroneous use of medicines. Other useful information is gathered, such as where the medicines are stored and the propensity of families to keep medicines beyond their expiration dates. Furthermore, in the context of the present cross-cultural study, even if it could not be implemented as intended in some particular cases, e.g., the researcher was not permitted to see the medicines *in situ* but the medicines were brought to the researcher, not only did the MCI capture most of the required information, it also served as a counter-check on the information collected by other instruments used in the project.

Caution should be used in interpreting the data reported from the locations in this study as representative of their respective countries. When the MCI was used in Chapel Hill, the average number of medicines found per household was 24, compared with seven found when the MCI was used in Washington, DC (Bush and Almarsdottir 1993). This large difference highlights the importance of using similar race and SES categories across as well as within the locations as these factors probably account for the large differences found in these two U.S. locations.

In contrast, the MCI data coming from the two Spanish locations were similar for all comparisons, probably because the families from both locations were chosen from very similar middle-class levels forming a homogeneous sample. In another study performed in Spain more than ten years ago (Puche et al. 1982) with a different methodology–students administered much simpler questionnaires– the average number of drugs was only seven per household, again suggesting that differences in methodology, sample selection, and temporality may yield quite different results within the same country.

The MCI compiles quantitative information on the number and characteristics of the drugs, but the administration of the MCI elicits additional information relative to the beliefs about, and attitudes toward, drugs in each family. While showing the medicines to the interviewer and reacting to the questions of the MCI, many respondents offered much more information than had been anticipated and for which codes were not provided on the form or elsewhere. Aside from providing standard details regarding purchase, use, and expiration dates, respondents discussed the perceived effectiveness of the medicines, their taste and/or side effects, and disclosed reasons for feelings about using medicines in general as well as about specific medicines. Sometimes these were in the context of attitudes toward the physicians who prescribed the drugs. It is the opinion of the investigators that, while the instrument can provide valuable information of a pharmacoepidemiological nature, it should also be used to elicit additional, more in-depth information. In homes where medicines were very numerous, simply recording them according to the MCI form took considerable effort and the interviewer may have failed to note the additional information offered by the respondent. Thus, more care should be taken in training interviewers to be attentive to other details not required on the MCI form and to expect to spend more time completing it. The use of an audiotape recorder would facilitate the task and enhance the amount of information being given informally.

Several explanations may account for the similarity in family size among the studies. First, the social pressures and economic conditions of the families predispose families to limit their size.

These pressures are present worldwide and seem to influence different populations similarly in developed countries. Another important reason is that all families had children of about seven or ten years of age. As the average number of children per family was low, this implies that the families were young and may be still growing. The presence of elderly persons (over 65 years) living in the same household was extremely uncommon in the samples. There are again two possible explanations: first, that the size of the homes is limited and, second, that most of the grandparents are young enough to live independently, perhaps still taking care of younger siblings of the parents in the studies (Sanz and Garcia 1993a).

The relatively high proportion of OTC drugs in Chapel Hill households may be in part related to the quite different system of promotion and distribution. OTCs are advertised widely and are sold in supermarkets, groceries, by mail order and catalog sales, etc., together with other home supplies, whereas on the other side of the Atlantic, the ability to purchase medicines in supermarkets and other stores simply does not exist. Although in Chapel Hill it was found that most of the OTC medicines had been purchased in pharmacies, drug advertising may account in part for the relatively high proportion. It is also the case that most people in the U.S. pay for prescribed medicines out of pocket, so there may be incentives to self-medicate with OTC medicines because they are less expensive. In addition, most U.S. pharmacies carry a much larger variety of merchandise than pharmacies in European countries, so that consumers are more likely to visit pharmacies for general purchases and to use these occasions to buy OTC medicines.

The Amsterdam/Groningen sample is distinguished in that it had a high proportion of OTCs, a high proportion of nonpharmacy sources, and a relatively high proportion of homeopathic remedies, vitamins, and topical preparations than other samples. These three variables may be related, but further information would be needed to confirm it. In Hamburg, 43 percent of the medicines were OTCs and the proportion of homeopathic remedies and vitamins was also high (18 percent), but as these substances are a normal part of the pharmacies' products, the amount of nonpharmacy products was negligible. Again, caution should be used in interpreting the data because the samples were very small in both of these locations.

Nevertheless, these data are in agreement with the published figures on the use of homeopathic products in Europe (Lewith and Aldridge 1991; Sermeus 1987), and reveal a trend that deserves a more intensive qualitative type of research.

Most of the medicines stored at home were acquired for a particular family member; the "good-for-all" medicine was uncommon. The vast majority of medicines were for family members. There were few elderly persons and few infants, thus limiting the amount of medicines that were found for persons in these age groups. In general, more medicines were allocated for adults than children, except in Hamburg and Madrid. Also, the number of medicines allocated for adult females was slightly higher than for adult males. In children this difference was not as evident. Most previous studies have found the use of drugs by female adults to be higher than by males, and for most locations, the data are consistent.

The most common medicines stored in the households were the kinds expected. From 60 to 75 percent of all drugs were analgesics, antipyretics, NSAIDs, cough/cold preparations, topical medicines, digestives, and vitamins/minerals. Antibiotics were very common in the Mediterranean locations, especially in Novi Sad, but also in Madrid, Tenerife, Athens, and Trieste, and homeopathy remedies were most common in the Central European locations, i.e., Amsterdam/Groningen and Hamburg. Notably, one-fourth of all drugs in the Dutch sample are considered to have no therapeutic value (homeopathic remedies and vitamins), although they may have important cultural meanings. A matter for discussion is whether the high presence of antibiotics is more or less rational than the high presence of "placebo-related" compounds (homeopathic or vitamins). Whereas, the first are active and efficacious drugs, they are frequently misused. On the other hand, homeopathic and vitamin remedies, which have none to little medical value, may have powerful cultural meanings and, despite not being used "rationally" according to therapeutical standards, are seldom dangerous.

The proportion of psychotropics was quite stable around one to three percent in all locations. In Jyväskylä, with its high proportion of OTCs, eye/ear/nose/throat and topical preparations ranked relatively high.

In the earlier Spanish study of Puche et al. (1982) of 1,548 families, the global distribution of medicines in the household was similar, with analgesic/ antipyretics/NSAID, cough/cold remedies and topical medication ranking in the first places. In agreement with the data found in the two Spanish locations, antibiotics were also very frequently stored in the homes surveyed (15 percent).

Sanz (1992) carried out a study on the medications given by parents to children, aged less than 14 years, attending an Emergency Service in Tenerife. More than 50 percent of the children received some treatment "prescribed" by their parents. Here again, analgesics were most frequent, accounting for more than 50 percent of all medications given by the parents. Antibiotics were seldom "self-administered" by parents to their children (<10 percent of all drugs given).

As for dosage forms, the results were quite similar with oral forms (both solid and liquid) ranking first everywhere. Only in the Spanish locations were injections and suppositories relatively common, a finding consistent with local traditions. The predominance of solid oral forms in Novi Sad probably reflects the pharmaceutical market in this country, with few liquid forms available.

Almost all of the children in all the locations stated that they have access to drugs at home. In Chapel Hill, the researchers visited only one home where medicines were kept locked up. In fact, drugs are spread all over the households, and when a family said that drugs are kept in only one place, this place is normally the kitchen, the bathroom, or the bedroom. However, the medicines may be in different locations in these rooms. It is evident that medicines are normally stored with foods and other hygienic supplies, mixed together and unprotected.

The proportion of expired drugs varied from 8 to 17 percent, except in Chapel Hill, where expired medicines accounted for almost 30 percent. In Chapel Hill, 31 percent of the drugs had been acquired more than one year before the time of the survey. Many of the Chapel Hill parents expressed disgust at the number of old medicines they were storing and used the occasion to discard them. In two other studies, Amsterdam/Groningen (33 percent) and Hamburg (29 percent), the percentage of drugs stored for more than a year was also almost double that in the rest of the locations, a situation undoubtedly related to the high proportion of homeopathic remedies, vitamins, etc., that either have no expiration dates or the expiration dates are longer than for other kinds of medicine. A problem associated with the packaging of topical medicines in tubes was observed. The expiration dates were stamped on the bottom of the tubes and were soon rolled out of view as the medicine was used.

The distinction between antibiotics and other medications used for the most common diseases of the upper respiratory tract was poorly understood in Spain. This kind of analysis was not done for the other locations but in the Greek National Report of the study to COMAC, it was also stated that antibiotics were the most misused medicines. They were used as decongestants, as "cold" medicines, and as prophylactic therapy. Similarly, the Dutch team commented upon the fact that, even if aspirin were not found at all in the medicine cabinet inventories, aspirins were frequently referred to in the interviews. The parents in the Amsterdam/Groningen study tended to use the word "aspirin" when referring to other analgesics/antipyretics in general, a situation that could lead to missuse. In Finland, the researchers explained that inappropriate use was not found, but this may relate to the methodology; when the parents themselves wrote the names of medicines on the medicine cabinet inventory forms, they could read the labels of the medicines. The indication and dosage of an OTC medicine is written on the label of the medicine package and thus the parents may have copied the indications from the labels.

It was remarkable that oral contraceptives appeared to be underreported in every location. It is difficult to explain the reason because no additional information was gathered that might provide an explanation. It is possible that some women may not view oral contraceptives as medicines, reserving this category for medicines that are viewed as curing or preventing disease. Also, oral contraceptives may have been stored in a private place away from other medicines and they simply were overlooked. It seems more likely, however, that women felt that use of contraceptives was too personal to reveal to the interviewer. For future use of the MCI, the investigators recommend asking specifically about oral contraceptives and perhaps other medications that might cause embarrassment or might not be viewed as medicines. In small sample qualitative research where the investigator forms a close relationship with the respondent through many visits over time, it is less likely that such medicines would be overlooked.

Previously it was found that children with more internal scores on the CHLC were less likely to perceive that medicines would help them for common illnesses than children scoring more externally (Bush and Iannotti 1990). Also mothers' health locus of control scores were positively correlated with older, but not younger, children's CHLC scores (Bush and Iannotti 1988; Sanz and Garcia 1993b). Some similar relationships were found in the present study, with locus of control scale scores correlated between mothers and the older children but not between mothers and the younger children.

In this study, the number of medicines in the home was not correlated with the CHLC scale, suggesting that the number of household medicines has no influence on the value of this variable in children, perhaps because they have little control over medicine acquisition and retention in the home. On the other hand, in Madrid, the more internal the MHLC scale scores of the parents, the more medicines stored in the household, and the greater the proportion of OTC drugs. These data suggest that an internal health locus of control represents the feelings of the parents that medicines are a personal tool they can use to preserve or achieve health quite independent of professional care.

CONCLUSIONS AND RECOMMENDATIONS

In addition to the use of the MCI to obtain information on the drugs stored at home, the investigators recommend using it as a focus to gather additional information about attitudes toward and beliefs about medicines via a qualitative as well as a quantitative methodology. The results suggest that efforts to encourage parents to keep medicines out of the reach of children of school age would be misplaced in any of the locations, because this is almost impossible in practice, and children already have a very structured knowledge about medicines and their risk (see Chapter 10, this volume). Therefore, efforts might better be spent teaching about appropriate storage and why and when it is important to discard expired medicines. We note that all medicines should have expiration dates and storage information that is directly on the medicine container and directly visible throughout the period of use of the medicine.

Most drugs kept at home are useful and appropriate options for the treatment of initial symptoms of normal viral infections and nonserious illnesses. It would not be practical for everyone to seek medical attention for every single, simple episode of influenza, headache, or bellyache. In this context, the contents of the home medicine cabinet can and should be used in a knowledgeable way for the promotion of health. Not only should recommendations be made about what medicines should be kept in the household on a regular basis, but health promotion campaigns and materials should emphasize information about self-treatment and related issues. Certainly, a medicine cabinet with a high number of drugs, (especially antibiotics), many of them expired and many of which will not and should not be used in the future, is to be avoided.

The MCI provided a mechanism to investigate cultural differences in household medicines among nine of the participating locations. The data provided information aiding the interpretation of other, more qualitative, data as well. We recommend this kind of instrument for future cross-cultural comparative studies that are performed with sociological and anthropological methods. Also, we encourage longitudinal and multigenerational studies to determine the stability of, and familial transmittal of, behaviors, attitudes, and beliefs relative to medicines.

NOTE

1. The COMAC Childhood and Medicines Project was funded through a European Economic Community (EEC) *Comité d'Action Concerté* (COMAC) contract, COMAC/HSR MR4*-CT90-0319, awarded to The Institute on Child Health, Athens, Greece, with Deanna J. Trakas as the Project Leader. The official title of the Contract was "Medicine Use, Behaviour and Children's Perceptions of Medicines and Health Care."

REFERENCES

Bergman, U. and Griffiths, R. R. 1986. "Relative abuse of diazepam and oxazepam: Prescription forgeries and theft/loss reports in Sweden." *Drug and Alcohol Dependence* 16:293-301.

Bush, P. J. and Almarsdottir, A. B. 1993. "Medicines in the home: Differences between two U.S. communities." Presented symposium: Children's Perceptions About Illness and Medicines. Athens, Greece. (December).

Bush, P. J. and Iannotti, R. J. 1988. "Origins and stability of children's health beliefs relative to medicine use." *Social Science and Medicine* 27 (4):345-352.

Bush, P. J. and Iannotti, R. J. 1990. "A children's health belief model." *Medical Care* 28 (1):69-86.

Bush, P. J., Parcel, G. S., and Davidson, F. R. 1982. "Reliability of a Shortened Children's Health Locus of Control Scale." *ERIC #ED 223354.*

Bush, P. J. and Rabin, D. L. 1976. "Who's using nonprescribed medicines?" *Medical Care* 14 (12):1014-1023.

Bush, P. J. and Rabin, D. L. 1977. "Medicines: Who's using them?" *Journal of the American Pharmaceutical Association* NS17 (4):117-230.

Chrischilles, E. A., Foley, D. J., Wallace, R. B., Lemke, J. H., Semla, T. P., Hanlon, J. T., Glynn, R. J., Ostfeld, A. M., and Guralnik, J. M. 1992. "Use of medications by persons 65 and over: Data from the established populations for epidemiologic studies of the elderly." *Journal of Gerontology* 47 (5):M137-M144.

Cunningham-Burley, S. and Irvine, S. 1987. "'And have you done anything so far?' An examination of lay treatment of children's symptoms." *British Medical Journal* 295 (September):700-702.

Gagnon, J. P., Salber, E. J., and Greene, S. B. 1978. "Patterns of prescription and nonprescription drug use in a Southern rural area. *Public Health Reports* 93 (5):433-437.

Helling, D. K., Lemke, J. H., Semla, T. P. Wallace, R. B., Lipson, D. P., and Cornoni-Huntley, J. 1987. "Medication use characteristics in the elderly: The Iowa 65+ rural health study." *Journal of the American Geriatric Society* 35 (1):4-12.

Jackson, J. D., Smith, M. C., Sharpe, T. R., Freeman, R. A., and Hy, R. 1982. "An investigation of prescribed and nonprescribed medicine use behavior within the household context." *Social Science and Medicine* 16:2009-2015.

Knapp, D. A. and Knapp, D. E. 1972. "Decision-making and self-medication: Preliminary findings." *American Journal of Hospital Pharmacy* 24 (December):1004-1012.

Kohn, R. and White, K. L. (editors). 1976. *Health Care: An International Study.* Oxford: Oxford University Press.

Lewith, G. and Aldridge, D. 1991. *Complementary Medicine and the European Community.* Essex: Saffron Walden. C. W. Daniel Company Ltd.

Maiman, L. A., Becker, M. H., and Katlic, A. W. 1985. "How mothers treat their children's physical symptoms." *Journal of Community Health* 10 (3):136-155.

Moore, T. S., Bush, P. J., and Iannotti, R. J. 1991a. "What's in the home medicine cabinet from one year to the next?" Presented Pharmacy World Congress. Washington, DC. (September).

Moore, T. S., Bush, P. J., and Iannotti, R. J. 1991b. "Families and medicines: A survey of household medicine cabinets." Presented 8th National Conference of the National Council on Patient Information and Education. Washington, DC. (April).

O'Brien, R. W, Bush, P. J., and Parcel, G. S. 1989. "Stability in a measure of children's health locus of control." *Journal of School Health* 59 (4):161-164.

Parcel, G. S. and Meyer, M. P. 1978. "Development of an instrument to measure children's health locus of control." *Health Education Monographs* 6 (2):149-159.

Puche, E., Saucedo, R., Morillas, M. G., Boloñas, J., and Vila, E. 1982. "A study of 1548 family medicine cupboards in Granada." *Medcina Clinca* (Barcelona) 79 (3):118-121.

Rabin, D. L. and Bush, P. J. 1975. "Who's using medicines?" *Journal of Community Health* 1 (2):106-117.

Sanz, E. J. 1992. "The hazards of medication in children." *Studying Childhood and Medicine Use* edited by D. J. Trakas and E. J. Sanz. Athens, Greece: ZHTA Medical Publications, pgs. 93-104.

Sanz, E. J., Bergman, U., and Dahlstrom, M. 1989. "Paediatric drug prescribing. A comparison of Tenerife (Canary Islands, Spain) and Sweden." *European Journal of Clinical Pharmacology* 37:65-68.

Sanz, E. J. and Boada, J. N. 1988. "Drug Utilization by Children in Tenerife Island." *European Journal of Clinical Pharmacology* 34:495-499.

Sanz, E. and Garcia, M. 1993a. "Cross-cultural results: Family medicine cabinets and their use." Presented symposium: Children's Perceptions about Illness and Medicines. Athens, Greece. (December).

Sanz, E. and Garcia, M., 1993b. "Autonomy in the use of drugs in children in Tenerife." Meeting of the WHO Drug Utilization Group. Oxford, UK. Abstract 83.

Segal, A. 1990. "A community survey of self-medication activities." *Medical Care* 28 (4):301-310.

Sermeus, G. 1987. Alternative Medicine in Europe: A Quantitative Comparison of the Use and Knowledge of Alternative Medicine and Patient Profiles in Nine European Countries. Brussels: Belgian Consumer's Association.

Serradell, J., Bjornson, D. C., and Hartzema, A. G. 1991. "Drug utilization studies: Sources and methods." *Pharmacoepidemiology. An Introduction*, edited by A. G. Hartzema, M. S. Porta and H. H. Tilson. Cincinnati, Ohio: Harvey Whitney Books, pgs. 101-119.

Van den Brandt, P. A., Petri, H., Dorant, E., Goldbohm, R. A., and Van de Crommert, S. 1991. "Comparison of questionnaire information and pharmacy data on drug use." *Pharmaceutisch Weekblad* (Scientific Edition) 13(2):91-96.

Wallston, K. A., Wallston, B. S., and DeVellis, R. 1978. "Development of the Multidimensional Health Locus of Control (MHLC) Scales." *Health Education Monographs* 6 (2):160-170.

WHO Collaborating Center for Drug Statistics Methodology. (January) 1993. *Anatomical Therapeutic Chemical (ATC) Classification Index*. Oslo.

Chapter 6

Perception and Treatment of Childhood Fever in Athens, Chapel Hill, Jyväskylä, Madrid, and Tenerife

Tuula Vaskilampi
Marcelino García
Emilio J. Sanz
Olli Kalpio

with Anna B. Almarsdottir, Pilar Aramburuzabala,
Chrysoula Botsis, Patricia J. Bush, and Deanna J. Trakas

Fever is one of the most common health problems during childhood (Chow et al. 1988), and it is also a common disorder during the entire life span of adults. As a common ailment, fever has been treated both at home according to "folk remedies" and traditions and in the professional medical arena. In other words, it is possible to identify two distinct historical traditions on coping with fever: the professional and the lay approach.

Fever has been defined, conceptualized, treated, and prevented, among the lay community. The lay (folk, popular) approach to sickness and care is primarily applied in the family context, but is also supported by social network and community activities. Moreover, most decisions about help seeking, consulting, complying, and evaluating the efficacy of treatment are made in the popular domain (Kleinman 1978). It can be argued that fever is a socially and culturally constructed health problem.

There exist very few empirical studies on lay belief models of fevers in Western societies. A reference point is the work by Cecil

Helman (1978) who studied the lay model of fever and cold in a middle-class urban neighborhood of London. The common English admonition to "Feed a cold, starve a fever" arises from a folk model and it relates to the conditions of a fever as an abnormal elevated body temperature, i.e., changes are perceived in the body temperature; it feels "warmer" or "hotter" than normal. Fever also has been seen as the expression of other somatic and physical causes. It is said to be due to the actions of entities known as "germs," "bugs," or "viruses;" terms which are not used in the strict biomedical sense. These terms are used as a hypothesized theory of causality. According to Helman's (1978) study, the cause is transmitted in social interaction and people themselves are not held responsible for it. Fluids are believed to "wash out" or liquefy the "germs." Also the reduction of food intake ("starve a fever") has been viewed as important. Germs are regarded as living entities–to starve their host is to starve the germs.

There has been a controversy in the professional sector for many centuries on the theoretical and practical treatment of fever. The question has been whether a physician ought to fight fever, ignore fever, or encourage it. For the ancient humeral pathologists, fever was the most important of the body's natural defense mechanism, when the amount of "phlegm" in the body increased. It was explained according to the theory that the heat of fever was designed to drive the excess phlegm out of the body. Then fevers were encouraged and celebrated (Schmitt 1980).

In the medical literature, some authors have defined fever as a rectal temperature above 38°C (100.4°F) (Schmitt 1984). Some pediatricians believe that temperatures lower than 41°C (105.8°F) are relatively harmless unless they are of long duration and are accompanied by dehydration (Casey et al. 1984), but there is no consensus on the temperature level that defines fever.

Most childhood fevers occur in response to infection and in most of these episodes the infecting agent is a virus (Fruthaler 1985). A febrile episode is produced when the infecting pathogen triggers receptors in the area of the hypothalamus that regulates body temperature. This interaction causes the body's "thermostat" to be reset so that a higher core body temperature is maintained. The elevation in body temperature activates other body defenses: increases T-lymphocyte production and the effectiveness of interferon in combating viral infections (Fruthaler 1985). Therefore, fever is one of the body's natural defense mechanisms against disease rather than merely an uncomfortable side effect of disease (Kilman 1987).

In most cases the professional medical sector does not consider moderate fever harmful to children; in fact most of the discomfort in a febrile patient is caused by chills as body temperature rises and sweating as the temperature returns to normal. Medical treatment of fever is directed toward the goals of reducing discomfort, preventing dehydration, and preventing febrile seizures in those children who are susceptible to them (Kilman 1987).

Some studies in the USA and Canada have shown that parents are concerned about their children's fever and seek medical treatments. From the professional medical viewpoint, this concern has been seen as fear, even "phobia," and parents' fever perceptions as misconceptions. Over concern and misconceptions, which were related to inappropriate physician contacts and medication errors, were found both in public health services and in private practices. These misconceptions were common in highly educated as well as in poorly educated parents (mothers) (Schmitt 1980; Casey et al. 1984; Kramer, Naimark, and Leduc 1985; Kilman 1987; Andersen 1988).

Kramer and his study group (1985) showed that in a Canadian private practice setting, parents of young infants had a higher threshold for what they considered as a fever than parents of older children. Also found was that parents of younger children favored the use of acetaminophen (paracetamol) over aspirin. No associations were found with the age of the responding parents or the presence of other children in the household. It was shown too, that parents of higher socioeconomic status were significantly more concerned about the risk of brain damage or seizures as the sequel of fever than parents of lower socioeconomic level.

Kilman's study indicated that most of the mothers believed that they could estimate the presence or absence of fever in their children by means of subjective methods. Palpation of parts of child's body (forehead, face, abdomen, neck, or arm) was the most commonly used method. Most of the mothers (96 percent) did not know what temperature is considered normal by medical professionals. In fact, many parents in the study treated "fever" when the child's body temperature was actually regarded within the normal range. In addition, the parents' interventions were often inappropriate according to the medical professionals (Kilman 1987). There also are observations that erroneously self-medicating childhood fever could lead to serious side effects and poisoning (Dusi et al. 1988). In contrast, a Norwegian study did not find fever "phobia" among Norwegian parents, but the findings did indicate a need for more definite and consistent information on fever and fever management (Eskerud 1992).

Studies on behavior and perceptions of childhood fever are based on individual opinions and statements that are evaluated only from the professional viewpoint neglecting lay beliefs and their degree of rationality. The data have mainly been collected by interviewing mothers. In sociological, as well as in health behavior studies, children have been seen, in general, as passive objects who are irrational and immature. But the new paradigm of childhood studies has brought children's own viewpoint to the focus, and according to it, children are able to create meanings and construct social reality (Bush and Davidson 1982; Bush, Iannotti, and Davidson 1985). They are part of social interaction representing cultural meanings and presenting their own subculture. They also participate with the adults in negotiating the sick role (Prout 1988, 1989; Prout and James 1990).

Bush and Iannotti (1988, 1990) have tested a Children's Health Belief Model to explain children's medicine use. Their studies indicated that mothers have a stronger influence on their children's health orientations than previously believed and that these orientations are relatively stable by school age. Strong similarities were observed between primary caretakers and their children in the health belief-based model to predict expected medicine use. Bush and Iannotti have brought both children and their primary caretakers (mainly mothers) to illustrate and explain children's socialization into medicine use.

This chapter reports on the "fever component" of the COMAC Childhood and Medicines Project.[1] In this component, the methods of coping with childhood fever were investigated through interviews with children and their primary caretakers. Fever was selected as the focus of the comparative investigation because it was believed that virtually every child in every study location would have had a fever at some time. Although most empirical studies on childhood fever have been performed in the USA and Canada, it is presumed that childhood fever is culturally structured and thus that intra- and cross-cultural variations exist. That is why international comparison is important.

The aim of this study was to describe and compare among some Western industrialized cultures, definitions of childhood fever, causal explanations, treatment, and the adaption of the sick role.

MATERIAL AND METHODS

The data were collected in two separate interviews by semi-structured questionnaires on the perceptions of childhood fever posed to both children and their primary caretakers (mainly mothers). The primary caretaker or caregiver was defined as the person most frequently responsible for taking care of the child during illness episodes. There were questions on perceptions and beliefs on the origins and prevention of fever and the characteristics of it, and on behavior, treatment, and medicine use during fever episodes.

The study communities were Chapel Hill, NC, USA (CH); Jyväskylä, Finland (Jy); Madrid, Spain (Ma); Tenerife, Spain (Te) and Athens, Greece (At). The questionnaires (one for the parent and one for the child) were designed by the working group, and the codes agreed upon in a coordinating session after piloting in three of the study locations: Chapel Hill, Madrid, and Tenerife. The same coding classification was applied in all study communities when it was possible. However, there were some minor local differences of coding in specific questions and some questions did not work in all of the study locations. The paper and pencil questionnaires were administrated at the families' homes by trained interviewers.

According to the general study design, the target groups were selected from middle-class neighborhoods. Excluded were minority groups and different ethnic groups. Participation in the study was voluntary. The study subjects in the five study communities were not selected randomly.

In Chapel Hill data were gathered in the summers of 1992 and 1993 in summer day camps. There were 103 schoolchildren and 102 primary caregivers in the study group. The summer day camps were chosen on the basis of convenience of location and consent of the camp administration. The sample size was selected to provide the same sensitivity as that in the Madrid and Tenerife studies. The refusal rate was low, about seven percent (Almarsdottir and Bush 1995).

In Madrid there were 100 school children and 100 primary caregivers in the study group in 1992. The sample was taken from four public elementary schools. The schools were randomly selected from middle-class neighborhoods in the center of the city. Some schools refused to participate in the study and in the schools that agreed to participate only a few teachers agreed (Aramburuzabala et al. 1995).

In Tenerife, there was a sample of 115 schoolchildren and 87 primary caregivers in 1993. The sample was selected from two public elementary schools which are representative of the middle class in the city. In contrast to Madrid, the refusal rate from schools, teachers, and for the interview with the children was negligible. However, after giving consent for the interview with the children, 32 parents refused to continue with the interviews at home, and did not take part in the study.

In Jyväskylä the interviews were conducted in two schools in 1991 and 1992. The sample consisted of 51 children and 46 primary caregivers. Two primary schools were chosen because they were in the middle-class area and the teachers agreed to participate. There were 12 children out of 49 children in one school who dropped out from the study and 24 children out of 57 children in the other school. In total, the study group consisted of 51 children who were selected on the basis of balancing the age and sex distribution. The refusal rate can be considered quite high; well-educated parents were more interested in participating in the study than less educated ones (Vaskilampi et al. 1995).

In Greece the data were gathered in 1992 from two public schools located in middle-class neighborhoods in the greater Athens area. No schools and no parents refused to participate in the study. The total sample was composed of 83 children and their parents. However the fever questionnaires were administered to only 32 of these children and their parents.

RESULTS

Concept of Fever

Definition

Large variations were found in the opinions of primary caregivers on the degree of temperature that they believed indicated fever (Figure 6.1). The "threshold" of fever was much higher in the Greek sample than in all other locations because almost 56 percent of parents thought that 38°C (100.4°F) is the lower limit of fever. The parents in the other locations were more conservative; two groups were observed that had lower and higher thresholds respectively: with lower thresholds, Jyväskylä and Tenerife, and with higher thresholds, Chapel Hill and Madrid.

Fever was commonly perceived as an independent disease by the Athenian parents in the study (53 percent). The opposite appeared to be true in other locations. In Chapel Hill (1 percent), in Madrid (10 percent), and in Tenerife (19 percent), the parents saw fever as a disease and considered the elevated temperature as a symptom of underlying disease. Jyväskylä parents were in a middle position: half of them viewed the fever as a disease.

In fact, the parents from Chapel Hill considered fever as a positive evolution of the disease and a defense mechanism in a great majority of the cases (95 percent). This opinion was more common than the answers from Athens and the two locations in Spain (61 to 65 percent), but was far more frequent than the answers obtained in Jyväskylä, where only 16 percent of the parents thought that fever has any positive aspects.

Etiology

One-third of the children in Chapel Hill, Madrid, and Tenerife did not know how they got their fever. The children attributed self-actions (for instance going out without a coat, jumping around too actively) as a cause. Almost half of the groups of children in Jyväskylä and Tenerife mentioned these as a cause, whereas in Athens and Chapel Hill most children (about 40 percent) regarded etiologic factors (e.g., vi-

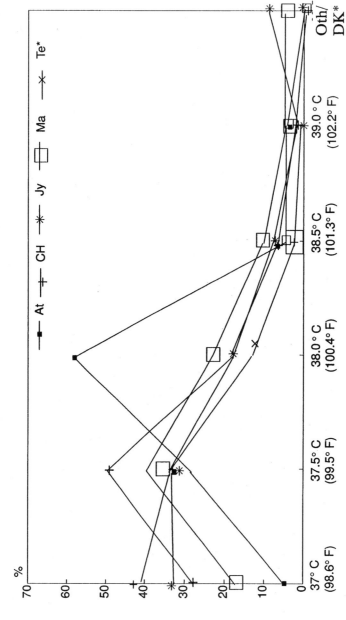

FIGURE 6.1. Parents' Fever Threshold for Children

— At   —+— CH   —*— Jy   —□— Ma   —×— Te*

* AT: Athens; CH: Chapel Hill; Jy: Jyväskylä; MA: Madrid; Te: Tenerife.
** Oth/DK: Other/Don't Know.

ruses and contagion) and their underlying disease (flu or grippe) as the cause of fever. In Madrid half of the children mentioned diseases and self-actions. Also environmental factors (rain, cold, heat) were mentioned in second or third place in all locations. In Chapel Hill, Jyväskylä, Madrid, and Tenerife, three to four percent of the children provided noncausal or tautological responses such as "just happens," "they gave me the thermometer and then the fever got up little by little," or "it was coming little by little. . . ." In Athens, one third of the children gave this kind of answer.

Diagnosis

In all five study locations it was the mother who most frequently first recognized that the child had fever. That came out both in the answers of the primary caregivers (55 to 84 percent) and in the answers of the children (57 to 69 percent).

The parents more often than the children said that the child was the first person to notice his/her own fever. The proportion of parents varied from four percent in Madrid to 23 percent in Chapel Hill, compared with the child respondents where the proportion varied from none in Tenerife to 16 percent in Athens. In Madrid and Tenerife, the two Spanish locations, 11 and 13 percent of fathers respectively were said to be the first person to notice the fever. The children in Chapel Hill (11 percent) were more likely than children in the other locations to mention a doctor as the first definer of their fevers (11 percent).

Physicians were consulted regarding the fever episode in about 70 percent of cases in Athens, Madrid, and Tenerife. In Chapel Hill almost half of the families had consulted a doctor and in Jyväskylä only 30 percent.

Although the measurement of fever by thermometer was not mentioned as the primary method, it was used by 90 percent or more of the families. Also about 90 percent of the children answered that their fever was measured by thermometer in all of the study groups. The diagnosis was made most often by the mother. In Finland almost one-fifth of the children said that they themselves had used the thermometer; whereas in other locations it was only two to four percent. In Chapel Hill, 5 percent of the children said that the doctor had measured their temperature, whereas very seldom was the measurement of temperature related to medical attention in other places.

In all five of the study groups, the parents mentioned warmth, tiredness or weakness, and changes in behavior as main indicators of fever, and only after that came the measurement by thermometer. The thermometer was not viewed as the main resource to diagnose fever. It was mentioned by 15 to 50 percent of children, but other symptoms such as touching the forehead, feeling bad or warm, or having a headache, accounted for a similar amount (40 to 60 percent). In Tenerife, for example, only 15 percent of children mentioned the thermometer measurement as the way to know that they had fever.

Seriousness

Various opinions existed on the seriousness of childhood fever. There were only a few parents in Athens, Madrid, and Tenerife who found childhood fever harmless whereas in Chapel Hill and Jyväskylä more respondents found it harmless. In Chapel Hill and Jyväskylä, the parents perceived the seriousness of fever to depend on the perceived cause of the fever and on the underlying disease; in Madrid and Tenerife on the level of the temperature. Perceptions of the seriousness of childhood fever were based on the same signs in almost all of the locations: high body temperature, dehydration, and seizures. It is remarkable that seizures were not mentioned at all in Athens.

But, in fact, when referring to the last episode of their child's fever instead of childhood fever in general, 72 to 86 percent of the parents in all locations said that it was not serious. However, the parents consulted with a doctor frequently (75 percent in Athens, Madrid, and Tenerife; 30 to 40 percent in Jyväskylä and Chapel Hill).

Treatment

Personal Care and Nonmedical Treatment

In all five study groups it was the mother who most often took care of the child during the last episode of fever. In Jyväskylä the father also was mentioned more often than in the other study groups. In Athens, Madrid, and Tenerife grandparents also cared for the child during the last fever episode. It was the mother who most often made the decision that the child should stay at home. However, this decision and the decision to give medicines represented two of the few occasions in which the father's opinion was consulted. Staying home from school and giving medications to the child were decisions taken by both the mother and the father in 25 to 36 percent of cases. In almost all other cases, the mother made the decisions alone. The primary caretakers lost, generally, one to two working days due to the child's fever.

Children themselves said more often than the parents that they stayed in bed during the last fever episode except in Madrid, where there were no discrepancies. Also in Jyväskylä, 88 percent of the children said they stayed in bed whereas in Chapel Hill comparable proportions were 59 percent and in Madrid 62 percent. Most often the children said it was the mother who had told them to go to bed during the fever episode. In Jyväskylä the children mentioned they went to bed out of their own initiative more often than the children in the other locations.

When asked about any special care given to the child during the child's last episode of fever, the vast majority of parents (80 to 100 percent) said that they helped make the child's fever go away: in Jyväskylä, 54 percent of the respondents mentioned putting the child in bed and 23 percent giving special liquids. In Chapel Hill, 96 percent mentioned administering medicines; and in Athens, Madrid, and Tenerife, over 60 percent cited medicines and 30 percent liquids, home remedies, or baths.

Surprisingly, the children did not see all these things as special, and when asked the same open question, only half of them said that they had received anything special. In Jyväskylä, drinks were mentioned by the children very frequently (67 percent), and in almost all other groups they were mentioned by more than 20 percent. Special food was mentioned only in Chapel Hill and Madrid and gifts were mentioned most often in Tenerife (30 percent).

Pharmacological Treatment

Almost all children and their parents mentioned medicines as a key tool in the treatment of fever. Direct mentions varied from 96 percent in Chapel Hill to 78 percent in Madrid. Jyväskylä deviated from this trend because only half of the parents and the children mentioned the use of any medicines during the last fever episode.

The pharmacological treatment was most frequently administered by the mother; the father was seldom mentioned. The children were not supposed to take the medicines by themselves, and only a few of them (one or two per location) said that they take the medicines themselves.

Paracetamol and aspirin (acetylsalicylic acid) were the most frequent pharmacological treatments for fever as expected. The most common treatment was paracetamol (acetaminophen), especially in Chapel Hill where almost 90 percent of treatments involved this compound. Aspirin was also extensively used in some locations, Madrid and Tenerife (32 percent) and Jyväskylä (26 percent). The use of antibiotics or other drugs (especially combination products) was very common in Athens (39 percent) whereas antibiotics were used less frequently in other places (about 5 to 26 percent) (Table 6.1).

Very frequently (more than 50 percent of the families), the medicines used for the treatment of the child's fever were already stored in the home. The figure is slightly lower in Jyväskylä (30 percent). The use of a medicine (the "prescription" of the fever medication) was a decision for parents (40 percent in Tenerife to 90 percent in Chapel Hill) more often than for doctors (9 percent in Chapel Hill to 52 percent in Madrid).

The direct opinion of the children as to "What made the fever go away?" is in contrast with the medical treatment of the ailment. In Chapel Hill, where almost all children were medicated (96 percent) and 89 percent of the parents gave medicines to the children, only 49 percent of the children attributed the lowering of the fever to the medication; the rest of the children thought that other kinds of care, such as special food or lying in bed was the real cause. A similar trend occurred in the two Spanish locations, where most children received medicines (82 to 86 percent) and only 70 percent referred to medicines as the cause of the curing.

Prevention

Parents in Chapel Hill and Madrid (90 percent) and Jyväskylä (60 percent) did not generally think that it is possible to prevent childhood fever. However, in Tenerife (50 percent) and Athens (70

TABLE 6.1. Percentage of Children Receiving Medicine for Fever

	Location*				
	At	CH	Jy	Ma	Te
N Children:	32	96	51	100	115
Received Medicine					
Yes	91%	96%	54%	86%	82%
No	9	4	45	12	11
Don't Know	0	0	0	2	6
Kind Received					
Aspirin	11%	3%	36%	31%	32%
Paracetomol	50	88	39	48	45
Antibiotic	14	6	21	3	9
Combination	25	2	0	2	5
Other	0	1	3	3	1
Don't Know	0	0	6	7	8

* At: Athens; CH: Chapel Hill; Jy: Jyväskylä; Ma: Madrid; Te: Tenerife.

percent) they mentioned actions such as "eating healthful food" or "getting fresh air" as able to prevent the fever.

Conversely, only three percent to 17 percent of the children thought that a fever cannot be prevented. What can a child do to prevent the fever? Most of the children mentioned avoidance of certain behaviors (e.g., "do not drink cold water," "not to sweat," "not to wear too light dresses"). Only in Jyväskylä did children mention prevention in a "positive" manner: over half of the children said that, for instance, "being properly dressed" and "eating properly" prevent fever. In all the five study groups self-care in behavioral terms was seen as the most important method. There were also some individual answers on direct medical action and taking medicines. However, there was a high proportion of "don't know" answers from the children, especially in Chapel Hill where over 30 percent of the children did not know any way to prevent a fever.

Changes in Behavior and Attitudes

Isolation, Restrictions, and Privileges

The children stayed in bed, mainly in their own bed, but as a privilege they could have stayed in their parents' bed too. Time in bed was spent, according to children's responses, mainly watching TV or listening to the radio, reading, playing, resting (sleeping) and having visitors. TV watching was a very popular activity in Chapel Hill where 60 percent mentioned it, whereas in the other communities it was mentioned by only about 40 percent of the children. Reading and sleeping (resting) were most common in Jyväskylä. In Athens, Madrid, and Tenerife, 10 to 20 percent mentioned having visitors. According to the caregivers in Athens, Madrid, and Tenerife, more children (45 to 60 percent) had visitors than in Chapel Hill and Jyväskylä (10 to 13 percent).

When the parents were asked whether the child was kept isolated from the rest of the family, from 0 to 13 percent of parents said that the child was isolated. The children experienced the last fever episode in a completely different way, because 9 to 39 percent of them felt some kind of isolation from the family. In Madrid and Tenerife this percentage was lowest (9 percent). It is possible that the children interpreted the question to mean general restrictions and their answers reflect feelings of loneliness in general (Table 6.2).

Restrictions are also a common feature associated with fever. Almost 90 percent of the children in Athens and Jyväskylä said that their parents had placed restrictions on their normal activities; in the other study groups this percentage varied from 60 to 80 percent. The most common restrictions were not to go to school and not to play with other children or alone.

School Absence

In Chapel Hill more children were absent from school than in the other groups during the last fever episode and in Madrid and Tenerife the fewest. The temperature determining whether the child stayed at home was 38°C (100.4°F) in most of the locations. In Jyväskylä the threshold was slightly lower, because more than one-

TABLE 6.2. Percentage of Children with Fever Isolated from their Families According to Caregivers and Children

	Location*				
	At	CH	Jy	Ma	Te
N Caregivers:	32	102	51	100	115
Response					
Yes	6%	13%	0%	3%	7%
No	94	87	100	95	86
Don't Know	0	0	0	2	6
N Children:	32	103	51	100	115
Response					
Yes	41%	22%	39%	9%	9%
No	59	77	61	89	86
Don't Know	0	1	0	2	5

* At: Athens; CH: Chapel Hill; Jy: Jyväskylä; Ma: Madrid; Te: Tenerife.

third of the parents indicated they would keep a child at home with 37°C (98.6°F) compared to eight to 18 percent of the parents in other locations.

DISCUSSION

In agreement with previous studies dealing with fever in childhood (Andersen 1988; Fruthaler 1985; Helman 1978; Kilman 1987; Kramer, Naimark, and Leduc 1985; Schmitt 1980, 1984) the results of this project showed that childhood fever is defined and treated at home. Fever creates a "caring community." It is an example of a lay health disorder that is treated both in the popular sector and in the professional medical sector. The parents themselves have perceptions and beliefs on the causes, treatments, and prevention as well as behavioral patterns related to fever.

But this study shows as well that the children themselves had their own opinions and that they perceived and experienced the signs of fever. They regarded themselves as having a role on the etiology and the prevention of the disease, and judged the medical and nonmedical treatment of the fever.

The parents in the samples had scientifically correct knowledge about fever, viewing it as a mechanism of defense, and a symptom of underlying disease. This has already been shown by Helman (1978) in a similar study. The diagnosis of fever is suggested by observation of symptoms (as the palpation of the forehead, tiredness, etc.) and is confirmed by signs (the objective measurement of the fever by a thermometer). The first is based on personal experience and perceptions, whereas the second establishes a bridge toward professional care. A similar approach is mentioned by Kilman (1987).

It is important to realize that the mother, being closer to the children and usually taking care of them, is the person who has a key role as definer of the condition, and it is she who makes the first decisions. But when a more serious action is needed, a second step of the treatment such as giving a medicine, consulting the doctor or being absent from school, both parents are likely to be involved. Only in these cases, is the father visible in the diagnosis, care, and prevention of childhood fever.

A big issue in the study of fever in children is the definition of the fever itself. The threshold from which the diagnosis of fever was made varied quite a lot from one location (and one culture) to another. As shown in Figure 6.1, there are two groups of locations in our study: Jyväskylä and Tenerife have a lower threshold (around 35 percent of the parents defined fever at 37°C (98.6°F), whereas in Chapel Hill and Madrid the limit is more frequently set at 37.5°C (99.5°F). In fact, 38°C (100.4°F) is the standard level of comparison. In a study of Canadian parents of 202 young febrile children, 48 percent of the parents considered temperature less than 38.0°C (100.4°F) to be a "fever" (Kramer, Naimark, and Leduc 1985). Similarly, in this study, between 57 to 67 percent of the parents set the definition of the lower limit for fever under 38°C (100.4°F). A remarkable difference was apparent in Athens, where 62 percent of the parents thought that fever is only present if the temperature is 38°C (100.4°F) or more. In fact, when the children had "fever" (i.e., the last episode of fever studied in this project), it was common that the child's fever was over 38°C (100.4°F). Only about 10 percent of the children had fever under 38°C (100.4°F) the last time they were diagnosed, except for Tenerife where the percentage was higher (34 percent).

The old beliefs about fever came out also in this study: fever was seen as good and bad. It was not regarded as a harmful ailment and it was not generally seen as a sickness. It was mainly considered as a mechanism of defense or as a mechanism to fight against sickness, making the recuperation quicker. When talking about the last episode, the parents in all locations (72 to 86 percent) said that it was not serious. However, that was not an obstacle to consulting the family physician frequently (sometimes by telephone): 75 percent in Athens, Madrid, and Tenerife, 45 percent in Chapel Hill, and 30 percent in Jyväskylä. It suggests that fear or worrying of parents is not out of control but is an expression of insecurity on the underlying cause, possible unknown sickness and also concern about the effects of long-lasting fever.

It was remarkable that the pharmacological approach was not in the frontline of the treatment of fever, and other nonmedical measurements such as resting, food, and drinks were viewed as important by the parents, and especially by the children. There were cultural differences. For example, in Chapel Hill, almost all children (96 percent) received some drugs: the treatment of fever is hardly describable separate from the technical approach or the magic of a pill. In the Nordic location, i.e., Jyväskylä, the treatment of fever was pharmacological in only half of the cases, and only 17 percent of the parents mentioned it as a main remedy. In the Mediterranean locations (Madrid, Tenerife, Athens), the use of medicines was also relatively high (about 80 percent), but other nonmedical treatments such as baths, or "hot-cloths" were very frequently mentioned, whereas these almost never were mentioned in the other locations.

Children indicated that they have a knowledge of fever. They learned by experience: they knew the symptoms, and could recognize by themselves when they have fever. They link the fever to their behavior more than to a disease. That is probably why the children think that fever can be prevented by self-care and especially by their own behavior. There is a difference in this respect between children and their parents. The parents seem to have a more structured and medicalized knowledge about fever and tend to see the fever as a nonpreventable event.

Most of the children thought that the relief of fever is due to the medical treatment (49 to 81 percent). Home remedies, special food, drinks, and baths, were also regarded as important in relief from fever, but many children did not think that this kind of care was anything "special." The beliefs about these approaches and relative weight given to them should be considered when promoting a more healthful treatment of fever.

There is a big discussion in the medical arena on the most appropriate treatment of fever in children. There is believed to be an increased risk of "Reye's Syndrome" in children suffering from a virus who have been treated with aspirin (Isselbacher and Podolsky 1991) and a campaign was launched against the use of aspirin in the treatment of fever in children. Despite the fact that there is scientific evidence of the increased risk of this serious central nervous system disease, the penetration of the campaign is very different from one country to another. In many places some physicians think that the risk of "Reye's Syndrome" is so low, that the increased risk is almost negligible in terms of the public's health. In any event, the treatment is being shifted from aspirin to paracetamol (which also is not without some risks and side effects) for the treatment of these viruses.

Differences in treating childhood fever with aspirin were clearly seen in the study. Whereas in the USA, where the campaign was initiated and is being fueled by the health authorities, the use of aspirin by the parents was very low (3 percent). On the contrary, in Jyväskylä and Madrid or Tenerife, the use of aspirin (when some medication was used) accounted for around one-third of all medications. The use of antibiotics is linked to the treatment of infectious diseases (which could produce fever), but not to the treatment of the fever itself. The percentage of antibiotics was low, in general, in the sample. The higher percentages were present in Athens (14 percent of all medication) and Jyväskylä (21 percent); but it is important to note that here the number of children treated with any drugs was relatively low (54 percent) and thus, the probability of a more serious disease and a medical prescription for antibiotics was higher. This is a very positive trend, deviating from the general data in other pharmacoepidemiological studies, where it has been shown that there is an overuse of medicines in general in the population, and specially antibiotics (Sanz 1992). In fact, some studies have shown that the prescription of medicines to children by their parents is sometimes more correct than the prescription to the same children by their doctors for common child disturbances (Boada, Duque, and Sanz 1989).

The children feel alone, restricted, and confined at home when suffering from fever. This feeling is not shared by their parents, because they think that their children are specially cared for when sick. The different experience of isolation was clearly shown. The children are restricted from their daily life activities: being out, playing with classmates, and, despite the extra care, they look forward to the "rights" of the everyday life. This fact, together with the real time alone at home, make the isolation the most vivid memory of the fever episodes. In a few places (Athens, Madrid, Tenerife) visitors and friends were commonly mentioned in the context of the fever episode. It can be concluded that the sickness role of the child includes the feeling of isolation.

CONCLUSIONS

All these data are relevant to what has been called in the literature "fever-phobia." Some authors think that the seriousness of fever is overestimated and that doctors are too easily consulted (Fruthaler, 1985; Kramer, Naimark, and Leduc 1985, Schmitt 1980, 1984). But a careful analysis could draw a quite different picture: parents perceive fever as a kind of "natural phenomenon," which can be dangerous, but which also can have good effects on health. They know how to treat a particular episode, but usually consult with the doctor in order to confirm an underlying cause and to be reinforced in the treatment already "prescribed" by themselves. This is hard to label "fever-phobia."

There were very many differences in the five locations regarding the definition of fever, the concept of fever, the percentage of children who used medicines for the treatment of fever, and who used nonmedical treatments. However, although each location presented a slightly different framework, each was internally coherent. When Eskerud (1992) stated that in the Nordic Countries it is not adequate to define "fever-phobia," the authors were probably referring to the same conclusion as here: "fever phobia" represents concern, but not fear in the face of childhood fever.

Any health project aiming to educate the population on the diagnosis and treatment of children's fever should not forget the main actor, i.e., the child. Children have their own experiences and ideas, which sometimes are more appropriate than their parent's prejudices, and could play an important role in rational behavior toward disease. Most of the chapters in this book deal with this idea.

NOTE

1. The COMAC Childhood and Medicines Project was funded through a European Economic Community (EEC) *Comité d'Action Concerté* (COMAC) contract, COMAC/HSR MR4*-CT90-0319, awarded to The Institute on Child Health, Athens, Greece, with Deanna J. Trakas as the Project Leader. The official title of the Contract was "Medicine Use, Behaviour and Children's Perceptions of Medicines and Health Care."

REFERENCES

Almarsdottir, A. B. and Bush, P. J. 1995. "Children's experience with illness in Chapel Hill, North Carolina, USA." *Childhood and Medicine Use in Cross-Cultural Perspective: A European Concerted Action* edited by D. J. Trakas and E. Sanz. Luxembourg: Office for Official Publications of the European Community, (EURO Report) pgs. 269-292.

Andersen, A. R. 1988. "Parental perception and management of school-age children's fever." *Nurse Practitioner* 13(5):8-9.

Aramburuzabala, P., Garcia, M., Polaino-Lorente, A., and Sanz, E. 1995. "Medicine Use, Behaviour, and Children's Perceptions of Medicines and Health Care in Madrid and Tenerife (Spain)." *Childhood and Medicine Use in Cross-Cultural Perspective: A European Concerted Action* edited by D.J. Trakas and E. Sanz. Luxembourg: Office for Official Publications of the European Community (EURO Report), pgs. 245-268.

Boada, J., Duque, J., and Sanz, E. 1989. "Parent drug prescription in children." IV World Conference on Clinical Pharmacology & Therapeutics. Mannheim-Heidelberg July 23-28. *European Journal of Clinical Pharmacology* 36(Suppl):A155.

Bush, P. J. and Davidson, F. R. 1982. "Medicines and 'drugs': What do children think?," *Health Education Quarterly* 9:113-128.

Bush, P. J. and Iannotti, R. J. 1988. "Origins and stability of children's health beliefs relative to medicine use." *Social Science and Medicine* 27(4):345-352.

Bush, P. J. and Iannotti, R. J. 1990. "A children's health belief model." *Medical Care* 28(1):60-86.

Bush, P. J., Iannotti, R. J., and Davidson, F. R. 1985. "A Longitudinal Study of Children and Medicines." *Topics in Pharmaceutical Sciences* edited by D. D. Breimer and P. Speiser. Amsterdam: Elsevier Sciences, pgs. 391-403.

Casey, R., McMahon, F., McCormick, M. C., Pasquariello, P. S., Zavod, W., and King, F. H. 1984. "Fever therapy: An educational intervention for parents." *Pediatrics* 73:600-605.

Chow, M. P., Durand, B. A., Feldman, M. N., and Mills, M. A. 1984. *Handbook of Pediatric Primary Care*. New York: John Wiley.

Dusi, A., Franco, D., Messi, G., Renier, S., and Marchi, A. G. 1988. "Study of analgesic-antipyretic drugs risk of poisoning in childhood." *Pediatria Medicae Chirurgica* 10:495-500.

Eskerud, J. R. 1992. "How do people perceive fever and what is done for it?" *Nordisk Medicin* 107(1) (Abstract).

Freidson, E. 1970. *Profession of Medicine. A Study of the Sociology of Applied Knowledge*. New York: Dodd, Mead.

Fruthaler, G. J. 1985. "Fever in children: Phobia versus facts." *Hospital Practice* 20(IIA):49-53.

Helman, C. G. 1978. "'Feed a cold, starve a fever': Folk models of infection in an English suburban community and their relation to medical treatment." *Culture, Medicine and Psychiatry* 2:107-137.

Isselbacher, K. J. and Podolsky, D. K. 1991. "Infiltrative and Metabolic Disease Affecting the Liver." *Harrison's Principles of Internal Medicine 12th edition*, edited by J. D. Wilson. New York: McGraw-Hill, pgs. 1353-1354.

Kilman, C. A. 1987. "Parents' knowledge and practices related to fever management." *Journal of Pediatric Health Care* 1(4):173-179.

Kleinman, A. 1978. "Concepts and a model for comparison of medical systems as cultural systems." *Social Science and Medicine* 12:85-93.

Kramer, M. S., Naimark, L., and Leduc, G. G. 1985. "Parental fever phobia and its correlates." *Pediatrics* 75:1110-1113.

Prout, A. 1988. "Off school sick: Mothers' accounts of negotiating sickness absence." *Sociological Review* 4(36):765-789.

Prout, A. 1989. "Sickness as a dominant symbol in life course. Transitions: An illustrated theoretical framework." *Sociology of Health and Illness* 4(11):336-359.

Prout, A. and James, A. 1990. "A New Paradigm for the Sociology of Childhood. . ?" *Constructing and Reconstructing Childhood: Contemporary Issues in the Sociological Study of Childhood* edited by A. James and A. Prout. London: Falmer Press, pgs. 7-34.

Sanz, E. J. 1992. "The hazards of medication in children." *Studying childhood and Medicine Use* edited by D. J. Trakas and E. J. Sanz. Athens, Greece: ZHTA Medical Publications, pgs. 93-104.

Schmitt, B. D. 1980. Fever phobia. Misconceptions of parents about fevers. *American Journal of Diseases of Children* 134:176-181.

Schmitt, B.D. 1984. "Fever in childhood." *Pediatrics* 74(Suppl):929-936.

Vaskilampi, T., Kalpio, O., Ahonen, R., and Hallia, O. 1995. "Finnish study on medicine use, health behaviour, and perceptions of medicines and health care." *Childhood and Medicine Use in Cross-Cultural Perspective: A European Concerted Action* edited by D. J. Trakas and E. Sanz. Luxembourg: Office for Official Publications of the European Community (EURO Report), pgs. 191-220.

Chapter 7

Children's Perceived Benefit of Medicines in Chapel Hill, Madrid, and Tenerife

Anna B. Almarsdottir
Pilar Aramburuzabala
Marcelino García
Emilio J. Sanz

Earlier studies have pointed to wide differences in medicine use across nations and population groups (Bergman 1979; Griffiths et al. 1986; King and Griffiths 1984; Moore, Geddes, and Patterson 1981; Sanz, Bergman, and Dahlstrom 1989; Svarstad et al. 1987; Wessling, Bergman, and Westerholm 1991; Zadoroznyj and Svarstad 1990). Morbidity has not been shown to account for this variation in medicine use. The amount of medicines as well as availability and preferences for medicines have also been shown to vary; although the research in this area is scant (Payer 1988). Chapter 4 in this book pointed out the variation in drug distribution systems with extremes ranging from a totally market-driven system to a tightly government-controlled system.

The meaning of sickness and treatment varies across cultures, as shown in other chapters of this book (see, for example, Chapters 3 and 9). Nations and cultures are known to possess different degrees of stoicism around illness and disease which means that some persons are more likely to seek treatment than others (Zborowski 1952; Zola 1973). Although it is important to study adults' interpretation and understanding of illness and treatment, it is paramount to follow how children are socialized into the adult world of help seeking and medication behavior.

Former research saw children as passive, incompetent, and asocial actors in medicine use. This claim is being contested by researchers who describe children as interpretive social actors (Bush, Iannotti, and Davidson 1985; Prout and James 1990). Bush and colleagues found that children had attitudes, beliefs, and expectations about medicines, and often had autonomy over their medicine taking without the knowledge of their parents. There is thus an emergence of the view that children have beliefs, attitudes, values, and behaviors toward treatment that are possibly distinct for each child, but are formed by the surrounding culture.

The research most conducive to the realization of the differences between cultural perceptions of sickness and treatment has been primarily qualitative. Ethnography was formerly mainly used as a means to understand cultures alien to the Western world. Lately, ethnography has become important in health care research in Western countries. The information from these studies has elicited important insights into the factors responsible for the above-mentioned differences in medicine use.

Ethnography is a multi-method approach that centers on participant observation; it aims at a contextualized account of social life. It can include interviews (and other methods such as document analysis) as long as they help to illuminate the context. Then there are interviews, sometimes known as ethnographic interviews, that are not accompanied by participant observation but do pay a great deal of attention to the social context of events. The ethnographic interview encompasses the goals of ethnography without going for a full-blown ethnographic approach. For example, some information formerly gained about medicine use and health using the ethnographic interview had informants talk open-ended about the experience of sickness instead of responding to questionnaires constructed a priori (Trakas 1990; Sachs 1990).

The COMAC Childhood and Medicines Project[1] had as its core, ethnographic (open-ended qualitative) interviews with children about a sickness episode at each study location (see Chapter 2). The results and interpretation of these ethnographic interviews may stand alone as information acquired through this method of inquiry, but are used here in association with other methods.

Researchers in health education have strongly advised the use of qualitative methodology as a precursor and complement to quantitative inquiry (Bauman and Adair 1992; Steckler et al. 1992). In addition, Chapter 2 of this volume focuses on the topic of triangulation. In this chapter, quantitative methods play a major role, but some of the information gained from the ethnographic interviews conducted at each site is used first to formulate hypotheses about children's perceptions and knowledge about medicines. Second, this information is used in triangulation to aid the explanation of the results of the quantitative model estimation.

RESULTS FROM THE ETHNOGRAPHIC INTERVIEWS

As mentioned in the introduction, ethnography may serve as a predecessor to quantitative assessment and as one cornerstone when triangulating methods. A brief description of the results of the ethnographic results in the Chapel Hill, Madrid, and Tenerife sites is provided here to illustrate how the findings influenced model building and testing. The results from the ethnographic interviews conducted simultaneously with the more quantitative assessment at the study sites of Chapel Hill, North Carolina, USA, and Madrid and Tenerife, Spain, showed that children have limited autonomy in declaring themselves sick and treating themselves in both countries (Almarsdottir and Bush 1995; Aramburuzabala et al. 1995). The mother was shown to be the primary caregiver to sick children in most instances. She was also the person who made most of the decisions about actions during the sickness episode in all three samples.

Age differences were seen in the Chapel Hill sample in the way children explained the concepts of illness and medicines. Older children described contagion as bacteria or "bugs," whereas younger children talked about the actual transmission routes. Older children talked about medicines using names (brand and generic). The younger children more frequently described color or taste when telling the interviewer about the medicines they were given. Older children indicated they believed more in their own power to overcome and prevent illness, whereas younger children relied more on external sources for help. Pronounced age differences were not observed in the ethnographic interviews with children in either of the Spanish samples.

Health care professionals were not very prominent in the Chapel Hill children's accounts of sickness. This may be caused by a health care system that does not encourage visits to medical doctors, uses telephones for consulting more frequently, and the fact that the area is saturated with health care professionals, which may make contacts with them a commonplace occurrence for the children. Conversely, there was more mention of doctors in the Spanish accounts.

The influence of the Western biomedical model could be seen clearly through the accounts of children at all three sites; comparing the body to a machine that has to be taken in for repair. This view of the body as something to be maintained and taken in for repair is an emic category in the American and Spanish ways of thinking about the body. The children had adopted this understanding. Furthermore, they had adopted the idea that medicines serve as part of the "repair" of what is wrong with the body. Children at all sites agreed that medicines are for "getting better." They seldom, however, viewed medicines as tools for maintaining the body's health.

It is possible to conclude that age is an important factor in children's thinking about health, illness, and medicines in at least one sample studied. Autonomy in medicine use seemed not to be an important factor influencing children's health beliefs at this stage, and may be omitted from a model explaining the perceptions. The influences of the environment (parents at all sites and media in Chapel Hill) were well documented in the interviews and need to be included in a quantitative investigation of the mediators of children's beliefs about medicines' role in restoring health.

Background for the Model

This chapter focuses on understanding the factors that influenced the children's perceptions about medicines. Children's Perceived Benefit of Medicines (KMEDBEN) as a construct has been shown to be one of the strongest influences on children's expectations to take medicines (Bush and Iannotti 1990), which in turn, indicates that understanding the influences on KMEDBEN aids in the study of the factors involved in medicine-taking behaviors.

A model was constructed to account for the influences of development and socialization on the outcome variable: the Children's Perceived Benefit of Medicines construct (KMEDBEN). The model built on information from ethnographic analysis, prior research on the Children's Health Belief Model (Bush and Iannotti 1990),

Social Cognitive Theory (Bandura 1986), and Cognitive Development Theory (Inhelder and Piaget 1958).

Bandura (1986) put forward the social cognitive theory (SCT) to explain the interaction of the person, the environment, and behaviors. According to Bandura, behaviors are acquired through the processes of attention, retention, production, and motivation. These processes operate in three domains: the personal, behavioral, and environmental. Personal factors include the child's own value system; expectations derive from observation and experience; behavioral factors include skills in performing the behaviors; environmental factors include peers, family members, and media, which both model and influence through expressed opinions. The model proposed in this chapter takes the value system, expectations, and environmental factors into account in seeking to explain children's perceptions about medicines.

Cognitive Development Theory (CDT) is attributed to the Swiss psychologist Piaget in the 1950s (Inhelder and Piaget 1958). The theory emphasizes stages for children's causal thinking from preoperational through concrete operational to formal operational. It suggests that stages of development, although influenced by personal experience, are not formed as the result of direct responses to parents, peers, or the child's own behavior, but result from the child's cognitive processes as they develop and operate within his or her environment. Piaget underlined the naturalness and universality of childhood. These ideas have been found useful in the arena of education wherein there are constraints on what types of information can be given to children according to their developmental stages.

The proposed model integrates the theories of SCT and CDT to explain influences on the important concept of Children's Perceived Benefit of Medicines. The model has components from SCT (value system, expectations, and environment). It also controls for developmental stage of the children (thus incorporating CDT).

It was hypothesized that the concept of Children's Perceived Benefit of Medicines (KMEDBEN) is a product of children's knowledge about medicines (observation and experience), the degree to which they find themselves in control of their health (value system), and the amount of drug advertising (environmental influences) to which they have been exposed, controlling for age, parental education, and whether parents are health professionals.

The concept of Children's Knowledge about Medicines arises from developmental as well as socialization considerations. The question that health policymakers grapple with is: When are children knowledgeable and developed enough to take responsibility for their medicine taking? Policymakers are also interested in understanding whether this knowledge is purely a function of development, or whether there are important social factors at work. Because there is little or no information given to children in schools about legal medicines, it is proposed in the hypothesized model that children's knowledge and understanding of medicines is a product of their development and the amount of influences from the environment in the form of parents and advertising (wherever advertising of medicines is legal).

The results of a simultaneous equation approach investigating influences on the construct of Children's Perceived Benefit of Medicines are presented in this chapter. This approach was taken due to the hypothesis that Children's Knowledge about Medicines (CKNOW) influences Children's Perceived Benefit of Medicines (KMEDBEN) and that CKNOW is also determined within the system and cannot be studied independent of KMEDBEN (Figure 7.1).

Research Goals

The goals of the analyses were

- to test a model of relationships between children's psychosocial and demographic factors and their knowledge and beliefs about medicines in two nationally and linguistically distinct samples;
- to compare the results of the two samples and suggest reasons for any differences observed; and
- to explore the role of ethnographic interview data in informing scale construction and model estimation.

FIGURE 7.1. Model to be estimated

a) Schematic view

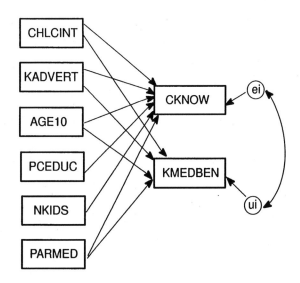

b) Equations

i. CKNOW = a_0 + a_1CHLCINT + a_2KADVERT* + a_3AGE 10 + a_4PCEDUC + a_5 NKIDS + a_6PARMED + e_i
ii. KMEDBEN = b_0 - b_1 CKNOW - b_2CHLCINT + b_3KADVERT* - b_4AGE10 - b_5PARMED + u_i

*Not in Madrid or Tenerife equations.

METHODS

Data Collection

The data employed in this chapter were gathered at three sites: Chapel Hill (CH), North Carolina USA; Madrid (MA), Spain; and Tenerife (TE), Canary Islands, Spain. The two Spanish samples (MA-TE) were combined for a more culture-specific comparison

(MA-TE). The methods of data collection at each site are described below.

Chapel Hill

Data were gathered in Chapel Hill during the summers of 1992 and 1993 from summer day camps in the urban and suburban area of Chapel Hill, North Carolina. These camps were chosen on the basis of convenience of location and the consent of camp coordinators.

The population targeted consisted of middle-class Caucasian Americans ages seven and ten and their Primary Caregivers (hereafter referred to as PCs). The PC, defined as the person most responsible for taking care of the child during illness episodes, was either the child's mother, father, or legal guardian. The PC was identified by asking the child at the time of interview: "Who takes most care of you when you are sick?"

The parents or guardians of children were approached as they picked up their children from camp and given a brief description of the study and a consent form to read. They were then asked whether they were interested in participating in the study.

The children (102) were interviewed during camp, in all camps but one. For one camp, the children were interviewed at home at the same time as their PC. Most PCs (99 of 102) were interviewed at home. Three PCs were interviewed at their workplace.

Very few people refused to participate in the study. In pilot studies conducted earlier it had been found that American parents and children were heavily scheduled around activities outside the home and thus had very little time for interviews. However, the participation rate was high with about 93 percent of those asked consenting. Two parents who originally consented to participate, later refused to be interviewed. The reasons given for nonparticipation were most often lack of time on behalf of the parents (N = 3); two children were unwilling to participate due to shyness, and two children were being tested extensively for medical problems and their parents were unwilling to subject them to more questioning.

The interviews were carried out by three young women, comparable in age to the camp counselors. During the first weeks of camp the interviewers spent a few hours almost every day there in order to recruit and familiarize themselves with the camp routines. Although the camps where the majority of respondents were had two week camps, most children were at camp almost all summer. The interviewers and the children did not know each other very well because the interviewers did not partake in the camp activities, but kept busy interviewing. They did however become familiar faces with the children who had already been interviewed.

The interviewers were trained first during the pilot study conducted before the summer camps started. In addition to familiarizing the interviewers with all items in the instruments, issues of confidentiality and how to treat respondents were discussed. Interviewers were taught how to record answers, how to read questions, and how and when to probe. After each interview the interviewers discussed problems they had with the instruments and with posing certain questions. This information was then used to improve the instruments (wording as well as general lay out). Each interviewer was observed during an interview in order to improve interviewing techniques. The reporting on interviews was continued during the study to solve problems that arose (e.g., how to treat children with behavioral problems).

Each respondent was interviewed once. The time each interview took was recorded, as well as the number of interruptions and privacy of the interview location. The mean interviewing time for children was 43.5 minutes; the range was 25 to 110 minutes.

The interview with the children started by asking them to draw a picture of a situation when they were sick or injured. After the picture was finished, the child was asked to describe the picture and the situation depicted there. The interviewers then prompted each child with questions about the situation in order to get him or her to describe it in more detail on the points relative to the overall research question. This section of the interview was tape recorded. The children were then interviewed using semi-structured questionnaires and scales. These were administered verbally to the child who responded, either verbally or by pointing at a visual Likert scale (bar graph).

Madrid and Tenerife

Researchers in Madrid and Tenerife gathered data during the school year of 1991-1992 from public elementary school children in grades two and five. Four schools were used in Madrid and two schools were used in Tenerife. The schools were a convenience sample of schools in middle class neighborhoods at each site. A middle-class neighborhood was defined as having a median income level.

Fifteen teachers refused to participate in Madrid (approximately 50 percent), and none refused in Tenerife. Of the children asked to participate in the study in Madrid, 75 refused (15 percent). Among the children who agreed to participate, 275 parents refused to let their children participate (73 percent). All the children approached in Tenerife consented to the study. They took home a letter informing the parents about the study and a consent form for them to sign. All parents signed the consent forms. There was a 28 percent drop-out rate in the Tenerife sample, but no dropouts in Madrid.

Eleven interviewers in both locations combined worked with the children for approximately two hours, divided into two or three sessions. Interviewers were not previously known to the children. In Madrid, the children were interviewed at home. Earlier, they had met in a small group with an interviewer at school to draw a picture of the last time they were sick. The home interview consisted of questionnaires and scales administered verbally to the child who answered either verbally or by pointing to a Likert scale.

In Tenerife, the children were interviewed individually twice: once at the school, where they drew the picture and were interviewed using ethnographic (or open-ended qualitative) interview methods and were administered some of the other instruments. The second interview was conducted at home, where the rest of the instruments were employed.

Operationalization of Variables

The endogenous variables in the proposed model were Children's Knowledge about Medicines (CKNOW) and Children's Perceived Benefit of Medicines (KMEDBEN). Knowledge was a construct describing children's understanding of the efficacy of medicines in relation to their chemical composition, formulation, and place of acquisition. Understanding these concepts reveals children's preparation in understanding issues in medicine use. Children's Knowledge about Medicines (CKNOW) was operationalized using an additive eight-item index. The index was composed of questions about whether color, taste, place of purchase, and dosage form account for differences between medicines. There were only right (coded 1) or wrong (coded 0) answers. An example of an item from the knowledge index was: "If you were sick, which would help you more, a big pill or a little pill?" If the child answered either "little" or "big pill," the item was coded as wrong; if the child answered "no difference" or "it depends," the item was coded as right. The other endogenous variable in the proposed model was the Children's Perceived Benefit of Medicines (KMEDBEN). It was a 16-item scale rated on a five-point Likert scale. Twelve statements about the benefit of medicines for each type of ailment and four control statements were read aloud to the child. An example of items in this scale were: "When I have a cold, medicine can help me." The child was then shown a bar graph on which there were five gradually increasing bars from left to right and asked to indicate the degree of agreement or disagreement with the statements in the instrument on the bar graph after the interviewer had made sure the child understood the scale. Four control statements were included to check for consistency of the child's answers. This was accomplished by reading two opposing statements at various points in the scale and seeing whether the child gave opposite ratings to these statements (e.g., by rating the statement "I love cats" as 5 and "I hate cats" as 1).

There were six exogenous in the model tested on the Chapel Hill sample: Children's Internal Health Locus of Control (CHLCINT), Children's Recognition of Medicine Advertising (KADVERT), Child's Age (AGE10), PC's educational level (PCEDUC), number of children in the household under the age of 14 (NKIDS), and whether any of the parents or guardians was a health professional (PARMED). KADVERT was excluded from the Madrid/Tenerife sample due to the fact that medicine advertising is very limited in Spain and thus was not measured there.

The concept of a three-dimensional health locus of control is well established (Wallston, Wallston, and DeVellis 1978). This concept means that people vary according to how much control they perceive they have over their health. Beliefs range from the notion that individuals can significantly affect the direction of their own health (Internal), to beliefs that they are helpless; that good or bad health is due to factors external to the person's control: either good or bad Luck or other persons more powerful or knowledgeable, such as parents or physicians (Powerful Others).

The degree of children's health locus of control (CHLC) was measured using the nine-item Children's Health Locus of Control scale shortened and adapted by Bush, Parcel, and Davidson (1982) from Parcel and Meyer (1978). The stability of the factor structure of the shortened nine-item version of the CHLC had been shown (O'Brien, Bush, and Parcel 1989). The child answered either yes (coded 1) or no (coded 0) to statements that each loaded on only one of the three dimensions (Internal, Luck, and Powerful Others). The degree of internal health locus of control (CHLCINT) was then measured by coding all items toward the Internal dimension.

Children's Recognition of Over-the-Counter Medicines (KAD-VERT) was tested in CH by showing children pictures of medicines that were frequently advertised in the month before the study was conducted (23 medicines). Generic or drugs not advertised in a corresponding category (18 medicines), were also shown to test correctness of the source indicated. Children were asked whether they had ever seen the medicine before. If they had, they were asked where they had seen the medicine, and told that they could indicate more than one source. The resulting index's composite number was the number of medicines recognized by the child from television (or other advertising).

The Child's Age (AGE10) was a dichotomous variable which equaled 1 if the child was ten years old or in fifth grade and 0 if seven years old or in second grade. PC's educational level (PCE-DUC) was measured in CH using a seven-point scale ranging from completion of elementary school to completion of graduate or professional training. In the Spanish samples, PCEDUC was measured on a six-point scale ranging from primary school to the completion of a university degree. NKIDS was the number of children under the age of 14 residing in the household. Whether any of the parents or guardians was a health professional (PARMED) was a dichotomous variable coded 1 if one or more were health professionals.

Confirmatory Factor Analysis and Instrument Reliability

Confirmatory factor analysis (CFA) was performed first to assess validity of all the scales administered; second, to test hypotheses about the underlying constructs to aid in understanding of the variables; and third, to facilitate data reduction by exploring the existence of subscales. These subscales were later subjected to internal reliability tests. The Children's Perceived Benefit of Medicines was tested for two dimensions (Perceived Benefit of Medicines for Physical versus Mental function). The Children's Health Locus of Control (CHLC) was tested for all three dimensions (Internal, Luck, and Powerful Others) as well as one dimension (Internal) after coding all answers toward that dimension.

Cronbach's alpha and Kuder-Richardson-20 reliability tests were performed on the (sub-) scales in the model after completing the CFA. These methods were used to determine the internal reliability of the scales and to eliminate items to achieve maximum reliability.

Model Estimation

The first equation of the model in Figure 7.1 (eq. i) does not include any endogenous variables on the right-hand side, and regular Ordinary Least Squares (OLS) can therefore be applied in its estimation. Conversely, equation ii cannot be estimated using regular OLS due to the assumption of the model that CKNOW is an endogenous variable on the right-hand side and that the covariance of the disturbance terms for the equations is nonzero. The system could be estimated using full information methods, such as structural equations modeling (SEM); or limited information methods, such as Two-Stage-Least-Squares (2SLS). The latter approach was taken due to computational ease and the fact that estimates in one equation will not be affected by specification errors in other equations.

Identification of the model was carried out using the rank and order conditions of simultaneous equations modeling. Identification is a topic relevant to simultaneous equations. The basic question posed when the identification of a model is investigated is: can all "unknown" parameters in the model be solved for by parameters that are "known"? If there is not enough information to solve the equation, it is unidentified and cannot be estimated. If there is exactly enough information for solving the equation, it is exactly (or just) identified. If there is more than enough information, i.e., the parameters can be solved for in more than one way–the equation is overidentified.

Equation i was found to be exactly identified and without an endogenous variable on the right-hand side; and therefore Ordinary Least Squares (OLS) estimation was a suitable method of estimation. Equation ii was found to be overidentified and Two-Stage Least Squares (2SLS) was used for its estimation.

The model was estimated using PC SAS. In the first step of the 2SLS, the equation containing CKNOW on the left-hand side (equation i) was estimated and the predicted values saved. In the second step, OLS was applied to equation ii using the predicted values of CKNOW from the first run (CKNOWHAT). In this way, the right-hand side variables of equation ii were not correlated with CKNOW, which otherwise would have led to biased estimates.

RESULTS

Table 7.1 shows the distribution of answers for variables in the model.[2]

There were 50 ten-year-old and 52 seven-year-old children in the CH sample, and seven children had at least one parent in a health profession. In MA/TE combined sample, there were 112 ten-year-old and 103 seven-year-old children. Of the Spanish children, 33 parents (15.3 percent) were health professionals.

Confirmatory Factor Analysis and Instrument Reliability

CFA of the Children's Perceived Benefit of Medicines (KMED-BEN) scale showed two dimensions of this construct: a physical and a mental dimension for both samples (Table 7.2). Each dimension, as well as the whole scale, were subjected to Cronbach's alpha reliability tests which showed that the mental dimension had a higher coefficient than the physical dimension and that the reliability of the whole scale was as high as the mental dimension alone. As a result, the scale as a whole was used in the estimation of the model after dropping items n and s.

TABLE 7.1. Descriptive Statistics for Variables in the Model

Variable*	Site**	Mean	Median	Mode	Range	Standard Deviation	Skewness	Kurtosis
KMEDBEN	CH	35.2	35	35	16 - 55	7.29	-0.19	0.11
	Ma/Te	36.7	37	33	0 - 55	8.63	-0.95	3.11
CKNOW	CH	3.97	4	3	0 - 7	1.67	0.07	-0.62
	Ma/Te	1.92	2	1	0 - 6	1.34	0.38	-0.54
CHLCINT	CH	2.84	3	3	0 - 4	1.07	-0.92	0.34
	Ma/Te	1.90	2	1	0 - 7	1.27	0.64	1.21
KADVERT	CH	4.52	3.5	0	0 - 18	4.59	0.94	0.17
	Ma/Te	N/A	N/A	N/A	N/A	N/A	N/A	N/A
PCEDUC	CH	5.97	6	6	3 - 7	0.95	-0.86	0.58
	Ma/Te	3.74	4	6	0 - 6	2.08	-0.17	-1.58
NKIDS	CH	1.82	2	2	1 - 3	0.59	0.06	-0.28
	Ma/Te	2.00	2	2	1 - 8	1.02	1.77	6.04

* KMEDBEN: Children's Perceived Benefit of Medicines.
CKNOW: Children's Knowledge about Medicines.
CHLCINT: Children's Internal Health Locus of Control.
KADVERT: Children's Recognition of Over-the-Counter Medicine Advertising.
AGE10: 1 for 10-year-old children, 0 for 7-year-old children.
PCEDUC: Primary caregiver's educational level.
NKIDS: Number of children under 14 living in the same household as the target child.
PARMED: 1 if 1 or more parents are health professionals, 0 otherwise.
** CH: Chapel Hill, Ma/Te: Madrid and Tenerife.

TABLE 7.2. Confirmatory Factor Analysis of the Children's Perceived Benefit of Medicine Scale

	Site							
	CH				Ma/Te			
	Physical Factor		Mental Factor		Physical Factor		Mental Factor	
Item	Loading	T-value	Loading	T-value	Loading	T-value	Loading	T-value
a	1.00*	N/A	**	**	1.00*	N/A	**	**
h	1.17	4.89	**	**	1.09	7.91	**	**
l	1.48	5.60	**	**	1.34	9.14	**	**
m	0.68	3.26	**	**	0.76	5.96	**	**
n	0.92	4.13	**	**	0.99	7.34	**	**
s	0.86	3.95	**	**	1.00	7.42 n.s.	**	**
b	**	**	1.00*	N/A	**	**	1.00*	N/A
c	**	**	0.75	5.58	**	**	0.62	7.34
f	**	**	0.29	2.10	**	**	0.21	2.39
g	**	**	0.81	6.02	**	**	0.83	10.29
j	**	**	0.73	5.44	**	**	0.82	10.22
k	**	**	0.36	2.64	**	**	0.53	6.15
$c^2 =$	327.12 (53 d.f.)				298.35 (53 d.f.)			

n.s. Not statistically significant.

* The loading of item a is set equal to 1.00 for the estimation of the whole scale; items a and b are set equal to 1.00 for the estimation of two-dimensions for scaling purposes.

** These items did not load on this dimension.

When the Children's Health Locus of Control (CHLC) was tested for all three dimensions (Internal, Luck, and Powerful Others), the model would not converge on a solution for either sample. Subgroups of children (according to age and sex) were tested to see whether one group was responsible for this result, but all four groups showed a lack of fit to the CFA model. The data were coded toward the Internal dimension and CFA run on Internal as the only dimension (or factor). The data did not fit this CFA model either. The Internal Health Locus of Control for children (CHLCINT) was tested for reliability using Kuder-Richardson-20. The scale showed low reliability for the CH sample as seen in Table 7.3. Four items were excluded from the scale to increase reliability for this sample (items 2, 4, 7, and 8). The combined sample from Spain (Madrid and Tenerife) showed a much higher KR-20 coefficient. Three items were dropped (items 5, 8, and 9). Only one item was dropped common to both samples. The KR-20 coefficient for the scale in the MA/TE sample dropping the same items as the CH sample was 0.5663. The scale reduced according to the CH specification was used.

Estimation of the Model

In the first equation (i), Children's Knowledge about Medicines (CKNOW) was regressed on the predetermined variables of the system (see Table 7.4). The results of the estimations for the two equations in the CH and MA/TE samples are shown in turn.

Equation i – Chapel Hill

Three coefficients were statistically significant: CHLCINT, AGE10, and PCEDUC. The more internal a child's health locus of control, the more knowledgeable he or she was about medicines. A one unit increase in CHLCINT led on average to a 0.44 unit increase in the CKNOW index, which was considerable considering the range of the CKNOW variable (Table 7.1). The ten-year-old children were more knowledgeable. Being ten years old led to a score that was 0.89 higher than for seven-year-old children, on average. Or, the ten-year-olds tended to answer right on roughly one question more than the seven-year-olds. Last, but not least, the

TABLE 7.3. Reliability Tests of Children's Perceived Benefit of Medicines (KMEDBEN) and Children's Internal Health of Locus of Control (CHLCINT)

Scale/Dimension (Reliability test)	Site*	Items dropped	Alpha**
KMEDBEN	CH	items, n, s	0.7905
	Ma/Te	no item	0.8072
KMEDBEN-PHYSICAL***	CH	no tiem	0.6889
	Ma/Te	item s	0.6289
KMEDBEN-MENTAL***	CH	no item	0.7923
	Ma/Te	no item	0.7951
CHLCINT	CH	items 2, 4, 7, 8	0.5644**
	Ma/Te	items 5, 8, 9	0.7100**

* CH: Chapel Hill; Ma/Te: Madrid and Tenerife.
** Kuder-Richardson 20 (KR-20) is reported for CHLCINT.
*** KMEDBEN-PHYSICAL = Physical dimension of the KMEDBEN scale.
    KMEDBEN-MENTAL = Mental dimension of the KMEDBEN scale.

TABLE 7.4. Results of Ordinary-Least-Squares Estimation of Equation i (Children's Knowledge about Medicines as a Dependent Variable)

| | Site | | | | |
| | CH | | Ma/Te | | |
Variable*	Coefficient	Prob >T	Coefficient	Prob >T
Intercept	0.178	0.3346	1.102	0.0006
CHLCINT	0.438	0.0014	0.141	0.0356
KADVERT	0.022	0.1840	N/A	N/A
AGE10	0.888	0.0021	1.195	0.0001
PCEDUC	0.381	0.0036	0.082	0.0401
NKIDS	−0.064	0.3052	−0.163	0.0801
PARMED	−0.050	0.3585	−0.234	0.1700
F-value	7.061		10.871	
(p-value)	(0.0001)		(0.0001)	
R^2	0.3107		0.2548	
Adjusted R^2	0.2667		0.2313	

* CHLCINT: Children's Internal Health Locus of Control.
KADVERT: Children's Recognition of Over-the-Counter Medicine Advertising.
AGE 10: 1 for 10-year-old children, 0 for 7-year-old children.
PCEDUC: Primary Caregiver's educational level.
NKIDS: Number of children under 14 living in the same household as the target child.
PARMED: 1 if 1 or more parents are health professionals, 0 otherwise.

145

degree of PC's education contributed to the child's knowledge. When PC's education increased by one level, the children's score on the CKNOW index increased on average by 0.38.

Equation i explained a significant amount of variation in the data compared to an intercept-only equation. The coefficient of determination of the equation explained 31 percent of the variation in the data.

Equation i – Madrid and Tenerife

The same variables were statistically significant for the sample from MA/TE as observed for the CH sample. The magnitude of the unstandardized coefficients were similar for AGE10, whereas the coefficients for PC's educational level (PCEDUC) and CHLCINT were lower for this sample. One has to bear in mind that the PCEDUC cannot be measured in exactly the same scale for two different educational systems (USA and Spain). CHLCINT was measured the same, but the items retained were items that favored the CH sample's reliability.

Table 7.5 shows the results of the test of equation ii.

Equation ii – Chapel Hill

The predicted values of CKNOW (CKNOWHAT) had a significant negative relationship with KMEDBEN in the estimation. This was consistent with the hypothesized model. A one-unit increase in the predicted value for CKNOW led to an estimated 4.01 unit decrease in the Perceived Benefit of Medicines (KMEDBEN). This is a considerable effect when the range of the additive scale (16-55) is considered. Other variables in the equation did not show a statistically significant relationship with KMEDBEN.

The goodness-of-fit for equation ii, as measured by R2 and adjusted R2, was not as high as for equation i (0.1225 and 0.0763, respectively).

Equation ii – Madrid and Tenerife

The model was not significantly different from the intercept-only model (α=0.05) according to the F-test. The predicted values of

TABLE 7.5. Results of Ordinary-Least-Squares and Two-Stage-Least-Squares Estimations of Equation ii (Children's Perceived Benefit of Medicines as a Dependent Variable)

	Site			
	CH		Ma/Te	
Variable*	Coefficient	Prob > T	Coefficient	Prob >T
Intercept	48.72	0.0001	42.62	0.0001
CHLCINT	0.365	0.2949	0.249	0.3182
KADVERT	0.207	0.0756	-	
CKNOWHAT	-4.010	0.0163	-3.270	0.0959
AGE10	2.126	0.1361	1.433	0.2984
PARMED	-1.331	0.2447	-2.259	0.0807
F-value	2.652		1.851	
(p-value)	(0.0274)		(0.1216)	
R^2	0.1225		0.0442	
Adjusted R^2	0.0763		0.0203	

* CHLCINT: Children's Internal Health Locus of Control.
KADVERT: Children's Recognition of Over-the-Counter Medicine Advertising.
CKNOWHAT: Predicted values of Children's Knowledge about Medicines from eq. i.
AGE10: 1 for 10-year-old children, 0 for 7-year-old children.
PARMED: 1 if 1 or more parents are health professionals, 0 otherwise.

CKNOW (CKNOWHAT) did not have a significant relationship with KMEDBEN, contrary to the Chapel Hill findings. The effect of CKNOW observed on the outcome variable was similar in magnitude and direction and was borderline significant ($\alpha=0.05$). Other variables were not significant as was the case in the Chapel Hill sample, but the coefficient for the number of children (NKIDS) had the right direction and verged on being significant. The goodness-of-fit is also much lower as would be expected.

CONCLUSIONS

Knowledge about medicines was explained to a great extent by the model, but not the Perceived Benefit of Medicines. Similar results were seen for the Chapel Hill sample and the combined Spanish sample in explaining Children's Knowledge about Medicines, but differences were found between the two samples in explaining Perceived Benefit of Medicines. These results thus cast doubts on the "universality" of models that explain beliefs and behavior. Although the second equation was not identical for both samples, when the CH sample was tested without the advertising variable, the equation remained significant. Therefore the equation differences did not account for the disparate findings.

The observed discrepancy may have more than one explanation. Although one assumes that health beliefs spring out of similar precursors, there are some limitations to this study that may help explain the results. No inter-interviewer reliability measures were used to confirm or refute bias in either the qualitative or the quantitative methods. Language is a very important issue here. The scales and indices were originally in English. The items were generated in English and tested for data reduction in English-speaking populations. These were then translated into Spanish by the researchers at the Madrid and Tenerife sites in cooperation. They were not translated back to English by an independent translator to test for changes in meaning.

Aside from the language issue–which certainly is cultural–there is the issue of cultural understanding of the items. The cultural meanings of the questions and statements in the scales may have been considerably different. There may even have been cultural prejudices against certain items in one sample and not other and vice versa. For example, one can speculate that the item in the CHLC scale asking whether the teacher should tell the child how to avoid accidents is not viewed by an American child as consistent with the rest of the items. An example of a culturally irrelevant item could probably be found for the Spanish children as well. These problems are illustrated by the variable analysis (factor analysis and reliability testing). Children's Perceived Benefit of Medicines showed a uniform factor pattern and similar reliability across settings. Children's Health Locus of Control defied earlier findings (O'Brien, Bush, and Parcel 1989) regarding its factor structure in both samples and the reliability testing revealed large differences between sites.

One other reason for dissimilar results could be that models do not transfer easily between cultures due to the embedded and relational quality of social action. This means that models are simplified structures describing beliefs, attitudes, and behaviors, but do not take into account the complexity of interactions within each cultural setting. Models improve as more knowledge is gained by research—using both qualitative and quantitative methods—making them more complex and nearer to describing the complex interactions between the individual and the environment.

Contrary to the qualitative results in the Spanish samples, age was found important in determining knowledge about medicines. Discrepancies like these can inform further investigation into the subject. Perhaps, the knowledge measured here is qualitatively different from that provided by the informant in the ethnographic interview. The CKNOW index was constructed to test how much of an adult understanding the child has gained. Spanish children may not be aware of what they are "supposed" to know about medicines, and therefore the information in the ethnographic interview is not elicited in the same way as the Chapel Hill children. However, the negative relationship found between children's knowledge of medicines and children's perceived benefit of medicines has been shown consistently in four different populations, two in Spain and two in very different populations in the United States (Bush and Almarsdottir 1993; Moore, Bush, and Iannotti 1991). It would be interesting to learn if this relationship exists in children in other locations, and whether this "cynicism" leads to improved medicine use.

Advertising of medicines may be an important factor in enhancing children's perceptions that medicines are beneficial, but not in increasing actual knowledge about them. Knowledge comes from other sources such as value systems and parental background. The question is: Should advertising of medicines be banned? Results from earlier studies on the issue conflict (for a review see Almarsdottir and Bush 1992), but these studies have not tested the influence of beliefs on the benefits of legal medicines. Whether the resulting use of medicines is "rational" or not cannot be determined by the results of this study, but it is very probable that drug advertising induces "irrational" beliefs about medicines without increasing factual knowledge or understanding of the benefits and limitations of legal medicines.

Age is important in determining knowledge. However, it does not seem to have a direct effect on Perceived Benefit of Medicines. It is most certainly possible to educate about children about medicines as early as the second grade. Children think about medicines and have already discovered the Western paradigm of the role of medicines in the repair of the body's malfunctions. They are ready to hear messages about what medicines may not be able to do yet (i.e., cure some diseases, prevent others) and that medicines are potentially harmful. The Chapel Hill children in this study seemed to make a great distinction between legal and illegal drugs, which may be good in some ways, but children should be warned that legal drugs also may be dangerous and should not be taken without restraints.

This study points to the importance of carrying out a careful qualitative analysis of the understanding of the meaning of medicines in the populations studied. This serves to strengthen the model building effort, as well as to point to ways of improvement in cross-cultural studies of children's perceptions of health, illness, and medicines.

NOTES

1. The COMAC Childhood and Medicines Project was funded through a European Economic Community (EEC) *Comité d'Action Concerté* (COMAC) con-

tract, COMAC/HSR MR4*-CT90-0319, awarded to The Institute on Child Health, Athens, Greece, with Deanna J. Trakas as the Project Leader. The official title of the Contract was "Medicine Use, Behaviour and Children's Perceptions of Medicines and Health Care." Additional funding for the study in Chapel Hill was provided by The United States Pharmacopeial Convention, Inc., and The American-Scandinavian Foundation, Inc.

2. Dichotomous variables (AGE10 and PARMED) are not included in Table 1.

REFERENCES

Almarsdottir, A. B. and Bush, P. J. 1992. "The influence of drug advertising on children's drug use attitudes and behaviors." *Journal of Drug Issues* 22(2): 361-376.

Almarsdottir, A. B. and Bush, P. J. 1995. "Children's experience with illness in Chapel Hill, North Carolina, USA." *Childhood and Medicine Use in Cross-Cultural Perspective: A European Concerted Action*, edited by D. J. Trakas and E. Sanz. Luxembourg: Office for Official Publications of the European Community, (EURO Report), pgs. 269-292.

Aramburuzabala, P., Garcia, M., Polaino-Lorente, A., and Sanz, E. 1995. "Medicine Use, Behaviour, and Children's Perceptions of Medicines and Health Care in Madrid and Tenerife (Spain)." *Childhood and Medicine Use in Cross-Cultural Perspective: A European Concerted Action*, edited by D. J. Trakas and E. Sanz. Luxembourg: Office for Official Publications of the European Community, (EURO Report), pgs. 245-268.

Bandura, A. 1986. *Social Foundations of Thought and Action: A Social Cognitive Theory.* Englewood Cliffs, NJ: Prentice-Hall.

Bauman, L. J. and Adair, E. G. 1992. "The use of ethnographic interviewing to inform questionnaire construction." *Health Education Quarterly* 19(1): 9-24.

Bergman, U. 1979. "International Comparisons of Drug Utilization: Use of Anti-diabetic Drugs in Seven European Countries." *Studies in Drug Utilization—Methods and Applications* edited by U. Bergman, A. Grimsson, A. H. W. Wahba and B. Westerholm. Copenhagen: World Health Organization Regional Office for Europe, pgs. 147-162.

Bush, P. J. and Almarsdottir, A. B. 1993. "Medicines in the home: Differences between two U.S. communities." Presented symposium: Children's Perceptions About Illness and Medicines. Athens, Greece. (December).

Bush, P. J. and Iannotti, R. J. 1990. "A children's health belief model." *Medical Care* 28: 69-86.

Bush, P. J., Iannotti, R. J., and Davidson, F. R. 1985. "A Longitudinal Study of Children and Medicines." *Topics in Pharmaceutical Sciences*, edited by D. D. Breimer and P. Speiser. Elsevier, pgs. 391-403.

Bush, P. J., Parcel, G. S., and Davidson, F. R. 1982. "Reliability of a shortened children's health locus of control scale." ERIC #ED 223354.

Griffiths, K., McDevitt, D. G., Andrew, M., Baksaas, I., Helgeland, A., Jervell, J., Lunde, P. K., Oydvin, K., Agenas, I., and Bergman, U. 1986. "Therapeutic traditions in Northern Ireland, Norway and Sweden: II. Hypertension." *European Journal of Clinical Pharmacology* 30: 513-519.

Inhelder, B. and Piaget, J. 1958. *The Growth of Logical Thinking from Childhood to Adolescence.* New York, NY: Basic Books.

King, D. J. and Griffiths, K. 1984. "Patterns in drug utilization–national and international aspects: Psychoactive drugs 1966-80." *Acta Medica Scand [Suppl]* 683: 71-77.

Moore, B. G., Geddes, G. L., and Patterson, A. W. 1981. "Prescribed doses of benzodiazepines." Unit for Research into Drug Usage, Heriot-Watt University, Edinburgh. Poster presentation at WHO Drug Utilization Research Group Meeting, Korcula, Yugoslavia, April 28-30.

Moore, T. S., Bush, P. J., and Iannotti, R. J. 1991. "Families and medicines: A survey of household medicine cabinets." Presented 8th National Conference of the National Council on Patient Information and Education. Washington, DC. (April).

O'Brien, R. W., Bush, P. J., and Parcel, G. S. 1989. "Stability in a measure of children's health locus of control." *Journal of School Health* 59(4): 161-164.

Parcel, G. S. and Meyer, M. P. 1978. "Development of an instrument to measure children's health locus of control." *Health Education Monographs* 6(2): 149-159.

Payer, L. 1988. *Medicine and Culture: Varieties of Treatment in the United States, England, West Germany, and France.* New York: H. Holt.

Prout, A. and James, A. 1990. "A New Paradigm for the Sociology of Childhood? Provenance, Promise and Problems." *Constructing and Reconstructing Childhood. Contemporary Issues in the Sociological Study of Childhood,* edited by A. Prout and A. James. Philadelphia, PA: The Falmer Press, pgs. 7-34.

Sachs, L. 1990. "The symbolic role of drugs in the socialization of illness behaviour among Swedish children." *Pharmaceutisch Weekblad Scientific* edition 12(3): 107-111.

Sanz, E. J., Bergman, U., and Dahlstrom, M. 1989. "Paediatric drug prescribing. A comparison of Tenerife (Canary Islands, Spain) and Sweden." *European Journal of Clinical Pharmacology* 37: 65-68.

Steckler, A., McLeroy, K. R., Goodman, R. M., Bird, S. T., and McCormick, L. 1992. "Toward integrating qualitative and quantitative methods: An introduction." *Health Education Quarterly* 19(1): 1-8.

Svarstad, B. L., Cleary, P. D., Mechanic, D. and Robers, P. A. 1987. "Gender differences in the acquisition of prescribed drugs: An epidemiological study." *Medical Care* 25(11): 1089-1098.

Trakas, D. J. 1990. "Greek children's perception of illness and drugs." *Pharmaceutisch Weekblad Scientific* edition 12(6): 247-251.

Wallston, K. A., Wallston, B. S., and DeVellis, R. 1978. "Development of the Multidimensional Health Locus of Control (MHLC) Scales." *Health Education Monographs* 6(2): 160-170.

Wessling, A., Bergman, U., and Westerholm, B. 1991. "On the differences in psychotropic drug use between the three major urban areas in Sweden." *European Journal of Clinical Pharmacology* 40(5): 495-500.

Zadoroznyj, M. and Svarstad, B. L. 1990. "Gender, employment and medication use." *Social Science and Medicine* 31(9): 971-978.

Zborowski, M. 1952. "Cultural components in response to pain." *Journal of Social Issues* 8: 16-30.

Zola, I. K. 1973. "Pathways to the doctor–From person to patient." *Social Science and Medicine* 7: 677-689.

Chapter 8

Decision Makers in the Treatment of Childhood Illness in Madrid, Tenerife, and Chapel Hill

Pilar Aramburuzabala
Marcelino García
Anna B. Almarsdottir
Emilio J. Sanz
Aquilino Polaino-Lorente

There are many studies relating to medicine use during childhood; however, most of them focus on structural factors such as the influence of drug advertising (Atkin 1978; Rossiter and Robertson 1980), the quantity and type of medicines prescribed to children (Fosarelli, Wilson, and DeAngelis 1987; Naqvi et al. 1979; Sanz, Bergman, and Dahlstrom 1989), the efficacy and innocuousness of medicines in children (Olive 1989; Rubio González et al. 1989), and adverse drug reactions (McKenzie et al. 1976; Mitchell, Lacouture, and Sheehan 1988). Some studies have been devoted to exploring the psychosocial components related to illness and medicine use in childhood. Among these, Bush and Iannotti (1992) pointed out that children have more autonomy in the use of medicines than most adults would expect, and Bush and Iannotti (1988) addressed the maternal influence on children's orientations toward medicines in childhood. Other studies have explored children's concepts about health and illness focusing on the children's capacity to make decisions (Lewis and Lewis 1982; 1989), and social learning and cognitive development (Campbell 1975). However, only a few studies explored conceptual and ideological factors related to medicine use as they are reported by children, placing such factors in the context of health and sickness behaviors within the larger cultural setting (Sachs 1990; Trakas 1990).

Our study is based on the idea that children's behaviors relating to health and medicines are developed early in life, and these behaviors are a reflection of their cultures. Therefore, differences in knowledge, behavior, and attitudes regarding treatment and the use of medicines during childhood illness should be expected across cultures.

This chapter focuses on the role of children and their caregivers regarding the use of medicines, home remedies, and medical services for the treatment of children's illnesses. Data gathered at the study sites of Madrid (Spain), Tenerife (Canary Islands, Spain), and Chapel Hill (North Carolina, USA) were used to draw out similarities and differences taking into account cultural factors.[1]

Some of the questions that were addressed are: Who decides when the child is sick? What type of therapy should be used? When is medication given? Who prescribes the medicines? The decision process is described from both the children and their parents' perspectives. Information about similarities and differences across cultures regarding the decision-making process in treatment and the roles played by the decision partners should help develop health education programs that take into account sociocultural factors.

METHODOLOGY

Methods of data collection in the three study sites have already been described in an earlier chapter (see Chapter 2, this volume). The following adds information about the samples studied:

Sample size:

- Madrid: 100 children (62 boys and 38 girls) from second and fifth grades and their primary caregivers.
- Tenerife: 115 children (63 girls and 52 boys) from second and fifth grades, and 88 primary caregivers.
- Chapel Hill: 103 children (51 boys and 52 girls) seven and ten years old, and 102 primary caregivers. Only 57 children (29 boys and 28 girls) participated in the drawing interview).

Number of primary caregivers who worked outside the home:

- Madrid: 66 (66.0 percent)
- Tenerife: 54 (61.3 percent)
- Chapel Hill: 88 (86.3 percent)

This chapter presents data gathered via drawing–ethnographic interviews with the children, fever questionnaires for children and parents, an autonomy index for children, and a questionnaire of health and medicine use for parents (not used in Chapel Hill). Missing data have been omitted for each question and each site; therefore, frequencies and percentages are based on available data.

Two approaches were used for the analysis of the data: (1) "triangulation" to compare information gained from a variety of research instruments, and from parents and children as participants; and (2) "cross-cultural comparison" using both qualitative and quantitative data from the three sites. These two approaches required the use of observational and basic statistical techniques (frequencies and percentages) for the analysis of the data.

RESULTS

In relation to the question, "Who decided that the child was sick?" the children in both Madrid and Chapel Hill identified three main figures: the mother, the doctor, and the child her/himself. (Data from Tenerife were not available.) Even though children in both Madrid and Chapel Hill considered the mother as the one who decides in most cases that the child is sick, this seems to be more obvious in the Madrid sample (45 percent) than in the Chapel Hill sample (33 percent). One child said, "My mother knows when I feel bad and she tells me if I have fever or not." Another child said, "My mother knew it first because she saw me coughing a lot." The doctor also plays an important role in this decision in both samples; however, this is more evident in the Chapel Hill sample. The percentage of children who identified themselves as the ones who recognize the illness state was larger in the Chapel Hill sample (25 percent) than in the Madrid sample (12 percent). In Madrid, sometimes the mother confirmed the child's own diagnosis as shown in the following ex-

TABLE 8.1. Person First Noticing Child Had Fever According to the Children

	Location*		
Person	Ma	Te	CH
Mother	61%	65%	56%
Father/both parents	18%	3%	8%
Other relative/various people	12%	6%	7%
Child	4%	11%	10%
Other	3%	11%	19%
Don't know	2%	4%	0%

* Ma: Madrid; Te: Tenerife; CH: Chapel Hill.

ample: "I told my mother that I was feeling sick, and she told me that I had a cold because she saw me coughing a lot."

The data from the fever instrument showed that in the three samples the mother was viewed by most children as the one who told them that they had a fever (Table 8.1). The father appeared to be more involved in the Madrid group than in the other two sites, and more children considered themselves as the ones who identified the fever in Chapel Hill and Tenerife than in Madrid.

As shown in Table 8.2, when a similar question was posed to the caregivers, their responses were consistent with the children's responses. More mothers in Madrid and Tenerife reported that they first noticed that the child had a fever, and more mothers in Chapel Hill than in the other two sites viewed the children as the ones who first noticed the fever.

Many children in the three samples stated that their parents noticed they had a fever by touching their foreheads and finding them warm (Madrid, 37 percent; Tenerife, 33 percent; Chapel Hill, 12 percent). Most parents and other caregivers agreed with the children in the way they noticed the child's fever (Madrid, 25 percent; Tenerife, 22 percent; Chapel Hill, 39 percent). Also, some parents reported that the child tells them that she or he has fever. The percentage was relatively high in the Chapel Hill sample (Madrid, 12 percent; Tenerife, 14 percent; Chapel Hill, 21 percent).

TABLE 8.2. Person First Noticing Child Had Fever According to the Caregivers

	Location*		
Person	Ma	Te	CH
Mother	72%	63%	55%
Child	11%	13%	23%
Father/grandparent	9%	15%	9%
Other	4%	2%	10%
Don't know	4%	7%	3%

* Ma: Madrid; Te: Tenerife; CH: Chapel Hill.

The majority of the children in the three sites recalled that the last time they had a fever, their mother measured their temperature with a thermometer (Madrid, 73 percent; Tenerife, 70 percent; Chapel Hill, 66 percent). Participation of the fathers was low (Madrid, 7 percent; Tenerife, 11 percent; Chapel Hill, 5 percent).

When the Madrid children talked about "Who helped them when they were sick?" 43 percent of them mentioned their mother together with the doctor, 21 percent reported both parents and the doctor, 17 percent only the mother, and 11 percent both parents. The children interviewed in Chapel Hill reported most frequently the mother (47 percent), followed by both parents (25 percent), but just a few of them (6 percent) mentioned the doctor or nurse as the one who helped them during the recorded illness episode. No data from Tenerife were available.

When questioned about who cared for the child when he last had a fever, most caregivers in the three samples named the mother (Madrid, 61 percent; Tenerife, 31 percent; Chapel Hill, 60 percent). The father seemed to be less involved in Madrid (16 percent) and in Tenerife (16 percent) than in Chapel Hill (33 percent). The main caregivers in Spain got help from relatives and other people such as friends and neighbors (Madrid, 19 percent; Tenerife, 43 percent), which did not seem to be the case in the Chapel Hill sample (6 percent).

Most interviewed parents in Madrid and Tenerife mentioned the mother as the main caretaker when the child is sick, followed by both parents (Table 8.3). In Madrid the father seemed to play a more important role as main health care provider than in Tenerife.

"The General Questionnaire on Health and Medicines for Parents" also revealed the importance of the role played by the mother in Madrid (43 percent) and Tenerife (37 percent) regarding the persons who take care of the child when she or he is sick, but it shows that mothers get help from the fathers (Madrid, 24 percent; Tenerife, 17 percent) and grandparents, other relatives, and other people (Madrid, 23 percent; Tenerife, 45 percent) in order to take care of a sick child when sick. No data from Chapel Hill were available.

Soon after the illness episode is identified, there are some decisions to be made. Should the child go to bed? Should the child stay home and not go to school? Should a doctor be called or visited? Will medicines and/or home remedies be used?

Eighty-five percent of the children from Tenerife stated that they stayed in bed the last time they had a fever. The percentage was lower in Madrid (62 percent) and Chapel Hill (55 percent). In the three samples it was clear that, according to children, this decision was mostly made by mothers (Madrid, 58 percent; Tenerife, 54 percent; Chapel Hill, 61 percent). In some cases, both parents (Madrid, 12 percent; Tenerife, 8 percent; Chapel Hill, 7 percent), or the father (Madrid, 7 percent; Tenerife, 11 percent; Chapel Hill, 2 percent) decided that the child should stay in bed. A significant percentage of children in the three sites considered themselves as the

TABLE 8.3. Main Health Care Provider According to the Caregivers

Person	Location*	
	Ma	Te
Mother	74%	67%
Father/both parents	23%	15%
Various people	1%	13%
Other	2%	5%

* Ma: Madrid; Te: Tenerife; No data from Chapel Hill available.

ones who made the decision to stay in bed; however, this percentage was higher in the Chapel Hill sample (Madrid, 12 percent; Tenerife, 11 percent; Chapel Hill, 19 percent).

Resting appeared to be the most frequent form of nonpharmacological therapy in the three samples according to the children's interviews (Madrid, 39 percent; Tenerife, 51 percent; Chapel Hill, 41 percent). Special diet as well as drinks were more popular among Madrid (42 percent) and Chapel Hill (28 percent) samples than the Tenerife sample (11 percent). The percentage of children who reported beverages as a therapeutic method was higher in Madrid (25 percent) than in Tenerife (3 percent) and Chapel Hill (16 percent). Honey for colds, water with lemon, and chamomile for upset stomach were among the most common home remedies used by Madrid families, as reported by children. Only 1 percent of the Madrid and 3 percent of the Chapel Hill children stated that home remedies were not used, while 22 percent of the children in Tenerife mentioned that this type of therapy was not used during the described illness episode.

According to the reports of caregivers in the three sites, the mother (Madrid, 50 percent; Tenerife, 29 percent; Chapel Hill, 59 percent), followed by both parents (Madrid, 23 percent; Tenerife, 27 percent; Chapel Hill, 18 percent), decided in most cases that the child with fever should stay home. More doctors made such decisions in Tenerife than in the other two sites (Madrid, 4 percent; Tenerife, 27 percent; Chapel Hill, 3 percent).

According to the children who were interviewed in the Madrid study, doctors were not consulted in 21 cases (21.0 percent). They explained that the mothers' knowledge and experience were the reasons for not seeking professional help, as seen in the following response: "My mother, as she knows what, she gave me aspirins."

When doctors were not consulted but children took medicines, mothers made the decision in all cases about what medicines to give them. Data from Tenerife and Chapel Hill were not available. However, in the general questionnaire for parents, most caregivers in Madrid (55 percent) and Tenerife (56 percent) agreed with the children's opinions from the Madrid sample; when the child is sick he or she usually is taken to the doctor. And when they are not taken, it is because the parents believe they know what medicines the children can take and what home remedies to use. Data from Chapel Hill were not available.

The majority of the children in the three sites took medicines during their last fever episode (Madrid, 78 percent; Tenerife, 89 percent; Chapel Hill, 85 percent). There was a difference of 11.0 percent between the highest (Tenerife) and the lowest percentage (Madrid).

Data obtained from the questionnaires about the child's last fever episode revealed that, according to the children in Madrid and Tenerife, the mother was the one who prescribed the medicines (Table 8.4). In most cases, doctors are perceived by children as the second major source of prescription. However, as shown in Table 8.5, according to the caregivers in both sites, the main prescribing source was the doctor, followed by the mother.

Both children and caregivers were questioned about "Who gave the medicines to the children the last time they had a fever?" In the children's questionnaires, the highest percentages identified the mothers in all three sites; however, this was significantly lower in Chapel Hill than in Madrid and Tenerife. On the other hand, more children in the Chapel Hill sample identified both parents and various persons as the ones who gave them the medicines. A very small percentage of children in the three samples recognized that they took the medicines by themselves.

Caregivers agreed with children in that the mothers are the ones in charge of giving the medication to the child (Tables 8.6 and 8.7); however, the percentages were higher than the ones in the children's responses. It was also interesting that for both the caregivers' and children's responses, in Chapel Hill the percentage naming mothers as in charge was lower, and the percentage naming both parents was higher, than in the Madrid and Tenerife samples.

The question about who gave the medicine to the child was posed in the same manner to both the children and the caregivers; a very small percentage of children mentioned themselves as the ones who took the medicine, and no caregivers identified the children as autonomous in this question. However, when a more specific question was posed to the parents, a small percentage recognized that children sometimes took the medicine on their own (Madrid, 7 percent; Tenerife, 8 percent; Chapel Hill, 6 percent).

TABLE 8.4. Person Prescribing Medicines for Fever According to the Children

	Location*	
Person	Ma	Te
Mother	42%	50%
Doctor	32%	29%
Father/both parents	12%	8%
Other	11%	8%
Don't know	3%	5%

* Ma: Madrid; Te: Tenerife; No data from Chapel Hill available.

TABLE 8.5. Person Prescribing Medicines for Fever According to the Caregivers

	Location*	
Person	Ma	Te
Doctor	50%	52%
Mother	41%	36%
Father/both parents/relatives	5%	6%
Don't know	4%	6%

*Ma: Madrid; Te: Tenerife; No data from Chapel Hill available.

The majority of the children in the three samples expressed that they never went to buy medicines by themselves (Madrid, 76 percent; Tenerife, 58 percent; Chapel Hill, 94 percent); the percentage was higher in the Chapel Hill sample, while the lowest corresponded to the Tenerife children. At the same time, a higher percentage of children in Chapel Hill stated that they have physical access to the medicines that are kept at home (Madrid, 74 percent; Tenerife, 65 percent; Chapel Hill, 77 percent), and more children in Chapel Hill (18 percent) than in Madrid (10 percent) and Tenerife

TABLE 8.6. Person Giving the Medicine for Fever to the Child According to the Children

	Location*		
Person	Ma	Te	CH
Mother	69%	72%	54%
Both parents	10%	7%	18%
Child/doctor/various people	6%	4%	15%
Father/a relative	12%	10%	11%
Don't know	3%	7%	2%

* Ma: Madrid; Te: Tenerife; CH: Chapel Hill.

(12 percent) indicated that they would take a medicine if they were home alone with a bad headache.

DISCUSSION

There are similarities as well as differences among the three samples (Madrid, Tenerife, and Chapel Hill) regarding the process of making decisions during children's illnesses. In general terms, there are more similarities than differences. However, a close look at the data gathered from both children and caregivers by various instruments shows important differences that require further analysis.

In terms of the similarities, it is clear that, in all three samples and according to both children and parents, the mother has the primary role as a caretaker during treatment. She is the one who makes most decisions regarding treatment, even though children and caregivers' responses to the following two questions show that doctors share the main responsibility with the mothers: "Who helped the child when she or he was sick?" and "Who prescribed the medicines?" Most parents in the three samples did not seem to realize that children perceive themselves as decision makers and active participants in this process. The children's participation is clearly active in certain cases, such as when they tell their mothers that they want to go to bed, or when they take the prescribed medicine on their own,

TABLE 8.7. Person Giving the Medicine for Fever to the Child According to the Caregivers

Person	Location*		
	Ma	Te	CH
Mother	83%	79%	64%
Both parents	7%	5%	22%
Other	6%	9%	14%
Don't know	4%	7%	N/A

* Ma: Madrid; Te: Tenerife; CH: Chapel Hill.

as allowed by the caregiver. In other situations, the children collaborate in the process of making decisions in more subtle ways; for example, by reminding caregivers about the time to take the medicine, or by telling their parents that they feel better and they want to go back to school. There is a specific question to which responses showed similarities across sites, but significant differences between children's and caretaker's responses ("Who gave you the medicine?" and "Who gave the child the medicine?"). The responses show that the percentage of caregivers who identified the mother as the one in charge of giving the medication is higher than the percentage of children who named the mother, even though there is agreement that mothers play the major role. Also in the three samples it was observed that caregivers did not spontaneously mention the children as the ones who took the medicine, while a small percentage of children identified themselves as the ones who took the medicine on their own.

Data from Madrid, Tenerife, and Chapel Hill indicate that fathers have a secondary role in this general picture drawn by children and primary caregivers. There was only one question in which, according to primary caregivers in the three sites, fathers play an important role, but after the mothers: "Who decided that the child should stay home and not go to school?" It would be easy to interpret that one possible reason for the fathers' participation in this decision is that routines and schedules change greatly when a sick child stays home.

As was already stated, children's and caregivers' responses coincide on most questions. However, a significant difference was observed across sites regarding the question "Who prescribed the medicine?" Most children pointed to the mother, followed by the doctor, while caregivers named the doctor, followed by the mother (data from Chapel Hill were not available). Who actually prescribes the medicine is not as important here as who children *perceive* as prescribers; and, in that sense their responses are clear: mothers first.

Most children in the three sites stated that they have physical access to the medicines, that they never went by themselves to buy medicines, and they would do something else instead of taking a medicine in the event they were home alone with a bad headache.

As was expected, there were more similarities between the data of Madrid and Tenerife than between the data of the United States and either of the Spanish sites. Data obtained at the two Spanish sites reflected many similarities, which indicates that cultural factors play a major role in the treatment of childhood illnesses.

Some of the major differences between Chapel Hill and the two Spanish sites are noted here. First, Chapel Hill children are more active partners in the decision-making process regarding treatment, and this fact is recognized by both children and caregivers. Also, more children in the Chapel Hill sample reported that if they were home alone with a bad headache they would take a medicine. However, surprisingly, when it comes to the actual fact of taking the medicine, the percentage of children that identified themselves as the ones who actually took the medicine during the fever episode was similarly low in all three sites, and according to parents, fewer children in Chapel Hill took medicines on their own, in spite of the fact that they have more physical access to medicines kept at home than Spanish children.

In general, Spanish children seem to be less active than Chapel Hill children in the process of making decisions about treatment; however, they have more autonomy than Chapel Hill children with respect to taking the medicines (according to parents), and buying medicines by themselves.

Caution should be taken, and health education programs should address the fact that Chapel Hill children recognize that they have physical access to the medicines, and that a significant percentage in the sample stated that they would take a medicine by themselves if they were home alone with a headache.

The role of the mother is more prominent in the Spanish sample than in the Chapel Hill sample. The traditional role played by Spanish mothers regarding health care is reflected in these data. This role has been kept in spite of the fact that more than half of the interviewed mothers in Madrid and Tenerife were working outside the home.

The greater autonomy of Chapel Hill children could be explained by factors such as: more primary caregivers work outside their homes (which means that when children are ill they have to care for themselves, since parental sick leave does not exist for the great majority of workers and working parents have to use their own sick days—usually two per month—when their child becomes ill); children are more exposed to medicines since medicines can be acquired in places outside drugstores; and there is more drug advertising.

More grandparents and other relatives are viewed as participants in the decision-making process in the Spanish sites than in the Chapel Hill site. Extended families are common in the Spanish culture, and physical closeness allows grandparents and other relatives to be active participants in the treatment of childhood illness. The family support network is usually not present for caregivers from the USA because middle-class people tend to move away from their families for employment.

Similarities among Madrid, Tenerife, and Chapel Hill in the process of making decisions regarding the use of medicines in childhood might be partially explained by the use of a similar Western biomedical model in all three sites. Differences might be explained by cultural factors, since it was observed that responses were more similar between Madrid and Tenerife than between either Spanish site and Chapel Hill.

The question is: What is the basis on which children and caregivers in Madrid, Tenerife, and Chapel Hill make decisions regarding the use of medicines and other types of treatment? In Spain, children's knowledge and attitudes relating to health and sickness and medicine use are developed almost exclusively through personal experience and family influence. There is no health education curriculum for children in the schools, and health education for adults is very limited and does not include instruction about medicine use. This means that there is no education about medicine use in the schools, and that the information that children get from their parents depends on what their parents know. Drug advertising is also very limited. In Chapel Hill children are more exposed to medicines; there is more advertising, and medicines are available in places commonly visited by children, such as supermarkets. Another factor that might help explain differences between countries is the fact that in Chapel Hill schools have health education programs that might make children more aware of their responsibilities in these matters, even though such programs do not include the topic of medicine use.

Therefore, environmental and cultural factors appear to be fundamental in explaining similarities and differences in the use of medicines during childhood and the process of making decisions about it.

IMPLICATIONS FOR HEALTH EDUCATION

In this final section, some suggestions for the development of health education programs based on the results of the study are presented.

Health Education programs should take into consideration that

1. the main figures involved in the process of making decisions regarding medicine use are the mother, the child, and the doctor;
2. the cognitive development of the child at the different stages allows him/her to comprehend and participate in such a process; and
3. environmental and cultural factors appear to play a major role in the process of making decisions about medicine use.

Children's attitudes and beliefs about medicine use are held together by an internal logic created by them. Parents and doctors should be aware that children seven to eleven years old begin to use the logic to solve problems, and to include internal physiological characteristics in their descriptions of illness causation and effects of medications.

Children's decision-making skills regarding medicine use can be developed through the use of strategies that take into account cultural factors. Some of these strategies are (1) role playing (e.g., recreating illness episodes and actions of caregivers such as parents, doctors, nurses) which can include recognition of symptoms that need to be conveyed to adults, steps involved in gaining adult permission to take medications, and noting specific amounts and methods of medication administration; (2) verbal persuasion which should be directed toward increasing parental self-efficacy regarding treatment, not only toward explaining the consequences of performing or not in a particular way. Persuasive efforts should also focus on giving children the opportunity to practice the desired behavior and therefore improving their skills and self-confidence (Nader 1985); (3) increase in doctor's role in promoting modeling behavior (e.g., involving children directly in their therapy, showing how to apply cream in appropriate amount, demonstrating how to measure amount of medication, or how to read a thermometer) (Nader 1985).

Children who are able to communicate with their health care providers will grow into adults who can do the same (Igoe 1987). Asking children to engage in the decision-making process related to their own care is evidence that caregivers–including doctors–believe that children are capable of mastering a situation. They have the opportunity to help children improve their self-image and to feel better about themselves (Lewis and Lewis 1990). As a result of this type of communication, children will be empowered to take part in their health maintenance and care into adulthood. Doctors and primary caregivers must make sure that children understand what is said to them–and for this reason, they must listen to the children.

NOTE

1. The COMAC Childhood and Medicines Project was funded through a European Economic Community (EEC) *Comité d'Action Concerté* (COMAC) contract, COMAC/HSR MR4*-CT90-0319, awarded to The Institute on Child Health, Athens, Greece, with Deanna J. Trakas as the Project Leader. The official title of the Contract was "Medicine Use, Behaviour and Children's Perceptions of Medicines and Health Care." Additional support was received for the study in Spain from The General Directorate for Scientific and Technical Research, The Ministry of Education and Science, and in the United States from The United States Pharmacopeial Convention, Inc., and The American-Scandinavian Foundation, Inc.

REFERENCES

Atkin, C. K. 1978. "Effects of drug commercials on young viewers." *Journal of Communication* 28: 71-79.

Bush, P. J. and Iannotti, R. J. 1988. "Origins and stability of children's health beliefs relative to medicine use." *Social Science and Medicine* 27: 345-352.

Bush, P. J. and Iannotti, R. J. 1992. "The socialization of children into medicine use." *Studying Childhood and Medicine Use* edited by D. J. Trakas and E. J. Sanz. Athens: ZHTA Medical Publications, pgs. 105-116.

Campbell, J. D. 1975. "Illness is a point of view: The development of children's concepts of illness." *Child Development* 46: 92-100.

Fosarelli, P., Wilson, M., and DeAngelis, C. 1987. "Prescription medications in infancy and early childhood." *American Journal of Diseases of Children* 141: 772-775.

Igoe, J. B. 1987. "Teaching youngsters to care about health care." *Hygiene* 6: 26-27.

Lewis, C. E. and Lewis, M. A. 1982. "Children's health-related decision making." *Health Education Quarterly* 9: 129-141.

Lewis, C. E. and Lewis, M. A. 1989. "Educational outcomes and illness behaviors of participants in a child-initiated care system: A 12-year follow-up study." *Pediatrics* 84: 845-850.

Lewis, M. A. and Lewis, C. E. 1990. "Consequences of empowering children to care for themselves." *Pediatrician* 17: 63-67.

McKenzie, M. W., Marchall, G. L., Netxloff, M. L., and Cluff, L. E. 1976. "Adverse drug reactions leading to hospitalization in children." *Journal of Pediatrics* 89: 487-490.

Mitchell, A. A., Lacouture, P. G., and Sheehan, J. E. 1988. "Adverse drug reactions in children leading to hospital admission." *Pediatrics* 82: 24-29.

Nader, P. R. 1985. "Improving the practice of pediatric patient education: A synthesis and selective review." *Preventive Medicine* 14: 688-701.

Naqvi, S. H., Dunkle, L. M., Timmerman, K. J., Reichley, R. M., Stanley, D. L., and O'Connor, D. 1979. "Antibiotic usage in a pediatric medical center." *Journal of the American Medicine Association* 242: 1981-1984.

Olive, G. 1989. "Pharmacovigilance chez l'enfant." *Therapie* 44: 141-144.

Rossiter, J. R and Robertson, T. S. 1980. "Children's dispositions toward proprietary drugs and the role of television drug advertising." *Public Opinion Quarterly* 44: 317-329.

Rubio González, A., Suárez Ochoa, J., Azanza Perea, J., and Honorato, Perez J. 1989. "Farmacología pediátrica: ¿Va la terapéutica infantil precedida de una adecuada investigación?" *Anales Espanoles de Pediatría* 30: 359-362.

Sachs, L. 1990. "The symbolic role of drugs in the socialization of illness behaviour among Swedish children." *Pharmaceutisch Weekblad Scientific Edition* 12: 107-111.

Sanz, E. J., Bergman, U., and Dahlstrom, M. 1989. "Paediatric drug prescribing. A comparison of Tenerife (Canary Island, Spain) and Sweden." *European Journal of Clinical Pharmacy* 37: 65-68.

Trakas, D. 1990. "Greek children's perception of illness and drugs." *Pharmaceutisch Weekblad Scientific Edition* 12: 247-251.

Zuckerman, D. M. and Zuckerman, B. S. 1985. "Television's impact on children." *Pediatrics* 75: 233-240.

Chapter 9

Sweet and Cozy or Bitter and Bored? Children's Anamneses of Illness Episodes and Medicines

Deanna J. Trakas
Chrysoula Botsis

Usually when I'm sick I stay in bed. I don't feel very happy, I feel a bit melancholy. And I'm jealous when I see the other children playing outside. I have to turn my face away from the window, so I don't have to see them being happy. (Narrative excerpt from a ten-year-old Greek child, Botsis and Trakas 1993.)

They spoiled me. They told me, "now you must rest in bed and I'll bring you some juice." And I said, "I don't want juice, I don't like it!" and I didn't have to drink it. (Narrative excerpt from a Spanish child, Aramburuzabala 1993.)

Narratives about illness were collected from more than 750 healthy seven- to 11-year-old children from ten countries as part of the COMAC Childhood and Medicines Project.[1] The above excerpts were selected to contrast two themes discussed by many of the children when recalling their experiences with a personal illness episode. One contrast consisted of boredom and social isolation versus nurturance and special privileges. The second involved recollections of medicines as being sweet or bitter, a contrast expressed not only according to their taste per se but to references such as good, necessary, and effective versus bad, dangerous, and not very helpful.

173

Similar contrasts were observed in the narratives of six- to eight-year olds in a 1988 three-country study about children's perceptions of illness and medicines. The children in the Swedish and Netherlands studies described their feelings during illness as "cozy" (e.g., protected, nurtured, pampered) and medicines as "sweet" (Sachs 1992; den Toom and Hardon 1992). In contrast, the children in the Greek study rarely spoke in these terms; rather, they described illness as a socially isolating and boring event, and medicines not particularly sweet but usually bitter (Trakas 1990, 1992).

Sweet-tasting medicines may be likened to candy, and offering candy, a confectionery, or something sweet seems to be an almost universal tactic used by adults to quiet a restless child. If medicines taste sweet, then the child may perceive that (s)he is being offered something to placate the trials and tribulations of illness; a "treat" that conveys security. However, memories of the sweet or bitter flavor of medicines may be related to the perceived seriousness of an illness. Thus, the more severe the illness, the more bitter the medicine (Sachs 1990); indeed, the entire recollection of the episode. Sour, bitter, or strong tasting medicines may be associated with their perceived effectiveness; e.g., only strong (tasting) medicines have therapeutic power. In this sense, the "taste" of medicine assumes a symbolic dimension, becoming a metaphor for the entire process of illness. On the "sweet" side, illness may provide the individual with the opportunity to gather the energy and concern of the immediate social environment, focusing it on him/herself; for children, the family and peer or playgroup would be a natural choice. Illness may serve to negate social expectations (of others) and responsibilities; but, on the "bitter" side, this negation is not always welcomed, leaving a sense of imposed isolation and boredom.

The narratives from the COMAC Childhood and Medicines Project provided material from a larger number of children in more European cultures to explore this framework. With few exceptions, all narratives were gathered using the Drawing-Interview technique described elsewhere in this volume (see Chapter 2). Local research teams provided information about categories developed for inter-study group comparisons, among them the categories of social isolation, special privileges, and the taste of medicines. This chapter has a dual objective: first to detail the way in which content analysis of the narratives was structured, and second to explore how children view medicines and illness using the constructs of sweet and bitter and cozy and bored. Its content is based upon information from two sources: (1) interpretative essays resulting from the local studies, and (2) specific steps in content analysis which were performed using the narratives from children in the Greek study.[2]

SEARCHING FOR THEMES IN NARRATIVES

Content analysis of narratives can be accomplished by (at least) two means. Categories can be constructed a priori to extract information woven into a narrative (etic categories), or they can be created through a process whereby the researcher allows the narrative itself to reveal them (emic categories). In both cases, the issue of researcher bias can be raised, more strongly in the first case (etic) where a grid of categories is imposed upon the data, but also present in the second (emic). This issue had already been raised with respect to some of the findings of the 1988 three-country study of children's perceptions of illness and medicines. The use of the sweet/bitter and cozy/isolated dichotomies prompted questions such as: Were there possible biases of the investigators which led them to arrive at the finding that children in the Swedish study tended to see illness as a cozy event whereby they were able to mobilize the attention the family whereas those in the Greek study did not discuss illness in this light at all? Were the researchers products of the culture they were studying, prone to interpret narratives using their own recollections of being ill during childhood?

The COMAC Childhood and Medicines Project data allowed us to reexamine the notions of sweet/bitter and cozy/bored in a wider study population. What follows is a description of the way that these data were handled at the project level (i.e., with comparative goals, using an agreed upon format by all research teams) and at the local level (i.e., further in-depth analysis of the Greek data). This attempt to excerpt information analyzed at both the project and the local level data is depicted schematically in Figure 9.1.

FIGURE 9.1. Levels of Analyzing Children's Narratives

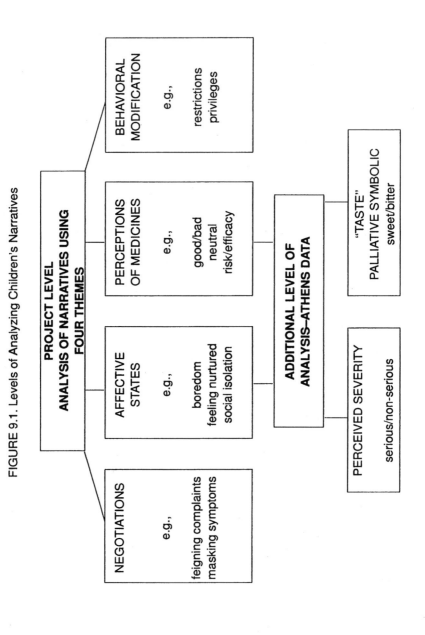

Project Level Methods

The strengths and weaknesses of qualitative, interpretative research methods reviewed elsewhere in this volume (Chapter 2) are relevant to the use of narrative content analysis. Here our discussion of methodological problems is confined to the way in which categories necessary for comparisons at the project level were developed for the children's interviews. Anthropologists and other scientists conducting cross-cultural comparative studies have become increasingly aware of the difficulties involved. Aside from the theoretical questions raised in such studies, at the level of interpretation a self-consciousness (in the positive sense) has developed about the shift from using emic terms of reference (informant centered) to etic ones (researcher centered). The members of the COMAC Project followed a lengthy process before reaching the analytic point at which they could begin attempting to define categories that would lend themselves to comparisons among study groups. In the development of etic categories for comparative purposes, it can be said with a fair degree of certainty, that categories were not imposed upon narrative contents.

In conformity with the COMAC Project protocol, the interviews with the children were designed to follow a format developed to elicit information about their attitudes and perceptions about illness (e.g., causation, bodily sensations, affective states) and means of becoming well again (e.g., behavior, medicines, home remedies). General thematic categories were determined by the interview format which was used in the first level of content analysis. Most interviews were audio-recorded and transcribed; thus, careful analysis of their content could be performed and re-performed if necessary. Some local teams entered verbatim narratives into computers and used keyword and phrase search programs; others carried out their search by the "naked eye," tabulating responses by hand.

In a consensus of the researchers in the concerted action, a second level of content analysis was conducted which refined thematics into categories. For example, the thematic of "affective states" was subdivided into:

1. feelings of social isolation and boredom, as evidenced by statements of "I had to stay at home," "I couldn't have any visitors," "I couldn't play with anyone," "I was bored."

2. feelings of being cozy and nurtured, as evidenced by statements such as "I was spoiled," "I felt pampered," "I got special treats," "My brothers and sisters read to me," "I got to sleep in Mommy's bed."

Additional categories about perceptions and understandings about medicines were added, such as their efficacy, their action within the body, their necessity, and their danger.

Analysis of the Greek Narratives

The narratives from the children in Athens underwent yet another level of analysis according to (1) the severity of the episode discussed; (2) the intensity of social isolation or boredom (vs. "coziness"); (3) concerns about the inability to continue with social responsibilities vs. "feigning" symptoms to avoid them; and (4) the "taste" of medicines. In assigning a "score" for each of the four dimensions, a certain number of "judgement calls"–subjective interpretations–were unavoidable, particularly in classifying the symbolic taste of medicines. However, with careful consideration of narrative contents, scoring for individual dimensions, and the creation of "nonclassifiable" or "intermediate" categories, subjective interpretations were reduced.

Severity of the Episode

A goal of the analyses was to pursue the suggestion that the perceived seriousness of the illness episode, as recounted by the children, might be related to their anamneses about the taste (real or symbolic) of medicines and the event as "cozy" (pleasant) or boring (unpleasant and isolating). The seriousness of the episode narrated by each child was evaluated according to:

1. the number of complaints and symptoms discussed;
2. the relative length of time spent in discussing the episode vis-à-vis the length of the interview;
3. the child's evaluation of seriousness;
4. the researcher's evaluation (related to reporting concrete events; e.g., a childhood illness, a hospitalization, a serious disease such as pneumonia, a surgical intervention).

Intensity of Coziness and Social Isolation

Expressions about social isolation were ranked in intensity from 0 (no mention) to 5 (feeling extremely isolated and worried). Intermediate scores were given for narratives characterized by feelings of being "pampered," being given many treats and special favors, and general feelings of being nurtured.

Social Responsibilities

The same was done for expressions about social responsibilities using scores of 0 to 4. Low scores were assigned to children who saw the episode as an opportunity to avoid responsibilities (e.g., school, an undesirable social event) and the highest for those who expressed worry and frustration about missing such responsibilities. That there are some problems with assigning a "0" to "not mentioned" has been appreciated by the authors, e.g., it is impossible to know if the topic was avoided on purpose (too difficult to remember, or too unhappy) or if the child was bored with the questions of the interviewer.

The Taste of Medicines

References to the "taste" of medicines were examined for both their "taste to the palate," (e.g., sweet, bitter, yummy, bleagh) and their symbolic or metaphorical meanings (e.g., necessary, not effective, bad for the body). The classification of responses about "taste" used the sweet/bitter dichotomy as umbrella categories.

1. Responses classified in the "sweet medicines" category included those which identified them as:

   • sweet or good according to actual taste;
   • good (e.g., for the body), nice, necessary, as indicated by expressions such as, "Good for you," "You need them to get well," and "They fight off the bad things in your body" ["things" described as microbes, bugs, bandits, ugly creatures].

2. Responses classified in the "bitter" category included those identified as:

- bitter (nasty) according actual taste, including verbal expressions interpreted in this way (e.g., "bleagh," "yuck");
- not good, not effective, not necessary, generally disliked and to be avoided, dangerous, as indicated by expression such as, "I don't like medicines; ever since I was a child I don't like them [!]," "You should never take them unless you really need them because they're bad for your body," and, "Sometimes medicines can make you sicker."

Neutral discussions about medicines formed a third category, and narratives which did not include any references to "taste" were assigned to a fourth category.

INTERPRETATION OF ANALYSES

As previously mentioned, the information examined for this chapter was provided from interpretative reports from local research teams as well as that gained from an additional level of analysis carried out with the narratives from the children in Athens. The former allowed for the formation of general impressions about the categories of sweet/bitter and cozy/bored; the latter provided more in-depth information about these themes, adding the dimension of the perceived severity of the episode.

Project Level Results

Research teams in the COMAC Childhood and Medicines Project developed interpretative essays, based on, among other data, the main themes that appeared in the interviews with the children in their local studies. The essays addressed the themes of children's feelings about social isolation and special nurture and privileges, as well as those of masking, feigning, and exaggerating symptoms (as indicators of children's role in avoiding the social isolation or eliciting the special care which they associate with illness). The following section contains information gained from the interpretative essays of the local research teams.

Coziness and Boredom

The topic of social isolation was most often and most dramatically expressed in the interviews from the children in Spain and Greece. Social isolation was also discussed by the children from The Netherlands through their comments related to restrictions (not being able to go out and play, not being allowed to go to school, not being able to do "fun things") even though having visitors was mentioned by half of them. Having visitors, a prominent part of the narratives in the Spanish and Greek studies, was rarely discussed by the children in the Chapel Hill, English, and Finnish studies in which feelings of social isolation were also not often mentioned. Perhaps the feeling of social isolation (or the need to express it) is less related to an actual loss of contact with the "outside world" and more to cultural context.

Some of the mechanisms involved in feelings of social isolation were discussed in the interpretative essay from the Spanish team:

> There are three types of feelings relating to sickness: boredom, sadness, and anxiety. Sickness means a journey from boredom to sadness and back [to health]. There is a reason for that. On the one hand the child has left activities which characterize him/her; his/her life is interrupted and s/he experiences sickness as something annoying because there are restrictions. Sickness is imposing "having to," "not being able to" and restrictive because it keeps the children from the school, his/her natural environment, and it limits social relations. This is the reason why there is also sadness and boredom. (Aramburuzabala 1993)

Children in all local studies also recounted having been granted special privileges while sick. However, the discussion of this topic usually required a probing or direct question from the interviewer, e.g., "Did anything nice happen?" and "Did you get any special privileges?" According to the interpretative essays provided by local researchers, the privileges most often mentioned were being able to watch extra television, being able to sleep on the sofa or in the parent's bed, getting gifts. In the Greek study, relatively more of the older children (compared to the younger ones, expressed disappointment about being absent from school when sick, because they wanted to be with playmates. They said that they worried about lessons missed, not being prepared for examinations, and the accumulation of school work that would be waiting for them upon their return. In other studies, the children discussed becoming sick during school holidays, expressing disappointment; others could remember the exact number of days they had taken school sick leave.

Feigning illness in negotiations to remain home from school was rarely discussed; it was raised primarily by children in only one local study in England, where some reported that initially their symptoms were regarded as feigned or exaggerated by their parents, and they were kept under observation (or "tested") until they were allowed to stay at home (Gelder 1993). In another local study, parents reported leniency in allowing children to stay home from school but stressed that children had to observe strict sickness behavior rules while allowed to be absent (Wirsing 1993). It may be that the issue of children's feigning symptoms in the negotiation of sickness was more of a parental concern than a construction of children.

It was unusual for children to raise the issue of trying to "control themselves," not appear ill, and mask symptoms, often in association with *not* wanting to be kept away from school or other social events. They may realize that they might be sick before informing an adult, trying to ignore their feelings, and their parents noticed signs of illness: "I didn't tell anyone; I held it in. My father asked if there was anything wrong with me" (Aramburuzabala 1993). Nevertheless, children rarely talked about trying to hide or conceal symptoms; to forget or ignore symptoms and "just relax" (e.g., Almarsdottir 1993; Botsis and Trakas 1993). In some narratives, there was, however, a great deal of talk about trying to find ways to function as normally as possible so that school studies would not accumulate. Many children talked about missing school as a negative part of illness; for example, one child said, "I don't like to miss school because the work collects and collects and then when I go back I have more work to do than before." Another said, "The last time I was sick, I was lucky; I didn't have to miss any school days" (Botsis and Trakas 1993).

The comparative information in the Final Scientific Report to COMAC (1993), a compilation of portions of the local study reports (Trakas 1993), indicates that children spoke more often about feelings of boredom and/or dimensions of social isolation than they did about coziness. In spite of references to gaining special privileges such as extra television hours, gifts, care, these are hardly trade-offs for loss of autonomy, lack of contact with friends, and worry associated with missing school assignments. In the case of acute, but nonserious states of disease children's reports about feelings of boredom or pleasant escapes from social responsibilities may be internally produced, but are also socially produced, e.g., disease as a family event, perhaps even strengthening the child's feeling of being cared for and protected by the family, versus one where the child is removed and isolated from social contacts.

Perceptions of Medicines

Children expressed varying degrees of confidence in medicines, as a curative necessity. Those in the English study rarely attributed recovery to medicines, but emphasized the care they received while sick (Gelder 1993). In Chapel Hill and Spain, recovery was usually attributed to medicines, and, in some cases to natural processes. An intermediate position was expressed by the children in the German, Dutch, and Greek studies; for example, "medicines help you get healthy faster" but they are not always necessary (Wirsing 1993) or even sufficient as they must be accompanied by other actions of care givers (Botsis and Trakas 1993). Finally, some brought up the point that some diseases can be cured without medicines; e.g., in the Italian study, intestinal flu, chicken pox, influenza, and headache were examples (Canciani et al. 1992). In a few local studies, children noted that there are some diseases for which no medicines exist and that medicines might not have the desired effect, as well as negative effects.

Negative effects were discussed by the children in all local studies, usually in response to direct questioning. Some comments reflected an ambiguous stance; for example, while medicines might have bad or unwanted effects, " . . . we need to use them anyway, sometimes" (Gerrits, Hardon, and Haaijer-Ruskamp 1993). In some studies, children gave more attention to not taking medicines often or when one is *not* ill (e.g., Vaskilampi et al. 1993; Wirsing 1993).

Some specific comments about effectiveness and risk of medicines from the children in the German study included:

> Medicines "make the disease (fever, rash) go away," "bring the belly in order," "make one healthy." They come in different strengths according to kind (i.e., name) or mode of application: penicillin is considered very strong, as well as injections ("injections go immediately into the blood"). Their color, however, is not indicative of strength, the same applies to their different forms. Some diseases (e.g., cancer), however, seem to be resistant against drugs, when e.g., "the disease does not go away." (Wirsing 1993)

The data from the Spanish study regarding efficacy and risk were summarized in the interpretative essay as follows:

> In general, the children perceived the benefits of taking medicines. Two-thirds of the children used the word "cure" to describe their effects. Others referred to them as "good." Some made comments such as "medicines are good when I have to take them and it is necessary; otherwise they are bad for you," and "they were going to give me the medicines and I knew I would go back to school." Only one child said "they can make you feel worse; I did not take any medicines." Most indicated that they felt better after taking medicine; only two explained that immediately after taking the medicine they did not feel any better, but did later. (Aramburuzabala 1993)

Most children in all local studies were unclear about how medicines actually work within the body, and some used metaphors to explain their action; e.g., medicines as policemen or warriors, helping rid the body of its enemies (Aramburuzabala 1993; Almarsdottir 1993).

It would appear that medicines are not seen as central in the healing process. The report from the English study summarizes this dimension:

> The medicines taken were not, on the whole, associated with getting better and their actions remained a mystery to the

children. I am suggesting that for the majority of the children, medicines are substances which are ritually prescribed by adults as part of the symbolic process of illness; they do not have any inherent meaning, only extrinsic meanings conferred upon them by the otherness and yet sameness in relation to foodstuffs which are ingested when healthy. (Gelder 1993)

Narratives from the Greek Children

In Greece, 80 children participated in the Drawing Interview, an equal number of boys and girls. Twenty-nine children were in the second grade (mostly seven years old) and 51 in the fifth grade (mostly ten years old). According to the perceived severity scale, 49 episodes were classified as relatively mild and 29, relatively serious.

Coziness/Boredom

The concepts of cozy or bored were used as umbrella terms for a range of positive (feeling pampered and nurtured) and negative (feeling isolated, worried about school commitments) recollections of illness. Proportionately, concepts about isolation and failing to uphold social responsibilities were more often a concern of the older children than the younger ones; feeling pampered more often expressed by younger ones. Nearly half of the children discussed feeling isolated and with few exceptions they were fifth graders. About twice as many girls felt isolated compared to boys. Seventeen children discussed receiving extra attention and feeling pampered, and with few exceptions they were second graders. Twenty-eight children did not discuss isolation at all or their narrative content could not be classified for this theme.

Having visitors during illness seemed to be important to Greek children; only nine did not introduce this topic. Nearly half did not recall having visitors and the rest mentioned having from one to six, too "many" visitors. Over half of the children did not address the topic of missing friends or feelings of failure in social life during their illness. When this topic was spontaneously introduced by the children, it was almost always by the older ones. Only two (fifth graders) were pleased to be allowed to stay at home or were ambivalent. The others discussed missing friends (even being jealous about others outside playing) (13), worrying about school (11), and both friends and school (10, all fifth graders).

The general sociocultural profile of the local study groups may help to account for differences in perceptions of illness as cozy or boring. For example, illness may be viewed as an opportunity to mobilize the extra attention of parents in cultures where both parents are usually employed outside the home, and/or where children have had a long experience with preschool day-care and after-school care by others than members of their immediate family. Employed parents may also see this as an opportunity to give extra time to a sick child; time which is usually spent outside of the home. Children raised in an extended family with care provided by several adults other than parents, and who are relatively overprotected even when well, (e.g., Greek children, as documented by Triandis, Vassiliou, and Nassiakou 1968), may not view illness as providing anything "extra," and may tend to be more concerned about social isolation and feeling bored.

Severity of Illness and the Taste of Medicines

References to pharmaceuticals were almost twice as common among the children in the severe illness group. Those with mild episodes were less likely to mention pharmaceuticals, and unlike their counterparts in the severe group, they mentioned alternative therapies and behavioral changes as important in their recovery. In the severe group of episodes, more than half of the children did not discuss the taste of medicines at all. Those who did talked about them as bitter, both bitter and sweet, or as neutral in taste. Only one child in the group referred to the sweet taste alone. Only a fourth of the children in the nonsevere group discussed the taste of medicines; however, very few of them used pharmacological therapies during their mild episodes. Their memory of taste was fairly equally divided between references to sweet, bitter, or both.

References to the "symbolic taste" of medicines (e.g., children's ideas about their efficacy, necessity, general "goodness" or "badness," and dangerousness) did not differ between the severe and nonsevere episode groups. In all cases they were approximately equal. However, the category of "don't like any medicines at all" was found only among the children discussing a severe episode.

That is, a slight tendency was observed for children recalling severe episode to also recall the symbolic taste of medicines as "bitter."

These findings suggest that the more severe the episode the more likely the memory of taste as bitter; sweet medicines are not very often associated with severe illnesses. In less severe episodes, the taste of medicines did not seem to be as important. Reasons for this need to be explored in further research to answer the questions: Do children repress talking about medicines they used when severely ill? Was the experience so "clouded" in their memory that they forget details such as taste?

FINAL THOUGHTS AND POLICY SUGGESTIONS

In this chapter we have tried to demonstrate how one dimension of the children's narratives were analyzed. There is still much more room for analysis of the more than 600 narratives from the COMAC Project, perhaps using the model applied to the Greek data. The general picture derived from the interpretative essays and the specific one from the additional levels of analysis using the Greek data show that children seem to feel the sense of social isolation, boredom, and even worry about missing social responsibilities, more often than they feel a sense of coziness. However, the intensity of these feelings (and the desire or freedom to express them) may be tempered by familial and cultural differences which need further in-depth exploration.

Children's recollections about the taste of medicine may have been influenced by adults; that is, the idea that medicine, by its association with disease is bad-tasting and seen negatively may be perceived by caregivers and passed on to their children (Sachs 1992). Parents are not likely to discuss that medicines are bitter per se, however, they may add sweeteners, or juice, or other rewards in order to coax children to take them. Children are aware of this, either through observation or being told.

Clearly there is a great deal of room for further investigation of the symbolic and metaphoric meanings that children attach to medicine and their place in the illness process. Expressions about medicines, pills, injections or "shots," and "a dose of" appear in references to the trials and tribulations of life; for example, "A little sugar helps the medicine go down," "It was a bitter pill to take," and "I'll give you a dose of something you'll not forget."

The more severely ill children tended to remember both the real and symbolic taste as bitter more often than sweet. This may be associated with anamneses of the entire episode being bitter—or with perceptions that unpleasant-tasting medicines are more potent, just as injections as opposed to oral preparations are often viewed in this way. To ensure that medicines are taken without fuss (and the memory of illness not bitter), parents often try to sweeten medicines by adding sugar to liquid preparations or crush tablets in juice. Such actions may be counter-productive and even dangerous: for example, some pills are designed for absorption in the lower intestine, not the stomach where their action could provoke peptic distress.

Recollections of childhood illness episodes can be carried into adulthood, shaping tenacious patterns of health behavior related to medicine use. The acceptance or rejection of medications as a "natural" and necessary part of the illness process is probably formed in childhood through personal encounters with illness. Perceptions of the self while experiencing illness (e.g., as isolated and weak, or nurtured and claiming attention) are suggested to be important in the development of "illness careers" which follow into adulthood. The processes involved in these phenomena are undoubtedly complex, involving an interaction between individual and sociocultural factors; e.g., severity of the episode, over- or under-medicating, care and concern expressed within the family environment.

Five policy recommendations can be made on the basis of our data:

1. While it is important that the social construction of sickness not be made into a haven of pampering for children, it is important to educate caregivers about the need for measures that will help take their minds away from their somatic and emotional symptoms and to help them gain their "balance" to prepare them for reentry into their normal persona.
2. In cultures where the main concern of children is with losing out on classroom educational activities and falling behind in studies, special attention should be given to both parents and children regarding "homework" that can be completed during

recovery at home. Ill children should not return to school for fear that they will fail a class.

3. With respect to the second policy suggestion, it goes without saying that when both parents are employed, parental leave should be extended for the care of a sick child. Regulations about this are not uniform through the European Union, and in some countries, they are almost lacking. This may result in parents sending their children to school before they are fully recovered from an illness.

4. Pharmaceutical products for children need not contain artificial sweeteners; medicines need not be so sweet that children are tempted to try them when not needed, especially, as it seems that sweet medicines are defined by qualities other than actual taste, at least for the age group in the Project.

5. Labelling of medicines to be used by children should include recommendations about ways to make them more palatable without interfering with their pharmacological properties. Family doctors, pediatricians, and pharmacists should be prepared to explain to parents how "doctoring" medicines (e.g., crushing pills in juice, adding sugar) may interfere with their intended pharmacological action.

* * *

Well, it was bad and good.
At the same time?
Yes.
How so?
There was at least lots of sugar.
What else then?
Well, it tasted bad anyway.

(Excerpt from a Finnish child's narrative;
Vaskilampi et al. 1993)

NOTES

1. Coordination of the Project was funded by the COMAC/HSR Contract MR4*-CT90-0319, organized through the Institute of Child Health, Athens. Addi-

tional funding for the study in Athens was provided by Glaxo Pharmaceutical, Inc.

2. National names are used to designate the local studies, which in reality took place in one or more localities within each of the ten countries in the COMAC Project. This does not reflect an attempt to generalize the findings to the entire country in which each local study took place; it was simply easier to use country names as reference points rather than abbreviations. Therefore, the reader should keep in mind that when the authors state, for example, "the Spanish children," the interpretations are not extended to all Spanish children. The same holds true for other methods of designating local studies; for example, when referring to, e.g., "the children in the Dutch study" the reference is only to those children who participated in the study in Amsterdam and Groningen.

REFERENCES

Almarsdottir, A. B. 1993. *Final Report to COMAC/HSR: Medicine Use, Health Behaviour, and Children's Perceptions of Medicines and Health Services.* (U.S.A.). University of North Carolina at Chapel Hill. (unpub)

Aramburuzabala, P. *Final Report to COMAC/HSR: Medicine Use, Health Behaviour, and Children's Perceptions of Medicines and Health Services.* (Spain). Complutense University, Madrid. (unpub)

Botsis, C., and Trakas, D. J. 1993. *Final Report to COMAC/HSR: Medicine Use, Health Behaviour, and Children's Perceptions of Medicines and Health Services.* (Greece). Child Health Institute, Athens. (unpub)

Canciani, G., Romito, P., Messi, G., and Marcellini, M. 1992. "Children and medicine use. COMAC project. The Italian experience." Presented International Public Health Conference. Paris, France (Sept 10-12).

den Toom, M. and Hardon, A. P. 1992. "Illness attitudes and perceptions of medicines in Dutch children" *Studying Medicine Use in Childhood: A Multidisciplinary Approach*, edited by D. J. Trakas and E. J. Sanz. ZHTA Medical Publications, Athens, pgs. 153-159.

Gelder, L. 1993. The Construction of Illness and the Use of Medicines among English Children (unpublished M.A. Thesis). Keele University, England.

Gerrits, T., Hardon, A. P., and Haaijer-Ruskamp. 1993. *Final Report to COMAC/ HSR: Medicine Use, Health Behaviour, and Children's Perceptions of Medicines and Health Services.* (Netherlands). Universities of Amsterdam and Groningen. (unpub)

Sachs, L. 1990. "The symbolic role of drugs in the socialization of illness behaviour among Swedish children." *Pharmaceutisch Weekblad Scientific Edition* 12: 107-111.

Sachs, E. J. 1992. "Sweet medicine: The symbolic role of medicines in the socialization of illness behaviour (Sweden)." *Studying Childhood and Medicine Use*, edited by D. J. Trakas and E. J. Sanz. Athens: ZHTA Medical Publications, pgs. 143-152.

Trakas, D. J. 1990. "Greek children's perceptions of illness and drugs." *Pharmaceutisch Weeksblad Scientific Edition* 39:147-151.

Trakas, D. J. 1992. "Heavy and light illnesses and medicines: Accounts from Greek children." *Studying Childhood and Medicine Use*, edited by D. J. Trakas and E. J. Sanz. Athens, Greece: ZHTA Medical Publications, pgs. 161-170.

Trakas D. J. 1993. *Final Report to COMAC/HSR: Medicine Use, Health Behaviour, and Children's Perceptions of Medicines and Health Services*. (Greece). Child Health Institute, Athens. (unpub)

Triandis, H. D., Vassiliou, V., and Nassiakou, M. 1968. "Three cross-cultural studies of subjective culture." *Journal of Personality and Social Psychology* (Monograph supplement):8(4).

Vaskilampi, T., Kalpio, A., Ahonen, R., and Hallia, O. 1993. *Final Report to COMAC/HSR: Medicine Use, Health Behaviour, and Children's Perceptions of Medicines and Health Services*. (Finland). University of Kuopio. (unpub)

Wirsing, R. 1993. *Final Report to COMAC/HSR: Medicine Use, Health Behaviour, and Children's Perceptions of Medicines and Health Services*. (Germany). University of Hamburg. (unpub)

Chapter 10

Concepts of Adverse Drug Reactions Among Children in Eight Countries

Marcelino García
Emilio J. Sanz
Pilar Aramburuzabala
Anna B. Almarsdottir

Very early in medicine, Hippocrates pointed out one of the main tenets of health care, "First, do no harm." Since then, the recognition of the harmful effects of medicines has been a constant throughout history and across countries and cultures. In modern days, adverse drug reactions (ADRs) and side effects of medicines which are supposed to preserve and promote health are well recognized and well evaluated.

In all cultures, socialization into the use of medicines, as well as an increase in knowledge and changes in attitudes toward medicines, are part of children's learning processes and cognitive development. A body of doctrine already has arisen on the changes and relationships of the "perceived benefit" of medicines with age and other environmental factors (Bush and Iannotti 1988), but little is known about the development of ideas about the risks and problems of medicines, as well as fears and negative attitudes toward them. In fact, one of the learned concepts that may influence the pharmacological behavior of children is the perception of risk and side effects that can be associated with medicines.

Children constitute a risk group for the inappropriate use of medicines. Within the multiple factors defining their risk are: immaturity of knowledge about drugs (see Chapter 7, this volume); mistaking drugs for candy or food (see Chapter 9, this volume); disagreement between children's perceived autonomy in the use of medicines and the autonomy perceived by their parents (Almarsdottir and Bush 1995; Sanz and Garcia 1993); and the availability and accessibility of drugs stored at home to the children (see Chapter 5, this volume).

It is difficult to determine whether the use of drugs in children is more extensive that it should be. The pharmacoepidemiological studies on the use of drugs in children, albeit rare, show that antibiotics, for example, account for almost one-third of all drugs prescribed to outpatient children in many places (e.g., Sweden, Spain, USA, Panama) (Sanz 1992a; Sanz, Bergman, and Dahlstrom 1989). Nevertheless, the total exposition of drugs in children does not seem to be greater than in other ages. The rate of adverse drug reactions (ADRs) in children is also low, especially in outpatient care, and lower than similar figures for adults (Sanz and Boada 1987; Sanz 1991, 1992b).

ADRs in children are normally mild, self-limiting, preventable, and judged inconsequential by both the parents and the doctor. Most frequently, they are attributed to antibiotics and NSAIDs, which are actually the drugs most habitually stored at home, and are most easily used by parents in the self-medication of children (Boada, Duque, and Sanz 1989; Sanz 1992a).

Children's concepts of diseases and of medicines have been studied previously; most often the studies have dealt with children suffering from chronic diseases such as asthma (Bernard-Bonnin et al. 1991; Donnelly, Donnelly, and Thong 1987; Seto, Wong, and Mitchell 1992; Yoon et al. 1991), diabetes (Follansbee 1989; Hackett et al. 1989), AIDS (Brown, Fritz, and Barone 1989), and other diseases (Cappelli et al. 1989; Chaney and Peterson 1989; Thompson et al. 1989). Most often, children have been considered to be passive recipients of health care, with the phenomenological and qualitative analysis of health traditions and uses in children based on parents' descriptions. Surprisingly enough, the influence of parental concepts and attitudes toward health care on their children is limited and accounts for only part of the development of health concepts (Bush and Iannotti 1990).

Using both qualitative and quantitative instruments developed in an international effort, i.e., within the framework of the "COMAC Childhood and Medicines Project,"[1] preliminary analysis of the beliefs and knowledge held by children on the risk of medicines was undertaken. This chapter is devoted to the description and evaluation of the perceived risk of drugs to children in the context of the "perceived benefit" of medicines and children's cognitive development.

CHILDREN'S PERCEPTIONS OF MEDICINE BENEFIT

The perceived beneficial effects of drugs by the children studied in the nine locations which participated in the COMAC Childhood and Medicines Project were explored through secondary analyses of the final reports of the participating studies: phenomenological analysis of the interviews, and qualitative information elicited during the interviews (see Chapter 2 for a description of these methods). From here forward, references to the final reports of the different locations participating in the study are made with the following abbreviations: D: Hamburg, Germany (Wirsing 1995); E: Madrid and Tenerife, Spain (Aramburuzabala et al. 1995); GR: Athens, Greece (Botsis and Trakas 1995); I: Trieste, Italy (Canciani and Romito 1995); NL: Amsterdam and Groningen, Netherlands (Gerrits, Haaijer-Ruskamp, and Hardon 1995); SF: Jyväskylä, Suomi-Finland (Vaskilampi et al. 1995); UK: Keele, United Kingdom (Gelder and Prout 1995); USA: Chapel Hill, United States of America (Almarsdottir and Bush 1995).

All children were familiar with medicines in the nine locations of the studies and the use of medicines was recognized very frequently by the children in some samples (D, E, NL, USA). In the two Spanish locations, for example, almost 90 percent of the children indicated they were taking some kind of medicine during the episode described in the drawing made by the child and up to 30 percent of the children actually drew some drugs. Conversely, in other locations, the use of drugs was very seldom mentioned spontaneously by the children (SF, UK).

Children recognized medicines as one of the first steps of the healing process, confirming that they see the use of medicines as a "normalizing" factor, that will positively influence the rapidity of the cure. But the children realized that medicines are neither the cause nor the only mechanism to cure illness. They also believed that their own behavior, e.g., eating, drinking, dressing, or "being wild," plays an important role both in the causation and in the prevention and recovery from illness (D, E, NL). For many children, in many instances, healthful behavior appeared to be more important than medication (UK).

Identification and description of drugs was based mainly upon external characteristics and not on "pharmacological" activity. Most children identified medicines by their form (mainly syrup) followed by the word "medicine," the generic name (mainly aspirin), the type of container, the route of administration, etc. When they described medicines, most of the children referred to the flavor, the color, the instructions for use, the form, and the type of container (D, E, GR, NL, SF, UK, USA).

In Madrid and Tenerife, a bag with 12 different containers of common children's medicines was given to the children who were asked to classify the medicines according to their own criteria. There were two different levels of knowledge and recognition: the containers were classified as medicines, (e.g., symptoms, indications, prior use, route of administration), or by their appearance, (e.g., as "colored funny packages") (Table 10.1). There was a statistically significant difference between the two age groups; older children tended to classify medicines according to symptoms, indications, use, etc., whereas the younger children tended to cluster containers on the basis of colors and shapes.

TABLE 10.1. Classification of 12 Medicine Containers by Children in Madrid and Tenerife

Classification Categories	Age	
	7 years (N=92)	10 years (N=93)
	%	%
Recognized as medicines[1]	15.2	33.3
Recognized as objects[2]	79.3	59.1
Others, unknown	5.4	7.5

Chi square 12.148; p = 0.016
[1] Symptoms, indications, previous use, route of administration.
[2] Form, color, size, container.

Together with the idea of medicines as a positive tool to achieve health, the majority of children were convinced that medicines should be taken only when sick (D, SF). Few of the children thought that drugs were always necessary for getting well, while a majority believed that, even though drugs may be helpful for this purpose, they are not always necessary for complete recovery. For instance, drugs may not be necessary for coughs or minor colds (e.g., a running nose), and not even for headaches or brain concussions (D). In the UK sample, for example, most of the children did not know the origin of illness amelioration and rarely attributed it to medicines, emphasizing, instead, the care they received while sick (UK). In contrast, children in Chapel Hill, Madrid, and Tenerife, rarely ascribed their recuperation to natural processes, but more often to medicines (E, USA). When children were asked about how they got cured from a specific illness, most mentioned the pharmacological treatment (e.g., "medicines go to that place and they cure you little by little"), but children also named other types of treatments such as diet, resting, and staying warm.

An intermediate position was seen among the Amsterdam-Groningen, Athens, and Hamburg children (D, NL, GR). As some of the Hamburg children said, "medicines help you get healthy faster," "makes the disease (fever, rash) go away," "brings the belly in order," "makes one healthy," but medicines were not always viewed as necessary. In the Amsterdam-Groningen sample, half of the children answered "sometimes yes, sometimes no" to a question on the perceived effectiveness of medicines (NL). According to the Athens children, medicines are not sufficient; they must be accompanied by other actions of caregivers (GR).

Finally, some children brought up the point that some illnesses can be cured without medicines. Among diseases or conditions in this group, the Trieste children cited intestinal flu, chicken pox, influenza, and headache (I). In a few local studies (D, NL, SF), some children noted that there are some diseases for which no medicine exists, i.e., "some things (illnesses) for which nothing has been found up to now" (NL) or that some diseases (e.g., cancer) seem to be resistant against drugs, when, e.g., "the disease does not go away" (D).

A number of these statements were elicited by use of one of the open-ended, direct questions asked in the children's fever instrument, "What makes the fever disappear?" The responses are shown in Table 10.2.

Three-quarters of all children in Madrid and Tenerife locations did not see the medicines as a preventive tool, but only as a curative one. The answer to a general question, "Do you think that if you received a medicine while healthy, this will keep you from getting ill?" was negative in 75 percent of cases (Table 10.3). When the children were asked to provide a reason for their response, up to one-third of the children mentioned the risk of side effects, without any perceived beneficial effect of medicines in healthy persons (Table 10.3). This selective recognition of the beneficial effects of medicines is of paramount importance in the socialization of children to the use of medicines.

CHILDREN'S PERCEPTIONS OF DRUG RISK

Negative effects were also discussed by the children, usually in response to direct questioning. Most of the Amsterdam-Groningen children in the study (NL) mentioned that they might have bad or unwanted effects, especially when you take too much of medicines, " . . . but we need to use them anyway, sometimes." The children could even distinguish between several ways of producing side effects: "when you take medicines for a (serious) disease that you do not have," "when a child takes medicines belonging to an adult," "when you are allergic to certain substances," "when you take it before having breakfast." One girl "knew" from the television that: "When you eat tablets you get pieces in your stomach, and you can get sick from it." Other children referred to side effects: one added that while a medicine can have side effects, "it will help for what it is needed" (NL).

When speaking of the negative aspects of medicine use, most of the children illustrated this with a concrete example. For example, a boy whose mother had a tumor in her head said that his mother took medicines that had positive and negative effects ("it gets better, but her teeth get rotten") and also referred to side effects of medicines

TABLE 10.2. Children's Beliefs about Fever Treatment

Question: "What makes the fever go away?"

Locaton:*	CH	Jy	Ma	Te
Response:	(%)	(%)	(%)	(%)
Medicines	83	17	68	65
Special food/drink	6	23	3	2
Resting/lying down	4	54	11	11
Others	7	6	18	22
Total	100	100	100	100

* CH: Chapel Hill; Jy: Jyväskylä; Ma: Madrid; Te: Tenerife.

TABLE 10.3. Children's Perceptions of Medicines as Preventive (Madrid and Tenerife)

Question: "Do you think if you took a medicine while healthy, it would keep you from getting ill?"

Response: (N = 212)	(%)	Reason: (N = 192)	(%)
No	75.0	Not useful[1]	32.3
Yes	14.2	Do not prevent and	
Don't know	10.8	may cause side effects	39.1
		Yes, vaccines for example	7.8
		Don't know	20.8
Total	100.0	Total	100.0

[1] e.g., not necessary to take medicines; only needed if you are sick.

in general ("a lot of medicines are not right; something gets better, but at the same moment something else gets worse") (NL).

The children in Jyväskylä said that one should not take medicines too often or when they are not ill; concrete side effects were mentioned by two children (tiredness due to antibiotics, stomach ache) and allergic reactions to penicillin by two (SF). On the other hand, those in Chapel Hill always related medicines to recovery, and none mentioned possible harmful effects (USA).

The children in the Spanish studies (Madrid and Tenerife) spoke about negative effects of medicines and expressed caution about their use, especially when asked about this aspect in a direct question. But some children made spontaneous comments such as "medicines are good when I have to take them and it is necessary; otherwise they are bad for you." Children's comments revealed that they know medicines can have negative effects, a response which might be related to other characteristics that also showed up during the interviews. For example, children perceived themselves as cautious about drug misuse; they follow instructions and, in most cases, they do not take the medicines by themselves (E).

Nevertheless, almost no children described a side effect that occurred to someone else or to them. Children in all the study locations knew about the possibility of drugs producing unwanted and harmful effects but they had not experienced them personally. This is in agreement with the published data on side effects and ADRs in children (Kramer et al. 1985; Sanz and Boada 1987; Sanz 1991). They are infrequent (about 1 percent of all consultations), and mild and self-limiting. Most of them are judged inconsequential by both parents and doctors (Kramer et al. 1985). Thus, the probability of having experienced an ADR is low in samples like ours, which are composed of healthy young children, with a low prevalence of drug use.

More than 50 percent of the children answered "no" to a general question, "Do you think that all medicines are good for health?" (see Table 10.4). When they were asked to explain their response, 40 percent of the children mentioned side effects as the main cause (Table 10.4). Again there were age differences in these beliefs about drugs. Older children were more prone to recognize that not all medicines are good for health because some of them can be dangerous. Thus, the perception of risk appears during cognitive development.

The answers of parents to similar questions in other instruments showed a similar trend in Madrid and Tenerife. About half of the parents mentioned side effects as the reason to be cautious and more than 60 percent expressed the need to be cautious with almost all available drugs.

TABLE 10.4. Children's Perceived Benefit of Medicines (Madrid and Tenerife)

Question: *"Do you think all medicines are good for health?"*

Age:	7 years		10 years	
Response:*	(N)	(%)	(N)	(%)
No	42	45.2	69	62.7
Yes	52	51.0	33	30.0
It depends	3	2.9	3	2.7
Don't know	5	4.9	5	4.5
Total[1]	102	100.0	110	100.0

Question: *"Why?" (do you think all medicines are good for health?)**

Age:	7 years		10 years	
Response:	(N)	(%)	(N)	(%)
No: e.g., some could be dangerous; could cause (ADR); could be "street drug";	27	29.0	50	48.5
Depends what "you have" and for what the medicine is intended.	6	6.5	8	7.8
Yes: e.g., all drugs cure; if the doctor prescribes them; they are good.	43	46.2	28	27.2
Don't know, other	17	18.2	17	16.5
Total[1]	93	100.0	103	100.0

* Chi square 10.528, p = 0.015.
**Chi square 11.337, p = 0.045.
[1] Percents do not always sum to 100.0 due to rounding errors.

The chronic use of a drug is not in the experience of healthy children and they tended to associate it with a serious disease and ADR (Table 10.5). Almost 50 percent mentioned side effects as the main risk of chronic treatment, and only 20 percent were convinced that chronic treatments are useful. The picture is probably quite different among children with chronic illnesses.

The concept of self-medication with OTC drugs was not a childhood idea either, 84 percent of the children indicated they believed that taking a drug without the prescription or recommendation of a physician is risky and should be avoided (Table 10.6).

FACTORS ASSOCIATED WITH CHILDREN'S PERCEPTIONS OF DRUG BENEFITS AND RISKS

The perception of the risk of medicines was associated with other variables such as the "perceived benefit of drugs" (explored using a 12-item questionnaire), and locus of control. The concept of locus of control means that individuals have beliefs along a continuum that varies from a conviction that one can significantly affect (or is responsible for) the state of one's health (internal) to the conviction that one is helpless, that the state of one's health is largely out of the individual's control (external). The health locus of control scale used for the children was the nine-item Children's Health Locus of Control (CHLC) Scale shortened and adapted by Bush, Parcel, and Davidson (1982) from a longer version developed by Parcel and Meyer (1978). The CHLC requires dichotomous (yes/no) responses. The stability of the factor structure of the nine-item version has been shown (O'Brien, Bush, and Parcel 1989). The Multidimensional Health Locus of Control (MHLC) Scale consisting of 18 items measured on a six-point Likert Scale (Wallston, Wallston, and DeVellis 1978) was administered to the children's parents.

The locus of control of children becomes more internal with age, (in the Spanish samples the ten-year-old children had more internal CHLC than the seven-year-old children: t-student = 4.64, $p < 0.0001$) (see Table 10.7). Also, the CHLC of children in Tenerife was correlated with the MHLC of their parents (Pearson r: 0.52, $p < 0.01$), but only in the oldest age group, whereas in younger children the relationship was negligible ($r\ 0.02$, $p > 0.05$).

TABLE 10.5. Children's Perception of the Risk of Medicines (Madrid and Tenerife)

*Question: "Could it be dangerous to take a medicine for a long
period of time?"*

Age:	7 years		10 years	
Response:*	(N)	(%)	(N)	(%)
No	23	22.5	18	16.4
Yes	71	69.6	70	63.6
Don't know	8	7.8	22	20.0
Total[1]	102	100.0	110	100.0

*Question: "Why?" (Could it be dangerous to take a medicine for a long
period of time?)*

Age:	7 years		10 years	
Response:	(N)	(%)	(N)	(%)
Side effect or ADR	41	46.1	39	44.3
No utility	12	13.5	8	9.1
Yes, they are useful	17	19.1	10	21.6
Don't know/Others	19	21.4	22	25.0

* Chi square 6.858, p = 0.032.
[1] Percents do not always sum to 100.0 due to rounding errors.

Children with more internal health locus of control were more
likely to realize that not all medicines are good for health and they
more frequently mentioned side effects as a risk of taking medicines. As the health locus of control was more internal among older
children, there were also important differences in the knowledge
and attitudes toward drugs (beneficial and dangerous effects) between seven-year-old and ten-year-old children (Table 10.7). The

TABLE 10.6. Children's Perception of the Benefits and Risks of Self-Medication (Madrid and Tenerife)

Question: "Could it be dangerous to take a drug without asking a doctor or being prescribed?"

Age:	7 years		10 years	
Response:	(N)	(%)	(N)	(%)
No	15	14.9	9	8.3
Yes	83	82.2	93	85.3
It depends	0	0.0	3	2.8
Don't know	3	3.0	4	3.7
Total[1]	101	100.0	109	100.0

[1] Percents do not always sume to 100.0 due to rounding errors.

differences were not statistically significant, but show a trend which should be further analyzed.

DISCUSSION AND CONCLUSIONS

Children seven and ten years old in this study did not have a very sophisticated knowledge of drugs, but all realized that medicines are important in the process of healing. The children located medicines at the same level as other nonpharmacological treatments and remedies, and perceived medicines as a tool to recuperate quicker and safer, especially if the illness seems to be serious. But healthy children rarely had a concept of self-medication, i.e., taking medicines without professional recommendations, or of taking medicines for prevention or chronic illnesses.

At the same time, almost all of the children recognized that medicines can cause side effects and ADRs even when used properly. This knowledge is "learned" and not normally experienced. This "healthy respect" for medicines did not appear to unduly worry children or prevent them from wanting to use medicines when required, but beneficially appeared to prevent them from taking drugs on their own.

TABLE 10.7. Correlation of Children's Health Locus of Control (CHLC) and Perceived Benefit of Medicines (Madrid and Tenerife)

Age:		7 years	10 years
Children's Health Locus of Control			
mean:		43	5.6
t-test:	4.64		
p-value:	< 0.001		

Question: "Why?" (Could it be dangerous to take a medicine for a long period of time?)

Response:			
No		4.78	6.04
Yes		3.94	5.21
t-test:		2.43	1.90
p-value:		0.017	0.060

Question: "Why?" ("Do you think all medicines are good for health?")

Response:			
Referred to Side Effects		4.77	5.77
Others		4.12	5.32
t-test:		1.61	0.96
p-value:		0.112	0.341

*Higher scores indicate more internal CHLC.

The more internal the locus of control of the parents (the more convinced that one can significantly affect or is responsible for the state of one's health), the more internal the locus of control of their children. But this relationship was only significant in children in the ten-year age group. This relationship is consistent with that previously observed between mothers and children (Bush and Iannotti 1988). Similarly, the negative relationship between children's perceptions of the benefits of medicine and a more internal health locus of control were found in this study and one undertaken earlier in Washington, DC (Bush and Iannotti 1990).

During childhood, education on the use of drugs needs to be strengthened to convey both the beneficial and risky aspects. This is critical because drugs were found to be accessible to children of seven years and ten years in all households of all families in all locations of the study. A proper education on the use of medicines and the restriction of them to their formal indications in the context of the whole family, will help toward building the concept of "rational use of drugs" in children, the future adults.

NOTE

1. The COMAC Childhood and Medicines Project was funded through a European Economic Community (EEC) *Comité d'Action Concerté* (COMAC) contract, COMAC/HSR MR4*-CT90-0319, awarded to The Institute on Child Health, Athens, Greece, with Deanna J. Trakas as the Project Leader. The official title of the Contract was "Medicine Use, Behaviour and Children's Perceptions of Medicines and Health Care."

REFERENCES

Almarsdottir, A. B. and Bush, P. J. 1995. "Children's experience with illness in Chapel Hill, North Carolina, USA." *Childhood and Medicine Use in Cross-Cultural Perspective: A European Concerted Action*, edited by D. J. Trakas and E. Sanz. Luxembourg: Office for Official Publications of the European Community, (EURO Report), pgs. 269-292.

Aramburuzabala, P., Garcia, M., Polaino-Lorente, A., and Sanz, E. 1995. "Medicine Use, Behaviour, and Children's Perceptions of Medicines and Health Care in Madrid and Tenerife (Spain)." *Childhood and Medicine Use in Cross-Cultural Perspective: A European Concerted Action*, edited by D. J. Trakas and E. Sanz. Luxembourg: Office for Official Publications of the European Community, (EURO Report), pgs. 245-268.

Bernard-Bonnin, A. C., Pelletier, H., Allard-Dansereau C., Chabot, G., Robert, M., Masson, P., Maheux, B., and Robitaille, N., 1991. "Parental knowledge about their asthmatic children." *Pediatrie* 46 (5):489-497.

Boada, J., Duque, J., and Sanz, E. 1989. "Parent drug prescription in children." IV World Conference on Clinical Pharmacology & Therapeutics. Mannheim-

Heidelberg July 23-28. *European Journal of Clinical Pharmacology*; 36 (Supp):A155.

Botsis, C. and Trakas, D. J. 1995. "Childhood and medicine use in Athens." *Childhood and Medicine Use in Cross-Cultural Perspective: A European Concerted Action*, edited by D. J. Trakas and E. Sanz. Luxembourg: Office for Official Publications of the European Community, (EURO Report), pgs. 221-224.

Brown, L. K., Fritz, G. K., and Barone, V. J. 1989. "The impact of AIDS education on junior and senior high school students. A pilot study." *Journal of Adolescent Health Care* 10 (5):386-392.

Bush, P. J. and Iannotti, R. J. 1988. "Origins and stability of children's health beliefs relative to medicine use." *Social Science and Medicine* 27:345-352.

Bush, P. J. and Iannotti, R. J. 1990. "A children's health belief model." *Medical Care* 28:69-86.

Bush, P. J., Parcel, G. S., and Davidson, F. R. 1982. "Reliability of a Shortened Children's Health Locus of Control Scale." ERIC No ED 223 354. Boulder Co.

Canciani, G. and Romito, P. 1995. "Children and medicine use: Situation and perspective from the Italian experience in the COMAC Project." *Childhood and Medicine Use in Cross-Cultural Perspective: A European Concerted Action*, edited by D. J. Trakas and E. Sanz. Luxembourg: Office for Official Publications of the European Community, (EURO Report), pgs. 177-190.

Cappelli, M., McGrath, P. J., MacDonald, N. E., Katsanis, J., and Lascelles, M. 1989. "Parental care and overprotection of children with cystic fibrosis." *British Journal of Medical Psychology* 62:281-289.

Chaney, J. M. and Peterson, L. 1989. "Family variables and disease management in juvenile rheumatoid arthritis." *Journal of Pediatric Psychology* 14:389-403.

Donnelly, J. E., Donnelly, W. J., and Thong, Y. H. 1987. "Parental perceptions and attitudes toward asthma and its treatment: A controlled study." *Social Science and Medicine* 24:431-437.

Follansbee, D. S. 1989. "Assuming responsibility for diabetes management: What age? What price?" *Diabetes Education* 15:347-353.

Gelder, L. and Prout, A. 1995. "Medicine use and sickness as cultural performance in childhood. Report of the UK for the COMAC Project." *Childhood and Medicine Use in Cross-Cultural Perspective: A European Concerted Action*, edited by D. J. Trakas and E. Sanz. Luxembourg: Office for Official Publications of the European Community, (EURO Report), pgs. (in press).

Gerrits, T., Haaijer-Ruskamp, F., and Hardon, A. 1995. "The perceptions and attitudes of Dutch children and their mothers about illness and the use of medicines." *Childhood and Medicine Use in Cross-Cultural Perspective: A European Concerted Action*, edited by D. J. Trakas and E. Sanz. Luxembourg: Office for Official Publications of the European Community, (EURO Report), pgs. 123-148.

Hackett, A. F., Court, S., Matthews, J. N., McCowen, C., and Parkin, J. M. 1989. "Do education groups help diabetics and their parents?" *Archives of Disease in Childhood* 64 (7):997-1003.

Kramer, M. S., Hutchinson, T. A., Flegel, K. M., Naimark, L., Contardi, R., and Leduc D, 1985. "Adverse drug reactions in general pediatric outpatients." *Journal of Pediatrics* 106:305-310.

O'Brien, R. W., Bush, P. J., and Parcel, G. S. 1989. "Stability in a measure of children's health locus of control." *Journal of School Health* 59 (4):161-164.

Parcel, G. S. and Meyer, M. P. 1978. "Development of an instrument to measure children's health locus of control." *Health Education Monographs* 6 (2):149-159.

Sanz, E. and Boada, J. 1987. "Adverse drugs reactions in paediatric outpatients." *International Journal of Clinical Pharmacology Research* 7(2):169-172.

Sanz, E., Bergman, U., and Dahlstrom, M. 1989. "Paediatric drug prescribing. A comparison of Tenerife (Canary Islands, Spain) and Sweden." *European Journal of Clinical Pharmacology* 37:65-68.

Sanz, E. 1991. "Methodological approaches to ADR detection in out-patient children." *Bratislavské Lekárske Listy* 92 (12):597-602.

Sanz, E. 1992a. "Drug use in nonhospitalized children." *Pharmaceutisch Weekblad* (Scientific Edition). 14(1):1-8.

Sanz, E. 1992b. "Hazards of Medication in Children." *Studying Childhood and Medicine Use. A Multidisciplinary Approach*, edited by D. J. Trakas and E. Sanz. Athens: ZHTA Medical Publications: pgs. 93-104.

Sanz, E. and Garcia, M. 1993. "Autonomy in the use of drugs in children in Tenerife." Meeting of the WHO Drug Utilization Group. Oxford, UK. Abstract 83.

Seto, W., Wong, M., and Mitchell, E. A. 1992. "Asthma knowledge and management in primary schools in south Auckland." *New Zealand Medical Journal* 105 (937).

Thompson, R. J., Kronenberger, W. G., Johnson, D. F., and Whiting, K. 1989. "The role of central nervous system functioning and family functioning in behavioral problems of children with myelodysplasia." *Journal of Developmental and Behavioral Pediatrics* 10:242-248.

Vaskilampi, T., Kalpio, O., Ahonen, R., and Hallia, O. 1995. "Finnish study on medicine use, health behavior, and perceptions of medicines and health care." *Childhood and Medicine Use in Cross-Cultural Perspective: A European Concerted Action*, edited by D. J. Trakas and E. Sanz. Luxembourg: Office for Official Publications of the European Community, (EURO Report), pgs. 191-220.

Wallston, K. A., Wallston, B. S., and DeVellis, R. 1978. "Development of the multidimensional health locus of control (MHLC) scales." *Health Education Monographs* 6 (2):160-170.

Wirsing, R. 1995. "Perceptions of German children and their parents about health, illness, and medicine use." *Childhood and Medicine Use in Cross-Cultural Perspective: A European Concerted Action*, edited by D. J. Trakas and E. Sanz. Luxembourg: Office for Official Publications of the European Community, (EURO Report), pgs. 149-176.

Yoon, R. McKenzie, D. K., Miles, D. A. and Bauman, A. 1991. "Characteristics of attenders and non-attenders at an asthma education program." *Thorax* 46 (12: 19-21.

SECTION III:
SINGLE CULTURE REPORTS

Chapter 11

"Preferably Half a Tablet": Health-Seeking Behavior When Dutch Children Get Ill

Trudie Gerrits
Flora Haaijer-Ruskamp
Anita P. Hardon

Findings are presented from an exploratory study on the perceptions and attitudes of Dutch children, and their caretakers, about health, illness, and the use of medicines.[1] The general objective of the study was to acquire more insight into the strategies that the children and their parents use when dealing with the children's common illnesses.

METHODS

The respondents were residents of Amsterdam, the Dutch capital, and Groningen, a rural provincial capital. They were contacted through neighborhood schools located in areas considered to be at the lower end of the socioeconomic scale, although not all informants interviewed belonged to this category. Most of the caregivers were in the low to middle level of education and employment. The proportion of people with only a primary school education was high: nine (47.4 percent) of the 19 caregivers.

The same interviewer (TG) collected the data by means of semistructured interviews with 19 caregivers (mostly mothers), and one of their healthy children in the 10- to 12-year age group. The Medicine Cabinet Inventory (MCI) was also used, wherein parents were asked to collect all the medicines present in their house so that information could be recorded about them (e.g., brand name, use, place acquired) (see Chapter 5).

RESULTS

From the information gathered, a model of parental therapeutic regimes was developed (Figure 11.1). The model defines the stages that emerged and the actions and decisions made by parents. The stages have much in common with what Hubley (1992) called "the classic stages in illness behavior." At each stage decisions are made and actions taken which have considerable implications for health. In the following sections are presented the caregivers' and the children's ideas and practices at each of these stages, and the caregivers' and the children's sources of information. These are followed by a description of the use of, and attitudes toward, medicine use.

Children's Perceptions of the Onset of Illness

The most common first step in the process of children's illness onset was where the children themselves indicated that they did not feel well. The children were aware of complaints or differences in their outward appearance, which some of them expressed as follows:

> . . . when you have belly-ache you feel itching; when you are queasy you don't feel like eating and when you have a fever you are really warm . . .

FIGURE 11.1. Parents' therapeutic regime

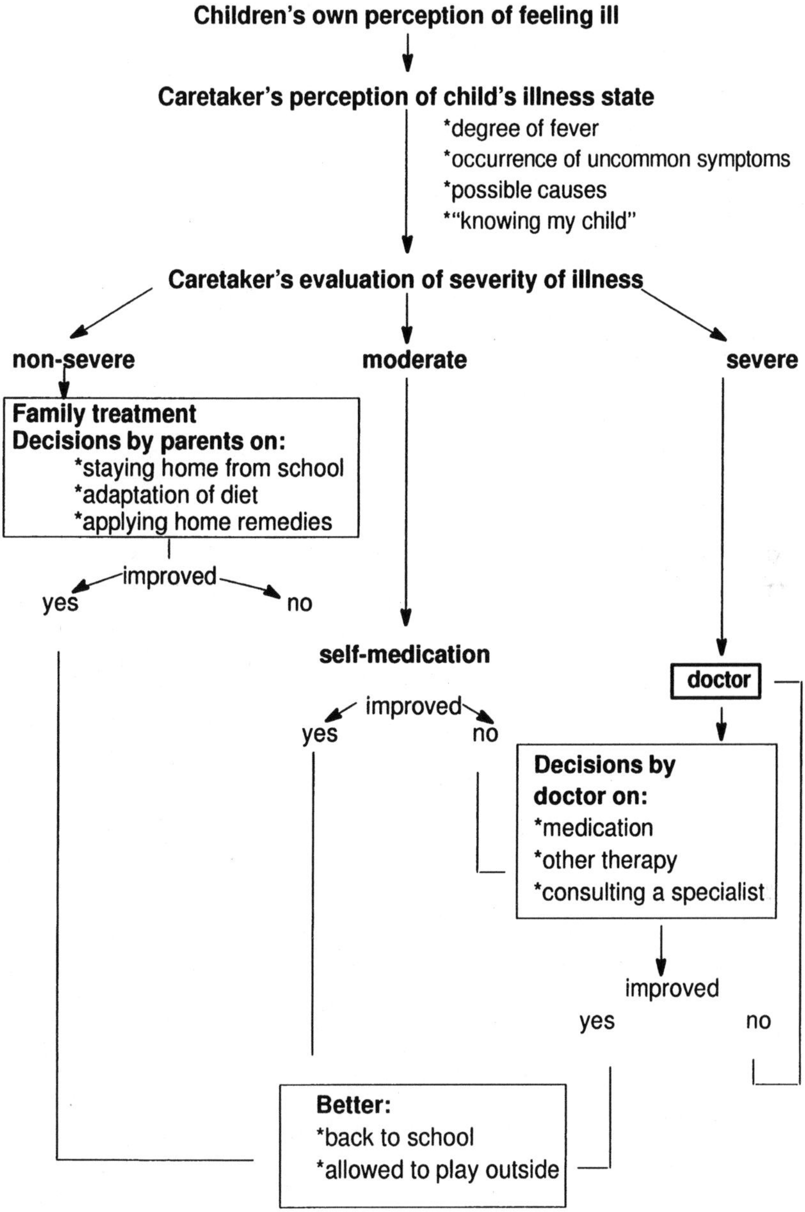

Children's own perception of feeling ill

↓

Caretaker's perception of child's illness state
*degree of fever
*occurrence of uncommon symptoms
*possible causes
*"knowing my child"

↓

Caretaker's evaluation of severity of illness

non-severe   **moderate**   **severe**

Family treatment
Decisions by parents on:
*staying home from school
*adaptation of diet
*applying home remedies

—improved—
yes   no

self-medication

improved
yes   no

doctor

Decisions by
doctor on:
*medication
*other therapy
*consulting a specialist

improved
yes   no

Better:
*back to school
*allowed to play outside

or:

> Then I look bad. Or my face is too red or too pale. When I'm
> too busy my ears become red and then I don't feel good. I look
> in the mirror and then it is red and I know I'm suffering from
> something.

The children communicated their concerns about not feeling well
to their parents or, sometimes, their teacher. Sometimes they did not
need to say anything at all as their parents already noticed that
something was wrong.

Caregiver's Perception of Child's Illness State

In general, the first detection of not feeling well led to a scrutiny
of the child by the principal caregiver, in most cases the mother. The
scrutiny consisted of surveillance and monitoring the child, trying
to detect complaints and their cause by posing questions. For some
caregivers, a change in the color of the face (getting red or pale)
another important signal. Very often the child's temperature was
taken. The results of this examination led to a provisional conclusion on the severity of the illness state. As one mother reported:

> When she is sick I'll watch her: how is she behaving . . . .Then,
> I'll watch her and take her temperature. In fact that is the first
> thing I do. . . . When it is over 38°C, I will let her stay at home.

As indicators for severity most parents mentioned the temperature level, the occurence, and duration of uncommon symptoms
such as headaches or coughing blood in combination with supposed
causes and "knowing my child."
Elevated body temperature (a fever) played a central role in the
caregiver's perception of severity and the therapeutic regime to be
applied. It influenced decisions such as whether the child is to stay
at home, what (s)he is to drink, whether (s)he is to be kept warm or
cool, which medicines are to be used, and whether a doctor's consultation is necessary. Some parents said that the degree of temperature or fever was the biggest help in the decision-making process:

I always do have that thermometer, that is the most important thing for me. When there is no fever, I say "You can go [to school]. . . ." It is an easy help to check whether to stay at home or not. . . . When you don't have fever, for me, you aren't sick.

Fever was seen as a clear indication that something was wrong in the body and was often positively valued as a means of fighting the disease and building resistance. Although fever played a particularly central role for all parents, they differed widely in their evaluation of when a fever is dangerous and a reason to call the doctor. This varied from 38.5 to 41.0°C (101.3 to 105.8°F) (see Chapter 6). Recent experiences with meningitis and convulsions in Groningen influenced parents' concern about high fever. The mode of taking the temperature differed as well. A few parents said that they did not always take the temperature with a thermometer but instead felt the child with their hand. Only when they thought it was needed did they use a thermometer. Some caregivers said that the child does not like having the temperature taken rectally. A few added that they do it nevertheless. Another said that if the child objected she took the temperature by mouth. Obviously the way of taking the temperature is a point of minor quarreling between parents and children. A small minority of the children reported that they are used to taking their own temperature.

Several times the caregivers referred to a specific severe illness episode of one of their own or other children, which alerted them to the importance of certain symptoms or signs. The caregivers continued to be alert for this special symptom. Half of the caregivers in Groningen and one in Amsterdam mentioned headache or high fever as such a symptom, relating this to meningitis or convulsions. When the symptom did persist after some days they called the doctor. The parents differed, as in the case of the level of fever, on how long they waited until calling the doctor. The caregivers also mentioned uncommon symptoms as factors which influenced their health seeking behavior. As one caregiver said of her son:

In the morning he didn't feel good and he had a fever. So, I let him stay at home. And then the fever got higher and he started to vomit. . . . And he had nosebleeds and vomited blood. And that frightened me. Then it is real for me.

Another example of such an uncommon symptom was a cough in combination with vomiting, subsequently diagnosed as tuberculosis.

The cause was derived from the presented symptoms, often in combination with "knowing my child." One mother, for example, explained the bellyache of her child as a result of "eating too much" and another as a result of problems at school. Another caregiver thought that her son used his bellyache as an excuse when he was reluctant to do something for the first time, like going to the sport club or swimming lessons:

> It is possible that he has bellyache, but . . . when he doesn't have any other illness symptoms, no fever or something like that, then I think it is psychological and then I try to find out what's the reason. And then he has to go to the sportclub.

The children as well as their parents mentioned several types of illness causation in children, as shown in Table 11.1.

Both parents and children mentioned several causes of illnesses related to the behavior: underdressing, sleeping too little, being too busy or eating in excess. It should not be considered remarkable that children refer to their own behaviors in discussing illness causation, as several mentioned that their parents had held these behaviors responsible (i.e., this is an idea which is socialized). Some of them gave the impression that they were doubting their caregivers' explanations.

"Motherly instinct" and "knowing my child" were often cited as important in decision making, stressing that these allowed parents to determine if symptoms were "real" or if the child was "making theatre." As one caregiver described: "It is important for me that I think that she is not playing theatre, and then she is allowed to stay at home. . . . I think it's your mother's instinct." Another parent learned from experience: "Since his appendix is removed I'm warned. He doesn't make theatre, I've learned. When he says it is hurting, I really can believe that he has pain."

TABLE 11.1. Illness Causation as Viewed by Children and Caregivers

Complaints related to:	Children's Views:	Caregivers' Views:
Eating/Drinking	* eating or drinking something wrong or poisonous * drinking too little or too much	* eating something wrong * eating too much
Contagion	* being infected by someone else * being caused by germs in general	* getting an influenza or virus going around * catching it somewhere
Behavioral factors	* going late to bed * using medicines when unnecessary * being underdressed (when cold outside)	* sleeping too little * being too busy
Psychological factors	* being nervous or anxious	* having problems at school * having "nerves" and needing attention
Physical environment	* catching cold * getting too much sun (leading to cancer) * breathing polluted or 'bad' air	* not mentioned
Physical factors	* not mentioned	* beginning menses * having eye problems

Caregiver's Evaluation of Severity of Illness

Perceived severity of the illness, based on the evaluation of the indicators discussed above, formed the basis for the following steps to be taken: allowing the child to stay at home from school, the application of home treatments, (self-)medication and/or consulting the doctor.

Mild Illness: Family Treatment

When the parent perceived the complaints of the child as rather common and *nonsevere* the children were treated at home. First, it was decided whether the child can stay home from school. Although most of the children felt they played a role in the decision-making process at the onset of the illness, actual permission to stay at home was invariably given by the principal caregiver, usually the mother. In three cases only was the father more or less equally involved in this decision.

Once at home, the children were usually free to choose where they wanted to be (e.g., sofa or in bed), provided they were not too active and engaged in sedentary diversions (e.g., reading, watching television). In the absence of a fever, they were allowed to play outside–again, with restriction on activity levels.

At this stage, parents adapted a "wait and see" attitude, perhaps modifying the child's diet. Eating was usually not insisted on by the mothers while drinking (tea and fruit juices) was considered to be very important. When the child's complaint (especially headache or bellyache) was perceived as caused by social problems, talking was mentioned as an important, and often the only, intervention.

Both children and caregivers referred to several home remedies, which were applied principally in case of this kind of common illnesses (see Table 11.2). Parents and children mentioned similar kinds of home remedies, (e.g., a hot water bottle, soda dissolved in hot water). Home remedies were used to comfort the child (e.g., rubbing or massage in case of back and belly pain) or to improve his or her health condition (give extra vitamins). Only four children said that their parents never used these kinds of home remedies. One emphatically stated: "My mother is not that type of person!"

TABLE 11.2. Home Remedies Mentioned by Children and Caregivers

Home Remedies	Used for:	Child Mentions	Caregiver Mentions
hot water bottle	bellyache	X	X
wet flannel on the forehead	refreshing when vomiting	X	X
teas/honey in tea	not specified	X	X
beetroot juice	extra vitamins	X	X
soda dissolved in hot water	cleaning small wounds	X	X
honey dissolved in warm milk	insomnia		X
salt water solution	nose cleaning		X
rubbing or massage	back and belly pain		X
onions with brown sugar/sugar water	coughing		X
ice cubes	bruised foot		X
ice water	sore throat		X
wet and/or warm flannel towels	not specified		X
amethyst stone	headache	X	
warmed oil	earache	X	
fresh orange juice	extra vitamins	X	
garlic	wart removal	X	

Moderate Illness: Self-Medication

When the complaints were considered a bit more serious *(moderate)* mothers often gave a medicine that they already had at home or which they bought over the counter. Half of the parents reported using medicines for their children in the two weeks prior to the interviews. Paracetamol and vitamins were mentioned three times. Vermicide, a preparation against warts, fluoride tablets, a penicillin (Acipen V), a cough-syrup, and a balsam were each mentioned once. Of these medicines, only the vermicide and penicillin were given on a doctor's prescription. When speaking in general about illness episodes where medicines were used, the caregivers referred more often to episodes of a cold or influenza than to bellyache or headache. For influenza, cough syrups, analgesics, nose drops, gargles, lozenges, a balsam and–in one case only–penicillin, were mentioned.

All children had at least some experience of medicine use and all but one were aware of the existence of the place (a cabinet, a first aid kit, a drawer) where medicines were kept at home. When they spoke about a medicine they named it or referred to the preparation's form and/or presumed purpose. Cough syrups and analgesics (aspirins and paracetamol) were most often mentioned.

Homeopathic medicines were not used by most of the parents for their children. One parent had previously used them, while three preferred (or sometimes used) them. The parents who preferred homeopathic medicines said that when painkillers were needed they had no other choice than to use allopathic medicines. The child of one of these parents was also very much in favor of homeopathic medicines, having brought the subject up himself.

The MCI showed that half of the household medicines were bought over the counter (OTC), without a prescription from the general practitioner.

In the absence of consultation with a doctor, the mother usually decided about the administration of medicines. The children were equally divided as to whether they asked for medicines. Of those who did not ask, some said they did not need to ask as their parents knew that when they were sick they needed medicines. One child expressed the contrary: "In general my mother doesn't know how I feel, so then I'll tell her. . . ." While most of the children did not report taking medicines out of their storage places without first asking for parental permission, a quarter said that they had taken medicines by themselves "now and then." In these cases, the exact medicines were remembered, e.g., vitamin C, iodine, antiseptic tablets, Sinaspril, cough syrup.

Caregivers as well as their children often expressed, quite explicitly, negative opinions about medicines. This attitude is discussed in a subsequent paragraph.

Severe Illness: Doctor's Consultation

Only in episodes when the home treatment and/or self-medication did not give any positive result or when the symptoms were considered very *severe* from the outset, was a general practitioner consulted. Some children were also aware of this sequence of events, as is illustrated by the following quotation:

> When my throat is hurting I take a Strepsil and when I have a cold I get a cough syrup. When I have something that isn't very common, then my mother goes to the doctor and fetches something at the pharmacy.

In general, the mother decided whether or not the doctor had to be consulted. Only in acute situations, especially in the weekends or at night, fathers seemed to also play a role. Once consulted, the doctor took over decisions on medicine use and some decisions on the therapeutic regime at home.

The majority of the caregivers explicitly stated that a doctor's consultation was not a common occurrence and only took place when really thought necessary. Almost all the caregivers said at least once during the interview that they only called the doctor when it was "really serious," "when I don't trust it," "as the headache or fever doesn't pass rapidly." As one mother put it: "I'm not sitting constantly with the doctor. And when I'm there, then it is really needed." Some caregivers immediately added that they did not, in fact, feel that they were taking any risk at all! One parent explained that he had learned this through experience. He once neglected the complaints of his son which later resulted in the removal of his appendix. Some of the children also referred to the fact that a doctor's visit is a rare thing, although others seemed to go there quite regularly.

The parents interviewed did not consult alternative healers for the health problems of their children. When referring to health care professionals they only spoke about representives of the allopathic health care system.

Medicine Use

When caregivers considered their child's illness as severe from the onset or when a preliminary parental evaluation of nonsevere or moderate condition was reevaluated as severe, they usually consulted a doctor (as is indicated in the model shown in Figure 11.1). The caregivers strongly voiced the attitude: "You should not bother your general practitioner with common diseases, but when the ailment is serious or uncommon then the doctor knows best." This attitude was accompanied by another one which can be summed up as follows: "Although 'wait and see' is a useful attitude in cases where the illness is not severe, you should not take any risk or let your children suffer." In general, the caregivers referred to experiences in the past, which taught them this lesson. When parents perceived illnesses as more severe, doctors were the most important, and often only, persons asked for advice. In general, parents were satisfied with the advice of their doctors. Several times they remarked that the doctor knows them and is not inclined to give medicines when they are not really needed. Although most parents seem to take the advice of the doctor for granted, some parents were critical of specific medical interventions or the conduct of a doctor. Critical remarks were made principally in relation to one or another more serious illness episodes as well as by parents whose child suffered a chronic disorder.

In general, parental (and sometimes children's) evaluation of the doctor's prescribed therapy (medicines or otherwise), depended on their previous experiences with doctors and medicines, and their sources of information, which led to a strongly developed attitude about medicines. These sources of information and their attitude about medicine use are discussed in the following paragraphs.

Sources of Information on Medicines

The caregivers' therapeutic regimes were based on a mixture of their own experiences and information gathered more or less consciously. Most caregivers did not actively search for information. None of them mentioned having been questioned about medicines by their children. Several caregivers added that they did not have questions because they have "healthy children." Medicine use was not considered a problem. Some of them remarked that they felt more need to talk about educational problems related to the onset of puberty. Only when something really serious or out of the ordinary occurred with their child which made them feel insecure, did they feel the need for more information and advice: "I consult the doctor when there are symptoms that I really can't understand." Another mother said: "When I do have questions, I'll ask my doctor, and when I'm not sure concerning medicines, I'll ask the pharmacist." Sometimes they consulted a medical handbook before contacting the general practitioner, but most often the doctor was seen as the only source of information. In general the parents felt satisfied with the answers to their questions. Several times parents remarked that the general practitioner knew them and was not inclined to give medicines when not really needed. Although caregivers spoke with others, particularly relatives, about the illness problems of their children, they did not usually ask for advice. They considered this more as "talking about" and "exchanging experiences." Some caregivers replied that they hardly ever ask others for advice. Two explained this by saying that they themselves attended a (basic) health care course. Another mother said that her child had nothing particular happen so she did not feel the need for advice.

The mass media were mentioned as another source of information on health and illness. Television programs were mentioned most often, followed by women's magazines, medical handbooks, and brochures. The frequency of watching television and reading varied widely. The information gathered in this manner seemed to serve more as general background information than as a guide for actual conduct in cases of (severe) illness. The decision to read an article or brochure or to watch a program was highly influenced by the perceived relevance of the presented subject. One mother said that, "when it is about children I can read it. . . . But I'm not interested in everything about illnesses." The relevance of a subject seemed to be determined principally by past experiences. For example, a mother who had lost three family members to cancer was more inclined to read everything about "how to detect it." Another mother read everything about hospital incubators because one of her daughters had been in an incubator when a baby. Some caregivers had been used to reading medical handbooks in the past, such as from Dr. Spock, but had now stopped doing this because they became "too anxious when reading what can happen" or did not consider the information very useful.

As one parent summarized it after answering the questions on sources of advice:

> You know, the fact that I do this, I've got it from booklets and a conversation here and there. Not from my parents, because they only gave pills. But . . . it is more based on experience and reading and then you combine your information. And then it functions reasonably on some things.

When children talked about their ideas on health, illness, and medicine use, they principally referred to their own illness experiences and on what they saw around them. Only a few of them referred to information received via the mass media and rarely to information at school.

Basic Attitude Toward Medicines: "Only a Half"

Our data indicated that the children did not play a very active role in the decision-making process surrounding their illness. However, they have already developed ideas and attitudes about health and illness, and especially on medicine use. Their parents' therapeutic regime seems to be guided by some basic attitudes, with the attitude about medicines being a dominant one. The caregivers often expressed, quite explicitly, negative opinions about medicines. They referred to possible side effects, e.g., on the kidneys or on the growth of children. And one mother said: "When you take too many medicines now, they will not work if you really need them." Some caregivers remarked that *when* the child took a medicine it was effective only because the child was not used to it, (e.g., a penicillin "cure"). Although they were all opposed to them most added that they could not avoid giving medicines sometimes. However, most saw themselves as persons who did not give medicines easily, "only when really needed, preferably only a *half*." Only one mother said that she changed her mind:

> In early times I thought you can do without medicines. But now I feel they are doing me good. When I have pain, I take a paracetamol. And it helps. So I give it to her also.

Three parents make the observation that Sinaspril is not good for children, one of them adding that several kinds of aspirins are bad. They heard about this and as one father said:

> Formerly we gave Sinaspril. But they are not allowed to use them anymore. It seems that it contains a certain kind of stuff. . . . .The doctor in the hospital told me that.

Although the parents expressed themselves to be firmly against frequent use of medicines, sometimes it was not quite clear what they perceived as "not using them frequently." For example, one caregiver said:

> I *never* have medicines. Now and then a Sinaspril, yes, that I have. When she can't sleep, I give her a half one, because she is saying that she has a headache and you can't check if it is true.

And another caregiver, after having stressed that she was strongly against medicines, added, "the doctor knows that our children hardly take any medicines. That is why I always have paracetamol at home. That is the only thing that I give, a half one." One mother at first said that she would give half an aspirin when her child really did not feel well. She then explained that the "aspirin" she used was a paracetamol and she continued: " When it doesn't pass, then I will wait some hours. And then I will give her another half one, but, I don't give it easily."

According to the children, medicines can be, but are not necessarily, effective. Half of them answered "sometimes yes, sometimes no" to a question on the perceived effectiveness of medicines. Some of them gave examples of their own experiences: "It is good when you have pain, but not always when you have a headache." Four children were convinced of the effectiveness of medicines in general. According to one, "because there are healthy things in it." Another added that there are, however, "some things [illnesses] for which nothing has been found up to now." The children considered taking medicines as less important for their recovery than resting. None mentioned it as a way to prevent illness.

Almost all the children thought you can get sick from medicines, especially when you take too much of them. You can also get sick from taking the "wrong" medicines. Medicines can be wrong in several ways: when you take medicines for a (serious) disease that you do not have; when a child takes medicines meant for an adult; when you are allergic to certain substances; when you take it before having breakfast. One girl "knew" from the television that: "When you eat tablets you get pieces in you stomach, and you can get sick from it." Two children referred to side effects. One added that while medicines can have side effects, "it will help for what it is needed." When speaking of the negative aspects of medicine use, most of the children illustrated this with a concrete example. For example, a boy whose mother had a tumor in her head said that his mother took medicines which had positive and negative effects ("it gets better, but her teeth get rotten") and also referred to side effects of medicines in general: "A lot of medicines are not right. Something gets better, but at the same moment something else gets worse."

DISCUSSION AND CONCLUSIONS

From the interviews with parents and children it can be concluded that for children of 10 to 12 years old, their parents (more often than not the mother) take the major role in the decision-making process in cases of illness. This conclusion was also reached by van den Bosch (1992) who studied the morbidity of younger Dutch children (zero to nine years of age). Several parents interviewed in this present study said that with their first child they were more often worried and insecure and were therefore more inclined to call the doctor than with their later children. This finding confirms Hugenholtz's (1992) observation that in the Netherlands, doctors' consultations on behalf of children are more based on parents' interpretations of their children's complaints than on those of the children themselves.

The children interviewed in the Netherlands seemed to have a less active role in the decision-making process surrounding illness than has been observed in studies carried out among American children (Bush and Davidson 1982; Bush, Iannotti, and Davidson 1985). In this American study it was shown that children even buy medicines themselves, something that never occurred with children in the Dutch study sample.

Furthermore, "perceived severity" was found to be basic for the steps to be taken to improve the ill health of the child. This is not a very surprising finding, for in the literature this factor is generally referred to as important in health care seeking behavior (e.g., Kleinman 1980). It is also a central element in the Children's Health Belief Model, developed by Bush and Iannotti (1992), who found it to be the strongest predictor of children's expectation of medicine use as well.

Fever played an important role in deciding on the severity of the illness. With fever parents are inclined to give medicines, principally analgesics. However, caregivers differed widely in at which temperature (ranging from 38.5° to 41.0°C) (101.3° to 105.8°F) they perceived fever as dangerous and whether medicines are needed or the doctor has to be consulted. Some did not feel quite so self-assured in their interpretation of and reaction to fever.

As the leading norm for caregivers about medicine use is found that, "Only when really needed, I may give a tablet to my child, preferably a *half* one." This attitude is strongly expressed by almost all parents. However, this also seems to mean different things to different people in daily life illness episodes. Parents have varying perceptions of "not too easily" and "when it is really serious." Although the norm toward medicine use is very clear, actual use seems to vary substantially between parents and is probably larger than the leading norm suggests. This idea is underlined once more by the results of the medicine cabinet inventory. Half of the medicines found in the cabinets were bought without prescription, indicating that self-medication plays an important role in the therapeutic regime of the parents.

Observations accompanying the Medicine Cabinet Inventory indicated that caregivers did not realize that they had so many medicines in their homes. To determine the relation between the perceived norm and actual behavior in medicine use, a follow-up study in a larger study population is needed. During a period of, for example, three months, the illness episodes of children and the therapeutic regimes should be followed and detailed data collected. Besides collecting information on complaints, medicines taken and doctor's consultations, the process of decision making in actual illness episodes should be carefully recorded. This will create a fuller picture of why the parents and/or the children take certain decisions and also make clear the meaning of certain concepts and expressions used by the parents.

One rationale for the study was related to the overconsumption of medicines, often cited as the most important problem related to medicine use in the industrialized countries (Haaijer-Ruskamp 1988; Sampers 1988), and the assumption that in this overuse unnecessary risks are taken. Although children are viewed as an important risk group, very little was—and still is—known about the beliefs and practices surrounding the use of medicines by children.

It is thought that people develop ideas and behavior on health, illness, health care, and medicine use during childhood. These ideas form the basis of behavioral patterns that are said to influence them in their later lives. It is therefore suggested that education to influence their health-seeking behavior, including medicine use, will be more effective when given at an early age (Bush and Davidson 1982). It is generally recognized that health education is more effective when the beliefs, practices, and perceived problems of the intended target group are taken into consideration (Green 1980). In the light of this rationale the finding that children are very well aware of the risks and side effects of medicines, especially when excessive quantities of the drug are used, or when they are the wrong medicines, is very important. The children mentioned almost all the causes for side effects as Fallsberg (1992) has observed in her study of Swedish informants on long-term drug regimes. However, despite the fact that most of the children viewed medicines critically, they saw them as an option to be taken when necessary. Furthermore, although the interviewed children were not using a great deal of medicines themselves, quite a few of them have observed a more frequent, sometimes daily, medicine use in their parents. This is particularly true of mothers, who are often seen taking medicines by their children. The children get ambiguous messages from their parents: parents say that medicine use is not good, but they themselves often use them. The fact that children are not frequent medicine users in this stage of life is most probably related to their limited experience of being ill. It is possible that the children's critical attitude toward medicine use will change to a more positive one if they experience more severe or chronic health problems at another stage in their lives.

The interviewed parents did not consider the medicine use of their children as a problem; neither did the children themselves. Children hardly get any information via school or the mass media, but they do not miss it at all (de Vries 1992). Few mothers actively looked for information. The decisions made by parents when dealing with the common illnesses of their children were based on a mixture of more or less consciously gathered information, and from past experience. Information from the mass media, in particular television, is mentioned by the caregivers, and seems to serve more as a provider of general background information than as a guide to conduct during actual cases of illness. In such cases the general practitioner is the most important, and often only, source of advice. Parents talk with relatives, friends, and colleagues about the illnesses of their children, but seldom ask for advice. They consider this to be more an exchange of ideas and experiences. The concept of *"consultation"* (in Dutch *"overleggen"*), as used by Verbeek-Heida (1992), would seem to be more appropriate than the concept of "advice" which seems to be too formal in this context. It is impossible to say how far this information-seeking behavior is related to the (low) educational background of the interviewed parents, due to the absence of a research group of more educated parents.

NOTE

1. The COMAC Childhood and Medicines Project was funded through a European Economic Community (EEC) *Comité d'Action Concerté* (COMAC) contract, COMAC/HSR MR4*-CT90-0319, awarded to The Institute on Child Health, Athens, Greece, with Deanna J. Trakas as the Project Leader. The official

228   *CHILDREN, MEDICINES, AND CULTURE*

title of the Contract was "Medicine Use, Behaviour and Children's Perceptions of Medicines and Health Care." In the Netherlands the study was also supported by The Ministry of Welfare, Public Health, and Culture and the Northern Centre of Health Care Research, University of Groningen.

REFERENCES

Bosch, W. J. H. M. van den. 1992. *Epidemiologische Aspecten van Morbiditeit bij Kinderen.* Nijmegen: Katholieke Universiteit.
Bush, P. J. and Davidson, F. R. 1982. "Medicines and 'drugs': What do children think?" *Health Education Quarterly* 9: 113-128.
Bush, P. J. and Iannotti, R. J. 1992. "The Socialization of Children into Medicine Use" *Studying Childhood and Medicine Use,* edited by D. J. Trakas and E. J. Sanz. Athens. Greece: ZHTA Medical Publications, Athens: ZHTA Medical Publications, pgs. 105-116.
Bush, P. J., Iannotti R. J., and Davidson, F. R. 1985. "A longitudinal study of children and medicines" *Topics in Pharmaceutical Sciences,* edited by Breimer, D. D. and Speiser, P. . Elsevier Science Publications, pgs. 391-403.
de Vries, T. 1992. "De dokter in de kinderboeken. Welk beeld van de dokter doen kinderen op uit hun literatuur?" *Medisch Contact* 42(47): 1226-1229.
Fallsberg, M. 1992. *Reflections on Medicines and Medications. A Qualitative Analysis Among People on Long Term Drug Regimens.* Linköping: Linköping University.
Green, L. W. 1980. *Health Education and Planning: A Diagnostic Approach.* Palo Alto: Mayfield Publishing Company.
Haaijer-Ruskamp, F. M. 1988. "Rational drug use; a view from the Netherlands in answer to the USA." *Journal of Social and Administrative Pharmacy* 5: 127-132.
Hubley, J. 1992. "Community drug use–Health education theoretical framework and lessons learnt." Paper presented Workshop on Community Drug Use. Amsterdam, May 22, 1992.
Hugenholtz, M. 1992. "Huisarts en kinderen (Commentaar)." *Huisarts en Wetenschap* (35)7: 265-266.
Kleinman, A. 1980. *Patients and Healers in the Context of Culture.* Berkeley: University of California Press.
Sampers, G. H. M. A. 1988. "Antimicrobiele middelen in de eerste lijn." *Nederlands Tijdschrift voor Gezondheidszorg* 132: 676-680.
Verbeek-Heida, P. 1992. *De Eigenwijsheid van de Patiënt. Alledaagse Overwegingen bij Geneesmiddelengebruik.* Amsterdam: Faculteit Politiek Sociaal-Culturele Wetenschappen.

Chapter 12

The Use of Conventional and Unconventional Medicines to Treat Illnesses of German Children

Rolf L. Wirsing

Payer (1988), in a comparative study of the therapeutic styles of medical doctors in four nations, reported that German physicians prescribe fewer antibiotics than their colleagues in France, Great Britain, and the United States. She also observed that German patients resort more frequently to unconventional medicine of the naturopathic, homeopathic, or anthroposophic kind. Even though she attributes such behavioral differences to differences in cultural tradition, she looks at them from the point of view of physicians rather than from those of their patients. Such a focus on physicians might leave us with the impression that patients play a negligible role in influencing their physician's decision. But a closer look at the behavior of German patients can show us that patients do play an active role in the negotiation of their prescriptions. It tells us how and why German patients often circumvent conventional physicians and their therapies and either self-treat or consult unconventional therapists (for literature on doctor-patient negotiations, c.f., Waissman 1990, Higginbotham 1977).

This chapter contains a discussion of the cultural context of medical care and the social conditions and personal justifications of German parents regarding the use and nonuse of either conventional treatment (in particular antibiotics) or unconventional therapies (in particular the homeopathic or anthroposophic kind) in treating the illnesses of their 7- to 11-year-old children. The discussion draws on data from a European-wide comparative research project on the perceptions and attitudes of children and their primary caretakers on health, illness, and the use of medicines.[1] Its only focus, however, is on data gathered in Germany.

During the course of our German study, we became increasingly aware that nearly all of the parents we talked to had some disdain for antibiotics and often a clear preference for therapies and medicines which are unconventional by scientific medical standards. Even though most of the parents had used antibiotics during the medical treatment of their children in the past at least once, they always seemed apologetic about having used them. In about half of the parents this disdain was coupled with a positive attitude toward unconventional medicine, including toward the doctors or healers that prescribe such medicines. In particular, these parents would not only consult "regular" general practitioners or pediatricians but would also accept treatment from those medical doctors or healers whose specialty or preferred mode of treatment is labelled "unscientific" by the scientific community. The medically trained yet "unscientific doctors" contacted by the parents of our sample happened to practice as homeopaths, or anthroposophic doctors. Two of our parents had consulted a naturopath ("Heilpraktiker") and one family admitted to having seen a faith-healer.

The surprising fact is that those parents of our sample who accept anthroposophic doctors, homeopaths, or faith healers are not lowly educated citizens or traditionally minded villagers but modern and well-educated cosmopolitans. There is nearly a perfect correlation between the high education of the mother (i.e., having at least Abitur, which is equivalent to two years of college) and the consultation of unconventional therapists (see Table 12.1). Since all of our parents viewed antibiotics with suspicion there is no comparable relationship between educational level and use of antibiotics, even though the more educated were more outspoken in their rejection of these drugs.

The study argues that the behavior of German parents concerning their choice of treatment of common childhood ailments can best be understood if we consider their behavior within sickness-relevant cultural contexts and the parents' position within these contexts. Sickness-relevant contexts in Germany center around either academically trained physicians working in hospitals or private

TABLE 12. 1. Parent's Education Level and Use of Therapies in the Treatment of Children's Illnesses

| | THERAPY | |
Education Level	Unconventional	Conventional Only
Abitur *	9	1**
Less than Abitur	0	5

* Equivalent to at least two years of college.
** The single case in the upper right cell may not be an exception—the mother herself uses a homeopathic medicine and gives an herbal immuno-stimulant to her child.

practice or are focused on certified naturopaths and sometimes even uncertified folk healers. These contexts also include corresponding therapeutic orientations and their materia medica. While physicians are generally associated with biomedical therapies, some of them also offer treatments based on homeopathy and anthroposophy that previously have been the domain of unconventional medical practitioners alone. Another context relevant to childhood illness centers around parents situated in the home where most of the lay management of illness is done on the basis of traditional cultural knowledge of diagnosis and care. The distinction between these three contexts centering around either academic physicians, certified naturopaths, or the parents at home corresponds roughly to Kleinman's (1980) three-part division of total health care systems into a professional, folk- and popular sector. The fit of Kleinman's three-sector model to the German health system can be shown to be loose since German physicians' behavior, as noted above, is not exclusively based in biomedicine but occasionally also borrows from unconventional medicine. The folk sector consisting of naturopaths and their unconventional therapies is also a German peculiarity. Most of its practices are legally institutionalized and most of its practitioners and clients share a common ideology that has its roots in German naturalism.

Parents participate in all sectors but in different roles. While their participation in the popular sector at home is in the role of an active health care provider, it shifts to the role of client as soon as they enter the professional or folk sector. But in their role of client they still have a number of options open to them: they not only have the choice of either entering the professional or folk sector but also the choice between different practitioners representing different therapeutic specialties available within each sector. Their options do not end here, since they still can influence the therapeutic encounter and the type of medication they get prescribed for their children. By thus carefully selecting their therapists, by skillfully negotiating the child's treatment, or even by occasionally refusing compliance with the therapists' recommendations, they are able to regain some of their autonomy and power in the treatment process.

The discussion is organized in three parts; the first is the shortest. It summarizes briefly the methodology used in the study by describing our instruments and by detailing our approach followed in the sampling of our respondents. The second part outlines relevant structural features of the German medical system. It focuses on the practitioners of conventional and unconventional medicine, their specialties and *materia medica*. The pluralistic German health system can tell us a lot about the availability and costs of health care professionals and the commercial medicines at their disposal. It also makes us aware of the philosophies, values, and justifications inherent in our cultural tradition, e.g., German naturalism, that help us understand why unconventional therapies still exist side by side with conventional therapies. The third part shows how the parents' knowledge and their evaluation of the child's symptoms of a selected number of common childhood diseases relates to health-seeking behavior and negotiation of therapy. It stresses that parents are rational social actors who act on the basis of their own convictions and their economic means.

METHODOLOGICAL APPROACH

The German team at the University of Hamburg translated, modified, and set out to test and use the following research instruments:

1. An interviewer's guide for a semistructured but informal interview with the children. In this interview we asked children to

draw a picture of their last illness episode and then to talk about their corresponding experiences.

2. A structured interview with the parent who was the main health care provider for the target child. It consisted of preformulated questions that focused on the parent's ideas and reported behavior concerning health practitioners and medicines during the treatment of children's diseases, regardless of whether their child had these diseases or not.

3. A highly structured questionnaire about the medicines kept in the home of the parents (the medicine cabinet form). This questionnaire asked about the brand name, dosage form, and therapeutic category of each medicine in the home.

Children were approached via their parents. We started by asking parents in Hamburg known to us personally and whose consent could be obtained by informal means. Four additional parents known to us personally came from a small town of about 10,000 inhabitants. Since in the small town only physicians practicing conventional medicine were available, the reported behavior of the parents residing there was expected to differ from the behavior of parents living in Hamburg.

We always asked consenting parents for the names and telephone numbers of additional parents who were known to have children between seven and 11 years who could possibly be won over to participate in our research. We are aware that such a snowball selection procedure was likely to heavily bias our sample in favor of those who were health conscious and those who were academically trained; 40 percent had attended a university.

Even though we managed to contact a total of 26 seemingly healthy school children between the ages of seven and 11 years from 25 families, we were able to transcribe word for word only 15 audiotaped interviews with children and 15 interviews with parents. We stored them as text files on a computer so that they could be analyzed by special text-analysis programs, such as Gofer. These 15 text files with both parents and children provided the most important data base for the analyses presented in this chapter.

Medicine cabinet inventories were recorded for 14 of the 25 families. About half of these were obtained by leaving the corresponding questionnaire with the parents together with the instruction that they be filled out conscientiously and mailed to us in a self-addressed stamped envelope. The data of the medicine cabinet inventory were then converted into a data-base computer file. Its information is also referred to occasionally in this report.

CONTEXT OF MEDICAL CARE

This section contains a discussion of the availability of therapists in the German context, stressing the range and variety available in medical specialties, modes of treatments, and pharmaceutical products in both conventional and unconventional medicine. The German health insurance system is also referenced because its criteria for which kind of therapy is refundable and which is not plays a large role in the choice of therapy. Next is presented the cultural phenomenon of unconventional medicine in the context of its popularity in Germany today. A case is made that it is one form of a recent cultural movement rooted in German naturalism.

Types of Practitioners

Germany owns a pluralistic but hierarchically ordered medical system. Its pluralism lies in the diversity of its academically trained physicians ("Ärzte") and its colorful array of state-certified naturopaths ("Heilpraktiker," i.e., healing practitioners) and noncertified folk-healers. In its hierarchy physicians rank highest, naturopaths next, and folk healers lowest. Physicians have the greatest authority, best legal recognition, and easiest access to health insurance money. The physicians' authority and power rests on their professional organizations' claim that only their members have the knowledge and experience to provide rational and scientific treatment of human diseases and that this knowledge can only be gained during a long and natural science oriented university education. Legally, physicians are subject to almost no restrictions related to medical treatment–quite in contrast to naturopaths. Naturopaths have been legally recognized since 1939 and are therefore allowed to treat diseases. In contrast to physicians naturopaths are legally prohibited from treating venereal diseases and a variety of reportable infectious diseases. They are also forbidden to treat teeth or assist during childbirth. As an emerging profession, they have little control over the training of their members (in fact, special schooling–even though available–is not a prerequisite for entering the profession). They cannot even decide who is allowed to practice. Their state certification and right to practice depends exclusively on passing an examination in front of a state-employed local public health physician. This examination mainly tests whether the applicants know the laws and restrictions applying to the practice of naturopathy. In contrast, folk healers in Germany, as long as they have not gained state certification as naturopaths, are only legally tolerated in the sickness domain as long as they do not call their interventions "medical treatment."[2]

Physicians in Germany already recognize more than 50 different medical specialties, general practice being considered one of them. Most of them practice conventional "scientific" medicine. Unconventional medical specialties rarely seen outside of Europe are homeopathic and anthroposophic medicine. These specialties, however, are not yet fully accepted parts of biomedicine and are subsequently not taught routinely at German medical schools. But the number of followers of these branches among physicians is increasing. They are already practicing in great numbers in every larger city.

There are about 2,000 physicians in Germany who specialize in homeopathy, a branch based on the teachings of the German doctor F. S. Hahnemann (1755-1843). Hahnemann was convinced that selected parts of plants or animals, including certain minerals, could be used in a highly diluted form as a medicine against those symptoms the same materials would have caused if applied in an undiluted form. During the course of his research Hahnemann tested higher and higher dilutions until he finally only had his patients sniff at his medicines. Today homeopathic medicines ("homeopathica") are produced by special pharmaceutical companies in the form of globuli and drops and are sold in pharmacies. True followers of homeopathy would never take homeopathica and conventional medicine (called "allopathica") at the same time.

There are also about 1,000 academically trained physicians in Germany who practice anthroposophic medicine. Anthroposophic medicine dates back to the philosophy of the Austrian Rudolph Steiner (1861-1925). In his philosophy, health constitutes a dynamic equilibrium between man's four body types (that also correspond to the planets): his physical body, ethereal body, astral body, and ego. Disease constitutes an abnormal relationship between the spiritual and bodily parts of the set above. Medical therapy should strengthen the patient's self-healing power and is hoped also to increase individuality and self-fulfillment. Medicines constitute only a minor part of therapy that also includes–among other things– diet, music therapy, dance therapy, or art therapy. Steiner's philosophy has attracted mostly the intellectual elite in Germany and has prompted some of them to send their children to private schools ("Waldorf Schools") that apply Steiner's ideas. Physicians with an anthroposophic orientation, like homeopaths, tailor their therapy to the individual characteristics of each patient. They prefer to prescribe special remedies (mostly plant-, mineral- or animal-based, but also synthetic drugs) modeled after Steiner's theories. These medicines are called "anthroposophica" and are available in pharmacies. A well-known anthroposophica used against cancer, for instance, is made of mistletoe (for a detailed description of anthroposophic medicine see Wolff 1982).

About 7,000 naturopaths are practicing in Germany. They trace their intellectual roots to German naturalism (see below), but they also borrowed much from the traditional folk medicines of Europe (especially in the form of herbs used for teas, compresses, or inhalations) and Asia (such as acupuncture or Ayurveda, [see Liebau 1988]). As a rule, they diagnose by uncommon and nonintrusive methods (e.g., homeopathic interview or iris-diagnosis) and treat by means of "natural," "complementary," or "alternative" medicine. In spite of legal restrictions, the scope of what they are legally allowed to do is still quite ample. For instance, they are allowed to give intravenous injections, to treat bone fractures and in principle could even perform operations or open a clinic (Commandeur and Neumann 1989). Our sample only discussed naturopaths who were homeopaths.

Finally, folk healers are usually formally untrained but naturally gifted individuals rooted firmly in the folk and Christian tradition of the rural area where they usually live and practice. They apply a

mixture of both traditional medical knowledge (such as phytothera-
py) and magical-religious procedures (such as prayers and laying
on of hands).

Materia Medica

The German pharmaceutical industry produces one of the greatest varieties of medicine in the world. The so-called "Rote Liste"
(Red List), an annual publication of all medicines produced and
sold by members of the BPI[3] in Germany, lists for 1993 a total of
8,195 different products in 10,755 different forms (as pills, injections, etc.) available in 23,431 different sizes and prices from a total
of 407 pharmaceutical companies. The Red List contains only conventional medicines and excludes homeopathica, anthroposophica,
and certain over-the-counter (OTC) drugs. Also not listed are medicines produced by non-BPI members.[4] All the products on the Red
List can only be sold in pharmacies or dispensed in hospitals. Other
stores, even drugstores are legally prohibited from selling any
single medicine listed in the Red List.

Pharmacies distinguish between two types of drugs: prescription
drugs and freely sold OTC drugs. Prescription drugs can only be
acquired with a prescription from a physician—and not from a naturopath. Antibiotics are an example of a prescription drug. OTC
drugs may be acquired with or without a prescription from a physician or naturopath. Examples of OTC drugs sold only in pharmacies
are such conventional drugs as aspirin and paracetamol (acetaminophen) and nearly all unconventional drugs such as homeopathica
and anthroposophica.

All medicines are sold packaged and have to come with a package insert. Exceptions are OTC drugs (see below), which can have
the main information on the package. The kind of information on
the inserts and the order it is presented are legally proscribed. The
inserts have to inform—among other things—about the frequency and
seriousness of side effects and have to include a warning to store the
medicine out of the reach of children. The information about side
effects in conjunction with the rising awareness of the German
public concerning the negative effects of physician-prescribed medicines has been blamed for high noncompliance rates and the rising
demand for "soft" and "natural" medicines.

Drugstores and other stores, in contrast to pharmacies, may sell a variety of other medicines not listed in the Red List. They do not sell drugs that include antibiotics, antihistamines, anticoagulants, or medicines having that effect. Add to this forbidden list hormones or drugs affecting the vegetative nervous system. The drugs sold in these stores also must never be in the form of injections, suppositories, aerosols, or vaginal or intrauterine inserts. They are more likely to be plant-based products, mineral waters, disinfecting gargles, vitamins, antacids, or tonics. They may be purgatives or swallowed against indigestion. They consist, e.g., of Baldrian (Valerianae radix) as sleeping pills, e.g., Baldrian-Dispert, ® of lozenges or syrups for colds and coughs, and of garlic pills for arteriosclerosis. They are the kind of medicines people may use in self-treatment or upon recommendation of a naturopath. These products always have to be paid for out of one's own pocket and their costs are not refunded by any health insurance.

Health Insurance

Since health-related costs play a large role in the choice of therapies, it is relevant to describe what kind of expenses are covered by either the State Health Insurance or private insurance and which ones are not.

The State Health Insurance in Germany is compulsory for all employed and unemployed people earning less than a specified amount (presently 5,400 DM per month before taxes). State Health Insurance demands a contribution of about 13 percent of one's income as a membership fee—with the employee and employer each paying half of it. Spouses and children up to a certain age are covered by the compulsory health insurance of the main breadwinner. Unemployed people get their monthly fees paid for by the state's unemployment insurance. All insured members have a legal right to the payment of nearly all costs for medical prevention and treatment,[5] but only if prescribed or performed by physicians. Members do not get reimbursed for the costs of naturopathic treatment and may even have difficulties having all of their expenses paid for if the insurance decides that the treatment prescribed by unconventional physicians is "unproved" or "unscientific." The costs of homeopathic or anthroposophic medicines, if prescribed by a physician, are, however, likely to be reimbursed.

Only a minority of people do not have to participate in the State Health Insurance scheme. To these belong all earners with a comfortable income. They can either enter the State Health Insurance as voluntary members or get private health insurance. Private health insurance presently insures only 5 percent of the population. Fees depend on the health risk of the insured person (i.e., on gender, age, health condition—but not on income). For young and substantial wage earners this usually means that they will have to pay considerably less per month than if they were insured voluntarily in the State Health Insurance.

Physicians love privately insured patients because they can charge about 2.3 times more for the same services they are allowed to charge for state insured patients. Also naturopaths are pleased about privately insured patients. As a matter of fact, they could hardly exist without them. Only privately insured patients get reimbursed for the costs of naturopaths and receive coverage for nearly all of their treatments. State Health Insurance does not. State insured patients visiting a naturopath have to pay all costs out of their own pockets. It is therefore no surprise if only the well-educated and thus better earning parents in our sample can afford both private insurance and/or the extra costs of a naturopath.

The Attraction of Alternative Therapies

There is no doubt that the majority of patients in Germany in search of medical treatment still prefer conventional physicians. This rule holds true for all patients regardless of where they live (urban or rural) or their level of education or social class. But it is equally true that interest in unconventional treatment among patients is rising—not only in Germany but also in Britain and the rest of Europe, as Sharma (1992) was able to demonstrate.

The main reasons for this rise in interest seem to be similar everywhere: first, there is a rising concern about the possible side effects of conventional treatment and the increasing medicalization of health. In Germany this trend started about 33 years ago with the so-called Contergan® catastrophe (Clemens 1983). The sleeping pill with the brand name Contergan® (with its ingredient thalidomide) caused disastrous deformities in the human embryo when it was used by pregnant women. About 7,000 babies (in Germany exactly 2,625, see Schott 1993:518) were born deformed–often with missing arms and legs. One-third of the babies were born dead or died early. Presently about 2,500 victims of this tragedy are still alive. This shock deeply shattered the trust people had in medicines and conventional therapies. People became increasingly critical toward the mechanical, inhuman, and seemingly meaningless portrayal of disease in conventional medicine and more and more fearful of its intrusive diagnostic procedures and seemingly aggressive treatments.

The dissatisfaction with conventional medicine that benefits unconventional therapists has to do with the greater prevalence of chronic diseases in our aging industrial populations for which modern medicine has little to offer but a chain of endless or intrusive diagnostic procedures and seemingly life-long, ineffective, or aggressive treatments. For some people unconventional medicine then becomes the source of revived hopes for a new interpretation of their illness and a soft and magical cure. People are also encouraged by popular stereotypes that view unconventional medicine as "soft," "safe," or "natural" without any serious side effects.[6] Other people see unconventional methods as an increase in their treatment options and eclectically try out the various options open to them (see also Sharma 1992).

Typical for Germany is the popularization of the ideology of "naturalism" in all segments of the German population. German naturalism today is characterized by a strong emotional tie toward "nature" and everything "natural." It shows a very deep-seated antipathy to the intrusion of technology and chemistry into most aspects of private life, especially into food production and medical practice. These attitudes have an old emotional and ideological base found in recurrent philosophical ideas criticizing contemporary civilization. Some of these ideas can already be traced to the classical Stoa, but it was the thinking of Rousseau (1712-1778) who evened the path to a naturalistic philosophy. Later the practice and preaching of so-called water-doctors (Prießnitz 1799-1851), vegetarians (Schroth) and others favoring a natural way of living (Rikli 1823-1906; Just 1859-1936) brought forward such movements as naturopathic healing (Kneipp 1821-1897; Felke 1856-1926), nudism, the German youth movement, and the life-reform movement. (For an excellent discussion of these ideas and movements see Rothschuh 1983 and also Velimirovic and Velimirovic 1983.) Naturopathic healing now is associated with the belief that one's health can be maintained or regained by exposing oneself to sunlight, fresh air, and cold water, by physical exercise, by eating raw or untreated vegetarian food, and by refraining from everything "unnatural," "artificial," or "chemical." Diseases and symptoms in this philosophy are seen as positive bodily regulatory processes in response to foreign and intruding material agents. Disease symptoms are not to be suppressed but should ideally be dealt with in a two-step procedure: first, by the removal and excretion ("Ausleitung") of the foreign material agents via skin and other body openings by means of, e.g., sweating, vomiting, cupping, blood-letting or enema. Second, by the active strengthening of the body and its self-healing powers by natural means, such as by means of a special diet in conjunction with herbal, mineral, or animal-based medicine and by naturally stimulating the organism by exposing it to warmth or cold, movement or rest, or light, air, sun, or water. Naturopaths claim that they are best trained to do just that.

At the outset it was stated that patients who consult homeopathic and anthroposophic doctors, naturopaths, or folk healers tend to come from the better-educated and better-to-do urban population. The question is therefore: what makes these unconventional therapists so attractive to this particular group? First, educated people are more familiar with the philosophies of homeopathy, anthroposophy, and naturalism and see them as additional treatment options. Educated people also feel attracted to more holistic and sometimes religious views of human nature and suffering. Second, better-educated people tend to occupy positions in society that grant them relative autonomy from the influence of others. They are likely to despise authority and passivity and to value independence and active personal initiative. By frequenting unconventional therapists they not only challenge the authority of physicians but also take over more control and responsibility over their treatment options. With unconventional therapists they demand (and are given) more time and freedom to discuss aspects of cause, meaning, and therapy and are more likely to see their own initiative during treatment encouraged. Third, educated people tend to be financially better off and thus to be able to personally carry (or be privately insured against) the costs of unconventional medicine. And fourth, unconventional therapists in Germany make themselves more accessible to the better educated by settling and offering their services in areas where the majority of the better-off work, reside, and send their children to school, namely in the greener and richer districts of larger cities.

PARENTS' KNOWLEDGE OF CHILDREN'S DISEASES AND EVALUATION OF SYMPTOMS

The following section presents more detail from our interviews with the parents. Described are the symptoms and signs parents were attentive to for different common childhood illnesses and how the parents thought and acted in relation to them. In particular, how parents rate the nature and severity of these diseases and how they choose and justify the treatment options known to them are discussed. The material also makes clear that children have little to say in most of these matters.

Infection of the Middle Ear

With few exceptions, all parents had experience with middle-ear infection among their children. The parents voiced concern about the pain their children suffered, felt disgust about the visible pus coming out of the child's affected ear, and were worried about the possible damages that might remain if it were left untreated. All these conditions made middle-ear infection a "serious" disease. Such a disease is thought to require swift action and the application of a "strong" rather than "soft" or slow-acting medicine. The first action for most therefore consisted of the consultation of a physician coupled with the expectation that an antibiotic, such as penicillin, would be prescribed. All of the parents knew that antibiotics help in this case. But many of them also pictured antibiotics to be "hammers" or "bombs," i.e., as extremely powerful and effective medicines with devastating and unwanted side effects. Such medicines are only to be used in cases of emergency. And since a middle-ear infection seems to be such an emergency, most thought that they had no other choice. For them it was like weighing the positive action of a medicine against its dangers. "I would consider using antibiotics in the case of middle-ear infection in spite of its side effects, since this seems to be a disease the body cannot overcome by itself," said one mother who would normally resort to unconventional medicine.

There is one exception to this generalization that seems worth mentioning. It is about one mother who valued naturopaths and preferred homeopathic treatment and about her only daughter that she raised alone. When her child succumbed to a middle-ear infection it so happened that her naturopath was away on vacation. She consulted an ear-nose-throat specialist. The physician prescribed two packages of antibiotics. The mother continued,

I did not give [the antibiotics] to her since I am of the opinion that such a treatment has to be preceded by the determination of the agent that caused the disease. Then we visited our pediatrician and told her that we had not administered the medicine prescribed by the specialist because it does not fit. And since the infection was already older than a week we wanted an exact analysis of the germs responsible in order to apply specific treatment. And then she did this test. In the meantime we went on vacation. The ear did not look so bad that we had to fear that the infection would pass on to other organs. Later we learned that the agent was harmless and that it is usually found on the skin. During vacation we also met a pediatrician who voiced the opinion that in this case he would not have given antibiotics. First, the infection has already gone on for quite a while and second, antibiotics would not be effective for such germs. These germs would disappear by themselves. Only if the disease were to continue for more than six months one should think of airing the ear. After vacation we consulted our naturopath. She gave her a [homeopathic] remedy and the infection disappeared after a week without our resorting to such strong medicine. Using antibiotics means impairing the whole body, provoking allergies and weakening the otherwise needed bodily resistance (Abwehrkräfte). This is also what the pediatrician had told us during vacation. (Mother of nine-year-old Lisa)

We can learn a number of things from this example. This mother, like other mothers, recognized the symptoms of the middle-ear infection and worried about their seriousness. Due to the temporary absence of her favorite naturopath, her worries made her do what she probably seldom does–she consulted a physician specialist unknown to her. This physician confirmed her lay diagnosis that she apparently accepted. But she did not accept the antibiotic treatment he prescribed. She thought that such an aggressive and allergy-provoking treatment is only justified if additional tests had determined the nature of the microorganisms responsible for the infection and if the tests proved the prescribed antibiotics' effectiveness against the germs. Since such tests were not done she preferred to be noncompliant, searched for a professional confirmation of her attitude from a pediatrician known to her, negotiated for the wanted tests to be done and achieved a (wanted?) delay in conventional treatment. Her suspicious attitude against antibiotics thus was stronger than the pain the child must have endured during the long time of waiting until the naturopath's return.

While it is hard to judge whether the girl involved (Lisa) also agreed with her mother's judgement, it is obvious that her illness had left a lasting impression on the child. She chose exactly this episode to talk to us about during the interview. On the drawing she made, she had painted a girl with a red and inflamed ear complete with yellow pus dripping out of it. She detailed it like this,

It always hurt when my mother removed the pus . . . . It got worse and worse and only improved when we went to Greece. I had to put some stuff into my ear so no water would enter. But when we returned home it got worse [again]. . . Then I went to my naturopath–I always go to her for my allergies–. . . and she looked into my ear . . . and prescribed white globuli and brown juice to swallow.

Measles

Measles, in the eyes of many parents, is another serious disease. Its seriousness lies in the long duration of the disease, in the danger of a "relapse" and in its possible secondary damages such as meningitis, pneumonia, or damages to the heart. But unlike a middle-ear infection it is not accompanied by pain or pus but only by fever or weakness and spots on the skin. All of the parents know that measles–unlike middle-ear infection–is a viral infection and they think that not much can be done about it. Most of those worrying about secondary damages tried to prevent the outbreak of measles in their children by having them vaccinated. Others, when faced with a case of measles, saw their physician and attempted to lower the accompanying fever by administering fever suppositories (Benuron® with its active ingredient paracetamol). Parents with a preference for unconventional treatment tended to be against vaccination and against "suppressing" the fever with analgesics. One common justification was that children's diseases, such as measles, are "normal" for children and strengthen rather than weaken them.

"They always wanted to vaccinate Manuel against measles. But I refused." "Why?"

> Because vaccinations are exactly the reason why diseases like measles progress so atypically nowadays. Vaccinations change the diseases and make children even more susceptible. Measles became more aggressive, also scarlet fever changed. One hears this a lot. . . . I agree with what anthroposophic doctors always say–that children's diseases belong to children and that they tend to strengthen rather than weaken them. When you want to evade these diseases by vaccinating the child or by suppressing these diseases' symptoms you are likely to take something away from the child that belongs to his development and that strengthens his immune system. (Mother of ten-year-old Manuel).

When their children had the measles most of them consulted their anthroposophic or homeopathic physician or naturopath and administered the prescribed homeopathic medicine–often accompanied with warnings and additional precautions:

Mother: "When [our son] Manuel had measles we treated him with medicines. He was the victim of a measles epidemic in Hannover in 1989. He was seven then and already went to school. [Our homeopathic] physician came to see him regularly because measles are said to be more aggressive now than scarlet fever."

Interviewer: "Did you lower the fever?"

Mother: "No, no. We accompanied the sickness homeopathically so no complications would arise, in order to prevent them right from the beginning. And since there is always the danger of meningitis we continuously observed him . . . . We accompanied his disease with homeopathic medicine since it does not act against the disease but supports the body to overcome it by itself . . . This measles epidemic was so dangerous that many homeopathic physicians even had to resort to antibiotics in the case of pneumonia or had to send the children to hospitals when meningitis was suspected." (Mother of 10-year-old Manuel)

What do the examples about measles illustrate? The parents judge measles a serious disease not because it is painful for the child but because they get alarmed by its high fever and presumed greater aggressiveness, and because they worry about its possible secondary damages. What makes them shun conventional symptomatic treatment in spite of these ideas is the parents' own experience with this illness during their own childhood, their belief that this experience is an important part of growing up, and their knowledge that little can be done against a viral disease that runs its course and goes away by itself. We also learn of a philosophy where measles vaccinations or symptomatic treatments are seen as unhealthful attempts to "suppress" a bodily experience that would have "strengthened" rather than weakened the child.

Fever

The last example shows how parental interpretations about the seriousness of an illness can shift over time. The interpretation of seriousness now seems to be based less on subjective impression or experience but more on the "objective" reading of a fever thermometer.

Because all parents had already had experience with fever personally and had seen it among their children, their earlier experiences facilitated diagnosis and influenced their reactions to it. They suspected fever if the child's body or forehead felt hot, if the child complained of being hot, or if his or her eyes looked "shiny" or "glassy." If parents got duly alarmed they usually measured the child's temperature by means of a thermometer. When reading the thermometer all of them made a distinction between "raised body temperature" (37 to 38°C/98.6 to 100.4°F), "fever" (38 to 39°C or 40°C/100.4 to 102.2°F or 104°F), and "high fever" (39° or 40°C/102.2° or 104°F and up).

This distinction is important for judging from what point the fever should be considered dangerous and whether or not any remedial or medical action is required. But to fully understand the parents' caregiving behavior we should be aware of the positive attitude they have toward fever. This especially holds true for parents favoring "soft" medicines. Fever as such is never considered a "disease," even though a child with fever is always labelled "sick." Fever is indicative of some underlying infection; it is a sign or symptom that an "immune reaction" is taking place. Its presumed function is the "fighting" of an underlying disease. It is therefore highly valued and should only be lowered or "suppressed" in the case of "high fever" or a fever lasting more than two days. Of secondary importance to our understanding may also be the parents' knowledge and evaluation of seriousness of the infection that may have caused their child's fever. Middle-ear infection, tonsillitis, and other bacterial infections–when accompanied by fever–are more likely to be attacked with medicines than colds, influenza, or other viral diseases and are more likely to be attacked earlier. Measles, because of its "seriousness" is another candidate for a possible early medical intervention.

A "raised body temperature" never causes any concern or action other than a raised eyebrow or increased parental vigilance. A "regular fever" that does not last longer than two to three days is also not considered dangerous but may lead to first remedial actions. Parents usually have their child go to bed or lie down on a sofa. Most parents would cook an herbal tea or prepare a juice made from boiled onions sweetened with honey. Sweating is looked upon favorably. Placing a cold washcloth on the child's forehead or leaving the child's feet in the bed uncovered is thought to prevent the fever from getting too high.

"Did you consult the physician or give her something?" "No, nothing except tea and our usual procedures; no medicines." "What are your usual procedures?" "First, I give tea and then I put a wet piece of cloth on her forehead. . . . These are our rituals." (Mother of Laura, 7 years)

> My children never got fever suppositories. This is because of my [homeopathic] pediatrician. He is against it and I am quite happy about that. I think that the children even benefit from the fever. . . . No, I don't give them anything. I cook them camomile or peppermint tea or prepare a juice from onions and honey. (Mother of Lia, 7 years)

If medicine is given it tends to be of the "natural" or homeopathic kind:

> "Manuel always had these infections of the tonsils until I had a breakthrough with the help of a homeopathic physician. When he had them again together with a high fever one day, the doctor said 'lets make a fever-kur.' And after that the infection never reappeared."
> "What is a fever kur?"
> "That was his system, he had a real plan. I can't recall each of his steps [and homeopathic medicines employed]. Retrospectively I have the impression that he wanted the fever and provoked it while accompanying it homeopathically with white globuli . . . Since then I can't remember that Manuel had tonsillitis again." (Mother of Manuel, 10 years)

Conventional interventions or the consultation of physicians are rare at the "regular fever" stage. They are more likely to be resorted to when the fever lasts longer than one or two days or when the treatment of a known underlying disease is of great concern. Also physician consultations appeared more frequently among those four parents who lived outside of Hamburg who only had access to conventional therapists. Conventional interventions were more likely to come into play the moment the child's body temperature passed the "high fever" mark, or when the child starts to fantasize. Then all parents become–as they freely admit–extremely anxious. At this point nearly all of them start wrapping towels dipped in cold water around the calves (Wadenwickel) or around the chest (Brustwickel) in order to cool the child's body. Fever-lowering medicine (usually left over from previous applications) is given from the medicine cabinet and the doctor is called. Medicines generally consist of the giving of aspirin or fever suppositories, or of an antibiotic juice (in our example in connection with tonsillitis).

> "When the temperature rises over 39°C [102.2°F] I start to worry."
> "What does that mean?"
> "That means that I consult a physician and wrap bandages around the calves." (Father of Felix, 7 years)

> When the fever approaches 40°C [104°F] I get nervous. I wrap bandages around the calves and call the doctor. Last time Sonja had high fever in conjunction with purulent tonsils our pediatrician visited us from [the other town] and prescribed fever-lowering medication and antibiotic juice. These I had to buy. Usually, I always have fever-lowering medication in the house, but no antibiotics. The antibiotics made the child "fit" fast; they abruptly lowered the fever. But I would like to use antibiotics as little as possible and only give them when necessary. (Mother of Sonja, 8 years)

THE ROLE OF CHILDREN

The children's perceptions and attitudes toward medicines never had any noticeable influence on their parent's choice of treatment. Once a medicine prescribed by a physician or naturopath has won the approval of the mother, nothing else (not even the child's refusal) could stop her from administering it to the child. If a child disliked his/her medicine, spit it out, or even refused to take it, parents (and prescribing physicians) found ingenious ways to literally "sweeten" the medicine intake or change the medicine's form of application (e.g., in the case of pills being hard to swallow or suppositories being too large to insert). Other strategies of parents to get their way include rational argument or force in order to achieve the child's compliance.

> "Did you ever have problems with the giving of medicines? Did he refuse them?"
> "Yes, in the case of penicillin. He had to take it but he did not like its taste . . . . But he had to take it anyhow . . . . I told him to close his nose. Then he had to pour it down his throat. I followed this procedure by giving him a spoonful of sugar. But the giving of penicillin was necessary. They only give it in serious cases." (Mother of Konny, 8 years)

Children's knowledge of medicine was less detailed but in general reflected that of their parents. Children rarely used the word "antibiotics" or "penicillin" and never mentioned the concepts "homeopathic" or "anthroposophic." A few knew that the medicine they took was "natural" or "plant-based" (anthroposophic doctors and naturopaths usually prescribe it) and this implied that the children had already been taught to differentiate between "natural" and "chemical" medicines. Aside from this they were more concerned with the form, color, and taste of medicine regardless of the source. Only when they talked about white globuli ("weiße Kügelchen") it was clear that they referred to homeopathic medicine. They did not object to drugs with a sweet taste, such as homeopathic globuli or conventional tablets and juices–provided they came in such flavors as orange, strawberry, or raspberry but hated drugs that tasted "bitter" (such as penicillin and "plant-based" medicines), "sour," or "like alcohol."

> "Do you like to take medicine?"
> "Well, as I told you, tablets or globuli . . . taste good. Only penicillin does not." (Konny, 8 years)

> "Sometimes my [probably anthroposophic] medicine consists of powder and sometimes of juice. But they are all plant-based medicines."
> "How do they taste?"

"Well, some of them taste horribly. They are made of plants and really taste catastrophically." (Maxi, 10 years)

Parents never granted their younger children autonomy in the taking of medicines. They only trusted their older children to take their medicine themselves, but were usually present when their children took it. Their cautious attitude and their repeated warning that medicine is equivalent to poison told children to be wary of even sweet-tasting medicine, and hopefully prevented them from misusing it in the future.

SUMMARY AND CONCLUSION

While children have little autonomy in the taking of medicines during a concrete sickness episode, parents act out their autonomy in a number of ways. First, it is parents who decide whether or not professional help is to be consulted. What they decide upon depends, among other things, on the parent's judgement of the seriousness of their child's disease, on previous experiences they had with its treatment, and on the availability in their home of folk remedies or conventional drugs that they think are appropriate. Second, if professional help is desired, parents protect their autonomy by selecting a particular type of therapist that fits their view. They might visit a conventional general practitioner or a specialist, consult an unconventional homeopathic or anthroposophic doctor, or go to a naturopath or faith healer. While preferences for either conventional or unconventional practitioners have been shown to correlate with the parent's educational level, they are more likely to be indicative of the degree of interest parents show in popularized "naturalism" and their willingness to pay extra for costs not covered by the state health insurance. Third, once a choice has been made, parents can exert influence on the prescriptions they are receiving or choose to be noncompliant. The parents in our sample did so by letting the doctor know what kind of medicine they would rather not give their children. Fourth, parents can either buy the medicine in the pharmacy–or, if they are uncertain about its appropriateness, visit or talk to another therapist and/or decide not to purchase it. Fifth, if they buy the medicine they still can opt for not giving it at all or for changing the dose or length of application.

> "What did the physician prescribe for Annika's ear infection?"
> "In the beginning ear drops and later always penicillin. I was told to give her the whole package. But one always hears that one should be cautious with penicillin. Therefore I gave it to her for only two to three days. When she got better I stopped giving it."
> (Mother of Annika, 11 years)

We have alluded to the general disdain for antibiotics and to the conditions under which antibiotics are acceptable to even those that favor homeopathic medicine. Even parents faithful toward homeopathy succumb to what they call "allopathic treatment," but only when they think that the seriousness of their child's disease leaves them no other choice.

> I have problems with allopathic medicine. Take antibiotics, for example. Before I give them I have to be really convinced [about them being necessary]. I am not against them principally. For instance, we had an emergency a few nights ago. I felt that way, because I could not reach my naturopath. And then I gave her a tranquillizer for children. She was so anxious; it was terrible. I did not know what to do. All the other things, like wet bandages and so did not help. That is why I gave it to her. As I said, I would use allopathic medicines if there are no other possibilities. It is not that I demonize them. If I do not have the appropriate medicine or if I cannot reach a naturopath I would put an antibiotic ointment on a seriously infected wound. (Mother of 9-year-old Lisa)

Those that use unconventional medicine make a conscious choice. They are well educated, knowledgeable, and critical about what they see as the strengths and weaknesses of modern medicine and are determined to take responsibility and initiative for health and recovery into their own hands. Their trust in the self-regulating powers of the body, and the health-stimulating powers of nature make them lean toward treatments that assumedly strengthen the body rather than suppress the symptoms the body creates to fight the disease. The availability of alternative treatment in large cities such as Hamburg where Germany's pluralistic medical system displays its greatest diversity, makes their choice easy. And private health insurance makes sure that the expense of unconventional doctors are covered.

NOTES

1. The COMAC Childhood and Medicines Project was funded through a European Economic Community (EEC) *Comité d'Action Concerté* (COMAC) contract, COMAC/HSR MR4*-CT90-0319, awarded to The Institute on Child Health, Athens, Greece, with Deanna J. Trakas as the Project Leader. The official title of the Contract was "Medicine Use, Behaviour and Children's Perceptions of Medicines and Health Care."

2. In our sample we ran across one folk healer (a faith healer) who was said to have successfully prayed over warts.

3. BPI = Bundesverband der Pharmazeutischen Industrie e.V., the most important organization representing the interests of the German pharmaceutical industry.

4. A total of 57,000 medicines has been officially registered since 1993 and may be legally sold in Germany.

5. Costs related to screening for cancer and diabetes, to preventive measures (e.g., vaccinations), to the treatment and hospital nursing care of diseases and accidents, to the provision of dental care and dentures, and to check-ups during pregnancy and childbirth.

6. That this is a popular misconception can be shown by pointing out that certain phytopharmaka (Weiss 1985) and even homeopathica in low dilutions, for instance, are anything but "soft" or "safe" but can be quite toxic–and that only a stretch of imagination would allow us to call such unconventional therapies as homeopathy, neural therapy, faith healing or Ayurveda "natural."

REFERENCES

Bundesverband der Pharmazeutischen Industrie e.V. 1993. *Pharma Jahresbericht 1992/93*. Frankfurt.

Clemens, C. 1983. "Arzneien: Ein goldenes Kapitel der Medizingeschichte." *Frau im Spiegel* 24.6.93:30-32.

Commandeur, W. and B. Neumann. 1989. *Heilpraktiker. Die Alternativen Mediziner*. München: Universitas.

Higginbotham, H. N. 1977. "Culture and the role of client expectancy." *Topics in Culture Learning* 5:107-124.

Kleinman, A. 1980. *Patients and Healers in the Context of Culture: An Explora-*

tion of the Borderland Between Anthropology, Medicine, and Psychiatry. Berkeley, CA: Berkeley University Press.

Liebau, K. F. 1988. *Handbuch für die Naturheilkunde.* München: Pflaum Verlag.

Payer, L. 1988. *Medicine and Culture. Varieties of Treatment in the United States, England, West Germany and France.* NY: Henry Holt.

Rothschuh, K. E. 1983. *Naturheilbewegung, Reformbewegung, Alternativbewegung.* Stuttgart: Hippokrates Verlag.

Schott, H. 1993. *Die Chronik der Medizin.* Dortmund: Chronik-Verlag.

Sharma, U. 1992. *Complementary Practitioners Today.* London: Routledge.

Velimirovic, H. and B. Velimirovic. 1983. "The European Region." *Traditional Medicine and Health Care Coverage: A Reader for Health Administrators* edited by R.H. Bannerman, Geneva: WHO, pgs. 240-251.

Waissman, R. 1990. "An analysis of doctor-parent interactions in the case of paediatric renal failure: The choice of home dialysis." *Sociology of Health and Illness 12* (4):422-451.

Weiss, R. F. 1985. *Lehrbuch der Phytotherapie.* Stuttgart: Hippokrates Verlag.

Wolff, O. 1982. *Anthroposophisch Orientierte Medizin und Ihre Heilmittel.* Stuttgart: Verlag Freies Geistesleben.

Chapter 13

Children's Perspectives on Illness and Medicines: Yugoslavia

Ronald J. Iannotti
Nila Kapor

Cross-sectional and longitudinal studies of preschool and school-age children in the United States indicate that factors predicting expectations to take action in response to illness include SES, age, family composition, health locus of control, autonomy, concern about illness, perceived vulnerability to illness, perceived severity of illness, and the perceived benefits of the health action (Bush and Iannotti 1985, 1988, 1990; Bush, Iannotti, and Davidson 1985; Iannotti and Bush 1992). Primary caretaker's beliefs and behaviors had but a small direct effect on the children's expected health behaviors but predicted children's health beliefs.

This research, performed as part of the COMAC[1] Childhood and Medicines Project, also suggests the importance of the child's interpretation of health and illness. The school-age children perceived themselves to have access to medicines and many indicated they independently had taken medicines for a common health problem or had given medicines to another child (Bush, Iannotti, and Davidson 1985; Iannotti and Bush 1992). Children perceive self-care as the most important determinant of health (Green and Bird 1986). Whether by themselves or with others, preadolescents take an active role in the treatment of their minor injuries and illness (Iannotti et al. 1990).

Parents differ in style, with some mothers emphasizing the child's control of health and illness (Iannotti and Bush 1992; Iannotti and O'Brien 1988). Mothers use occasions of minor illness to teach children as young as two about health and illness, varying in the extent to which they attribute responsibility for health and illness to the child or to themselves. Responsibility of the patient in health care and maintenance has not received much attention (Maiman, Becker, and Katlic 1985, 1986) and the role of children in this process needs to be considered (Lewis and Lewis 1982; NCPIE 1989). It is common practice for pediatricians to direct their recommendations for prevention and treatment to parents, not children (Pantell et al. 1982). Further study is needed of the role of children in their own health care and of children's perceptions of illness and health care.

The health belief model, social learning theory, and cognitive developmental theory are the dominant models applied to health behavior and health behavior change (Bush and Iannotti 1985, 1990; Leventhal and Cameron 1987). In their review of the pediatric literature, Burbach and Peterson (1986) conclude that the development of children's understanding of health and illness is consistent with Piaget's theory (Inhelder and Piaget 1964; Piaget 1932) suggesting that there is systematic development in a predictable sequence of stages similar to those proposed by Bibace and Walsh (1979, 1980, 1981). The six stages parallel the preoperational, concrete operational, and formal operational stages of development. In the early stages, children interpret the world in terms of familiar events and experiences. A mixture of physiological, social, and mechanical explanations are combined in novel ways in the middle stages. In the later stages children are willing to speculate on the necessary processes, dealing with them in increasingly more complex ways, until a majority of children arrive at somewhat scientific explanations of birth, conception, illness, or death. There is no evidence of gender differences in any of these studies.

More recently, Iannotti and his colleagues (Iannotti and O'Brien 1993; Iannotti et al. 1993; Obeidallah et al. 1993) interviewed a diverse sample of 600 elementary school children aged six, eight, and ten. The children were interviewed about their understanding of colds, cuts, heart disease, and AIDS and the children's responses were coded using an adaptation of the Bibace and Walsh system. The investigators found a developmental progression but also identified within-child differences depending on the illness. In a related study, understanding of health and illness was unrelated to recent incidents of illness or injury, but was related to children's health attitudes and to efficacy of their response to common health problems (Iannotti et al. 1990).

The current study examines children's health beliefs in a sample of children from Novi Sad. In addition to questions about the children's perceptions of the illness experience, their role in health care, and the use of medicines, the interviews were coded using the Bibace and Walsh categories (1979, 1980, 1981).

METHODS

One preschool and one primary school were randomly selected from the directory of all preschools and primary schools in the city of Novi Sad to participate in the study. A balanced sample of 50 children in each of the three age groups, four, seven, and 11 years of age, were recruited. Children who had symptoms of an existing illness were excluded from the sample.

All interviews were completed in the child's preschool or primary school by two trained graduate students in 1991-1992. Children were asked to think about the last time they needed to stay home from school or could not go outside and play because they were not feeling well. They were then asked to draw what it was like the last time they were ill. After they completed the drawing, children were asked the core interview questions including: How did you know you were ill? What did you do first when you realized you were ill? How do children feel when they are ill? What causes illness? What do children do to get well? Who decides what they should do to get well fast? Coding of the interviews was completed by the second author.

RESULTS

The answers to all but three questions have been classified. The age of the children is an independent variable (four, seven, and 11 years), crossed with 22 dependent variables.

Analysis of the Children's Drawings

The children generally were happy to make the drawings. However, regardless of their sex or age, some showed signs of bewilderment, saying things such as "that can't be drawn." The drawings were very impressive. Some children drew only a point, representing a measles spot. Some drew a huge medical instrument, but most of them drew self-portraits. Forty-two percent of the children presented themselves as lying in bed alone at home.

The drawings were classified as belonging to one of four categories (see Table 13.1). The first category included the drawings in which children were alone (at home, in the hospital, or in some unusual place). The second category comprised drawings in which children were together with their mothers (at home, in the hospital, etc.). The drawings in the third category represented children as being together with their fathers or grandparents. The fourth category included drawings of medicines and medical instruments in isolation or in a context (e.g., a large medicine bottle in a pharmacist's shop).

A chi-square test rejected the null hypothesis at the level of .01. Children made different kinds of drawings depending on their age. The older the children, the more often they drew themselves as being alone and ill. There were no statistically significant differences between the boys and the girls, regardless of their age. It appears that children in all three age groups experienced being alone as something negative. Nine children aged four years drew themselves as being alone at home, and ten as being alone in the hospital. This indicates that the children felt alone wherever they were. They also drew toys (toys were prominent in 14 drawings), and only four children drew their mothers.

Fathers were drawn mostly by four-year-olds. The older the child, the less often a father appeared in the drawings. Fathers appeared in only four drawings made by 11-year-olds. Fathers, as well as third persons—mostly grandparents, sisters and neighbors—were drawn by only 15.3 percent of the children. Fourteen percent of the children made drawings dominated by a medical instrument or a medicine. Most of these drawings were made by seven-year-olds.

TABLE 13.1. Content of Children's Drawings of "What it Was Like the Last Time I Was Sick"*

| | Age in Years | | | |
Drawing Category	Four	Seven	Eleven	Total
1. Alone	22	26	39	87
2. With mother	9	4	6	19
3. With father/ grandparent	11	11	4	23
4. Medicines/ instruments	8	12	1	21
Total Children	50	50	50	150

* Chi-square = 19.52; p < 0.01

It is interesting to note that the four-year-olds often drew pharmacies (beautiful and in bright colors). Their explanations of their drawings were dominated by the attribution of magic importance to pharmacies. It appears from their accounts that they like to be taken to a pharmacy by their parents. They want to be involved in the process of medical treatment (dispensing of medicines). Doctors did not dominate the drawings made by children in this age group. If doctors appeared in the drawings at all (in hospitals and waiting rooms only), they were presented as small round colorful figures. This could mean that four-year-old children are not afraid of doctors. The children described doctors as kind to "their sweet little patients," and the walls in the waiting rooms as covered with posters of cartoon characters. The older the child, the less colorful the waiting room and the less kind the doctors appeared in the drawings. The doctors described by older children often lost their patience, not bothering to explain the disease to the child.

Analysis of the Answers to the Questions

How did you know you were ill?

Answers to the question "How did you know you were ill?" were divided into two categories (see Table 13.2). The first category included answers indicating that it was the child who noticed he or she was ill. The second category included answers indicating that someone else told the child that he or she was ill, e.g., "mama told me." Of the 150 children interviewed, 93.3 percent said they were aware they had fallen ill without being told so by anyone else.

The children knew they were ill by the condition of their throats, nervousness, fever, or "blackened teeth." Eleven-year-olds knew it by their "bad mood," "sleeplessness" and "shivering." Six children replied that they had known they were sick because they were "under stress."

Only 5.3 percent said they knew they were ill because their mother, father, grandmother, or a doctor had told them so; 1.3 percent of the children (four-year-olds) gave vague answers, such as "by a flat tire."

None of the seven-year-old children said they found out about their illness from other people. One 11-year-old boy said he learned he was ill from his grandmother. There was a significant association between age and the categorization of the responses; older children were less likely to say they knew they were sick from somebody else, but significantly more children at each age said they used their own judgement.

Of the four-year-olds, nine had to be told by others that they were ill. Even at this age, most children feel that something is wrong, although their parents usually think they are the ones to notice their child's illness first. This behavior is particularly characteristic of mothers. Some of the children said they had been asked by their mothers how they felt but these mothers did not even listen to their answers because they had already told neighbors about their child's illness.

What did you do first when you realized you were ill?

Children appeared to know exactly what to do first when they discovered they were ill: 56 percent sought help from others, and 44 percent tried to cope with their problem on their own (see Table 13.3). The latter usually went to bed, made themselves a cup of tea, or even took aspirin. The children who were unable to deal with their illness on their own mostly asked their parents to take them to the hospital.

TABLE 13.2. Children's Perceptions of Who Decided They are Sick*

	Age in Years			
Decision maker	Four	Seven	Eleven	Total
Child's Own Judgment	41	50	49	140
Someone Else	9	0	1	10
Total Children	50	50	50	150

* Chi-square = 12.24, p < 0.01

Twenty-two four-year-olds said they had tried to deal with the problem on their own. This answer was provided by 20 seven-year-olds and by 24 11-year-olds. Differences between the three age groups were not striking. Table 13.3 shows no statistical significance. That means that the children saw themselves as reacting well to other illness regardless of their age.

The four-year-olds answered the question by saying "I lay in bed," "I didn't get up," "I cleared my nose" and they all believed they had coped with their illness successfully. Some of them even said they had gone to see a doctor all by themselves. The children were asked additional questions in order to categorize their answers.

Four percent of all the children mentioned a specific emotion as their first reaction to their illness. It is interesting to note that not all emotions mentioned were negative. The children also gave answers such as "I was happy," "I kept jumping up to the ceiling," or "I went to a video outlet right away, rented six videos and felt good about it."

Most of the children, particularly the seven-year-olds, did not know what to do when they realized they were ill. These children felt extremely insecure. They said that they were afraid "I could do something wrong" or that "I didn't know which medicine to take." Some of the answers indicated that the children saw their illness as a temporary respite, a way out of the everyday bustle.

The most elaborate answers were provided by the 11-year-olds. Their reactions depended on their own estimates of their illness. If they thought it was "serious," they sought help. If they thought it

TABLE 13.3. Children's Response to First Realization is Sick*

Response	Age in Years			
	Four	Seven	Eleven	Total
Child Takes Action	22	20	24	66
Child Asks for Help	28	30	26	84
Total Children	50	50	50	150

* Chi-square = 0.65, $p < 0.05$

was an "ordinary" disease, they did not for some time. Children also answered this question at the end of the interview when they were asked "Is there anything else you want to tell me?"

How did you feel when you were ill?

The children gave very different answers to the question depending on their age. The four-year-olds often understood the question as "What were you doing when you were ill?" This question was asked at the end of the interview, by which time the children were capable of identifying with their illness.

Of all the interviewed children, 12 percent said they felt well while they were ill. Fourteen children age four said they felt well even though they were ill. They stuck to this answer no matter what questions were asked. The younger the children, the more "feel well" answers they gave, suggesting that children learn not to feel well from those around them.

Sixteen four-year-olds mentioned unpleasant reactions. Their usual answers were "I vomited" or "there was a lump in my throat." Nine four-year-old children said that they were "terrified" by their illness. Some of the answers suggested that the children were afraid their parents would leave them alone while they were ill. Eleven four-year-old children gave completely vague answers.

Eleven-year-old children were more likely to say they felt "bad," "uncomfortable," "sick," or "sad" while they were ill. Eight of them were afraid, mostly of possible complications and of being sent to the hospital for an operation. Their answers were often difficult to classify as belonging either to the two types; therefore they were categorized on the basis of the overall impression left by the child–whether he or she was really afraid of something (second type) or felt uncomfortable (first type). The chi-square obtained from Table 13.4 indicated that differences related to the age of the respondents were statistically significant. Few 11-year-olds felt good, and eight of them gave vague answers (see Table 13.4).

Children's Beliefs about Illness Cause Relative to Cognitive Development

Studies conducted by Bibace and Walsh (1980, 1981) suggest that children's interpretations of their illness depend on the level of their cognitive development. These interpretations follow certain patterns. Children's answers to the question, "What causes illness?" were classified as belonging to one of seven different categories:

1. *Puzzlement*–when a child does not know what causes illness, says nothing or knows nothing, or knows the cause but is unable to explicate it.
2. *Phenomenism*–when a child says that illness is caused by a concrete external phenomenon. This interpretation of illness is characteristic of children at the preoperational stage of development, aged two to six.
3. *Infection*–when a child sees the cause of illness in people or things he or she comes into contact with (not necessarily physical contact); this explanation is characteristic of older children at the preoperational stage.
4. *Contamination*–when a child differentiates between the cause of illness and the way in which it manifests itself. The child sees the cause of illness in a person, thing, or action regarded as external to the child. There is always an aspect to this cause that is bad or detrimental to the body of the child. The child believes that illness is the result of physical contact with a person or thing or his or her own participation in harmful activities. This interpretation is characteristic of children at the concrete operational stage (approximately age seven to nine).

5. *Internalization*–illness is explained as something internal, although caused by external agents. A person or thing is associated with the internal effects of illness. Children are extremely confused about the functioning of their internal organs. This interpretation is provided by older children at the concrete operational stage.

6. *Physiological Interpretation*–illness is explained in terms of the physiological structure and functioning of internal organs. The cause of illness can be an external event, but its source lies in the malfunctioning of the body. This interpretation is characteristic of children at the formal operational state (11 years).

7. *Psycho-Physiological Interpretation*–is the most mature one. It resembles number six above, but children also quote alternative causes which are of a psychological nature. Children become aware that someone's thoughts and feelings can affect the course of an illness.

The four-year-olds usually provided phenomenist interpretations, claiming that illness is caused by "air," "popcorn," "fingers," etc. Ten children described illness as something "infectious." They said their friends from kindergarten passed on their illness to them, although they did not know how. Four children said participation in harmful activities leads to being ill. They noticed a difference between the cause of an illness and its manifestation.

TABLE 13.4. Children's Feelings When They Are Sick*

Feelings	Age in Years			
	Four	Seven	Eleven	Total
Unpleasant	16	28	32	76
Scared	9	13	8	30
Well	14	2	2	18
No Reply	11	7	8	26
Total Children	50	50	50	150

* Chi-square = 23.87; $p < 0.001$

Twenty seven-year-old children provided "contamination" interpretations, saying, for instance, that "you fall ill if you don't wear warm clothes or if you drink cold water and your kidneys get too cold." They often said they had fallen ill because they had not "listened to mama." When asked to be more specific, they said their mothers took care of their health by, for instance, not allowing them to drink cold water after physical exercise or walk without their socks on. Seven children in this age group provided type-five interpretations (see Table 13.5). The terms they used were often completely inappropriate. Five children gave phenomenist interpretations, saying, for instance, that the cause of illness was a "dirty planet" or "dirty water." One explanation of this response is that some of the children learned about ecology in school. The children seem to have missed the meaning of most of what the teacher said. Their answers were not clear enough. They could say what causes illness, but they failed to say how.

The thirty 11-year-olds who provided contamination and internalization interpretations were equally divided between the two categories. Physiological interpretations, which were expected to be more prevalent in this age group, were provided by six children. Only three children explained illness by referring to a person's

TABLE 13.5. Developmental Categories of Children's Understanding of the Cause of Illness*

Category	Age in Years			Total
	Four	Seven	Eleven	
Phenomenism	34	19	5	58
Contamination/ Internalization	4	27	30	61
Physiological/ Psychophysiological	0	0	9	9
Did Not Understand	12	4	6	22
Total Children	50	50	50	150

* Chi-square = 56.42; $p < 0.001$

psychological state, saying, for instance, that a person who is always in a bad mood is more likely to be taken ill than a person who laughs often. Some of the children emphasized healthful living styles as a precondition for not falling ill.

Assuming that interpretations in terms of phenomenology and proximity to an infectious agent are characteristic of the preoperational stage, interpretations referring to contamination and internalization are characteristic of the concrete operational stage, and physiological and psycho-physiological interpretations are characteristic of the formal operational stage, the children's responses could be categorized as follows:

- 34 four-year-olds were at the preoperational stage, and four were at the concrete operational stage (12 children could not be classified);
- 19 seven-year-olds were at the preoperational stage, and 27 were at the concrete operational stage (four children could not be classified);
- 30 11-year-olds were at the concrete operational stage and nine at the formal operational stage (11 children could not be classified).

As indicated in Table 13.5, the responses followed an age-dependent pattern; Chi-square = 56.419; p < .01. Responses were significantly more sophisticated in older children. Sixty-eight percent of the four-year-olds provided phenomenist and infection-type explanations of illness. Fifty-four percent of the seven-year-olds provided contamination and internalization type explanations. Eighteen percent of the eleven-year-olds explained illness as physiological and psycho-physiological.

What Children Do to Get Well and Who Decides What They Should Do

The questionnaires also contained the question: "How did you get well and what did you do to get well?" Children provided similar answers regardless of age. An attempt was made to divide the children's answers into two categories: one comprised of answers emphasizing conventional methods for treating illness, e.g.,

"I drank medicines to get well," the other included answers emphasizing alternative methods. However, the children mixed conventional and alternative methods in 89 percent of the cases.

The most interesting answers were provided by the youngest children, who said things such as "I drank tea," or "I lay in bed and took
medicines." Some of the children dwelt on this question more than
on any other one, describing details of their medical treatment at
length. Changes in diet were of utmost importance to them. This is
characteristic of this region, where it is believed that "health enters
the body through the mouth." The children said their mothers and
grandmothers were the best experts on this. Many of the children
stressed the importance of tea, even attributing a magic component to
it. Tea was followed on the list of foods with medical properties by
soup, farina, and mashed potatoes. These child-raising practices are
certainly determined by the culture in which a child lives.

The children often said that medicines could never be as good as
the above-mentioned foods. Some of the children spoke of compresses and "wet handkerchiefs" as something "strangling but
helpful." A relatively large number of children said that they had
been to practitioners of alternative medical techniques. All four-
year-olds said lying in bed was necessary.

The answers provided by the seven-year-olds were similar to
each other. All of the children mentioned lying in bed and taking
medicines and a few children mentioned drinking tea. The situation
was the same with the 11-year-olds, although their answers were
often accompanied by explanations of medicines. Children at this
age understand that the outcome of their medical treatment depends
primarily on the medicine they use (the adjectives used by the
respondents were "bad," "good," "universal," etc.).

In 40.7 percent of the cases, the children said that a doctor decided which medicine they were to take, and in 35.3 percent the
mother was said to make the decision. Although overall there was
little difference between mothers and doctors, the following observations deserve attention:

• the older the child, the less influence the mother has in deciding which medicine should be taken;

TABLE 13.6. Children's Perceptions of Who Decided What Treatment They Should Have*

Decision Maker	Age in Years			
	Four	Seven	Eleven	Total
Doctor	8	20	33	61
Mother	23	20	10	53
Father/Somebody Else	15	8	3	26
Child	4	2	4	10
Total Children	50	50	50	150

* Chi-square = 25.82, p < 0.001

- it is exactly the opposite with doctors. Eight four-year-olds believed that the doctor made the decision. This view was held by 20 seven-year-olds and 33 eleven-year-olds (66 percent). (See Table 13.6.)

A small number of children (6.7 percent) believed they themselves decided what medical treatment they should be given. As for the father's role, the older the child, the less important the father. Fifteen fathers made decisions on medical treatment in the four-year-old group, and three fathers in the eleven-year-old group.

DISCUSSION

There were statistically significant age differences in children's drawings on the theme "what it was like the last time I was ill." The younger children drew themselves as being together with their mothers (and fathers), and the older children usually presented themselves as being alone. The inclusion of fathers in the drawings was unexpected because it does not conform with the Serbian culture's prevailing image of fathers. Specifically, it is believed that fathers become interested in their parental role only after their children are older. However, the fathers in this sample were all young fathers from urban communities, where fathers are expected to participate in child care. This pattern of behavior is almost un-known in rural communities, where the results would probably be different.

However, fathers and others appeared in only a small percentage of the drawings. This could mean that fathers play only a minor role in caring for sick children. We can only make limited inferences on the basis of these drawings; it could simply mean that children rarely draw their fathers when representing their own illness graphically.

Seven-year-old children often drew medical instruments when representing a recent illness. Children at this age may be upset by or perhaps even afraid of medical instruments. (Most of the children drew injections.) They appear to identify an illness with its treat-ment. This response was more prevalent in seven-year-olds than four- or 11-year-olds. However, that does not necessarily mean that four-year-olds are less afraid of injections than seven-year-olds. It may be that four-year-olds draw what they know or can, rather than what is really happening. Or it may be that the fear of these proce-dures deter four-year-olds from drawing them.

Consistent with the results of previous studies, children thought that they were aware of being ill and played a role in their own treatment (Bush, Iannotti, and Davidson 1985; Green and Bird 1986; Iannotti and Bush 1992; Iannotti et al. 1990). The results illustrated in Tables 13.2 and 13.3 seem unlikely to have been a coincidence. They could be applied to most children in Yugoslavia. Children seem to know they are sick even before those around them do. As in the interpretation of the answers provided by the four-year-olds, it is questionable to what extent the children were aware of what was really happening. However, their answers must not be rejected outright.

The feeling of discomfort during illness was more pronounced in older children, i.e., the older the children, the less well they said they felt. Most seven-year-old children felt fear. Again, there is the question of interpreting the answers provided by the youngest chil-dren (especially the "feel good" answers). The four-year-olds re-garded illness as something external. It was completely outside them, and therefore they had nothing to be afraid of, i.e., you cannot be afraid of something you do not know. Older children regarded illness as localized inside the body. Their fear was as concrete as their illness.

The categorization of the children's responses into levels corresponding with cognitive stages (Bibace and Walsh, 1980, 1981) suggests that most four-year-olds were at the preoperational stage, most seven-year-olds at the concrete operational stage, and, contrary to our expectations, most eleven-year-olds were still not at the formal operational stage. Why? Two possible answers to this question are:

- our children really enter the formal operational stage later (after age 11);
- a question about an abstract illness may not have provoked physiological and psycho-physiological interpretations from the children. Perhaps children would have provided different answers and more of them would have been classified as being at the formal operational stage if they had been asked what causes a cold or a heart attack.

However, these results are consistent with those found by Iannotti in a large sample of six-, eight-, and ten-year-olds (Iannotti and O'Brien 1993; Iannotti et al. 1993; Obeidallah et al. 1993). Iannotti asked questions about specific health problems, colds, cuts, heart disease, and AIDS, and found a considerable range within age groups. Most of the ten-year-old children did not demonstrate reasoning at the formal operational level. More important Iannotti interviewed approximately 500 parents and found that many of the parents did not think about illness (AIDS) in a manner consistent with formal operational reasoning, the highest level in the Bibace and Walsh (1980) system. Therefore, it appears that the results are consistent with similar work in the USA and may reflect either that different levels of thought are applied to health issues or that children may not reach formal operational levels in all content areas at the same time.

There may have been methodological problems with the categorization of children's responses using the system developed by Bibace and Walsh (1980). Some 11-year-olds listened to other children's answers or agreed among themselves what answers they would give. They may have observed that the interviewer dwelt on this question particularly long and inferred that this must have been one of the most important questions. This may have happened because five 11-year-olds were questioned on the first day and the rest of the children from this age group were questioned a week later. In the intervening period (Easter holidays), the children may have agreed among themselves on how to answer this question because they were all from the same neighborhood. In future studies, an effort should be made to interview children within the same period. However, in the studies conducted by Iannotti (Iannotti and O'Brien 1993; Iannotti et al. 1993; Obeidallah et al. 1993) an effort was made to interview all children within a grade on the same day or within a period of three days. It could be that children's discussion of answers with peers may not have a significant short-term effect on their understanding of health and illness.

The levels of understanding may also help to explain the response to the other questions. Older children appear to take a more active role in their own health. They also place more emphasis on physiological causes and cures. For example, it is now possible to understand the children's answers to the question about what they do to get well. The four-year-olds attached importance to the mother and her medicines, the seven-year-olds found the mother and the doctor equally important, while the eleven-year-olds thought the doctor and medicines were more important. The results from Table 13.6 are not random. There is a significant difference among different age groups regarding decisions on medical treatment.

The comparison with the results of studies conducted by Iannotti and Bush would suggest that the pattern of older children playing a more active role in their own care is consistent across cultures. Cross-cultural difference may be more evident in the affective responses to illness and in the roles of different caregivers, i.e., mothers, fathers, doctors, etc. Further research should examine transcultural elements in child-raising regarding health.

NOTE

1. The COMAC Childhood and Medicines Project was funded through a European Economic Community (EEC) *Comité d'Action Concerté* (COMAC) contract, COMAC/HSR MR4*-CT90-0319, awarded to The Institute on Child Health, Athens, Greece, with Deanna J. Trakas as the Project Leader. The official

title of the Contract was "Medicine Use, Behaviour and Children's Perceptions of Medicines and Health Care." In addition, portions of this research were supported by a grant to the first author from the USA NIH National Institute of Mental Health (MH47252).

REFERENCES

Bibace, R. and Walsh, M. E. 1979. "Developmental stages in children's conceptions of illness." *Health Psychology*, edited by G. Stone, F. Cohen, and N. Adlert. Washington: Jossey-Bass, pgs. 285-301.

Bibace, R. and Walsh, M. 1980. "Development of children's concepts of illness." *Pediatrics* 66:913-917.

Bibace, R. and Walsh, M. E. 1981. Children's conceptions of illness. *Children's Conceptions of Health, Illness, and Bodily Functions*, edited by R. Bibace and M. E. Walsh. San Francisco: Jossey-Bass, pgs. 31-48.

Burbach, D. J. and Peterson, L. 1986. "Children's concepts of physical illness: A review and critique of the cognitive developmental literature." *Health Psychology* 5:307-325.

Bush, P. J. and Iannotti, R. J. 1985. "The development of children's health orientations and behaviors: Lessons for substance abuse prevention." *The Etiology of Drug Abuse*, edited by C. L. Jones and R. J. Battjes. National Institute on Drug Abuse Monograph 56, DHHS Pub. No. (ADM)85-1335. Washington, DC. Supt. of Docs., U.S. Govt Print. Off., pgs. 45-54.

Bush, P. J. and Iannotti, R. J. 1988. "The origins and stability of children's health beliefs relative to medicine use." *Social Science and Medicine* 27: 345-355.

Bush, P. J. and Iannotti, R. J. 1990. "A children's health belief model." *Medical Care* 28:69-86.

Bush, P. J., Iannotti, R. J., and Davidson, F. R. 1985. "A longitudinal study of children and medicines." *Topics in Pharmaceutical Sciences*, edited by D. D. Breimer and P. Speiser. Elsevier Science Publishers B. V., pgs. 391-403.

Green, K. E. and Bird, J. E. 1986. "The structure of children's beliefs about health and illness." *Journal of School Health* 56:325-328.

Iannotti, R. J. and Bush, P. J. 1992. "The development of autonomy in children's health behaviors." *Emotion, Cognition, Health, and Development in Children and Adolescents: A Two-Way Street*, edited by E.J. Susman, L. V. Feagans, and W. Ray. Hillsdale, NJ: Lawrence Erlbaum, pgs. 53-74.

Iannotti, R. J. and O'Brien, R. W. 1988 (November). "Parental and peer influences on the health practices of urban black preschool children." Presented Annual Meeting American Public Health Association, Boston.

Iannotti, R. J. and O'Brien, R. W. 1993 (March). "A cognitive-developmental approach to children's and parents' understanding of AIDS." Presented Annual Meeting Society for Research in Child Development, New Orleans.

Iannotti, R. J., O'Brien, R. W., Cowen, E., and Wilson, K. 1990 (March). "Understanding and response to minor injury and illness among pre-adolescents." Presented Conference on Human Development, Richmond.

Iannotti, R. J., O'Brien, R. W., Obeidallah, D., and Turner, P. 1993 (March). "AIDS: Relations between understanding and knowledge in children and parents." Presented Annual Meeting Society for Research in Child Development, New Orleans.

Inhelder, B. and Piaget, J. 1964. *The Early Growth of Logic in the Child*, translated by E. A. Lunzer and D. Papert. London: Routledge and Kegan Paul.

Lewis, C. E. and Lewis, M. A. 1982. "Children's health-related decision making." *Health Education Quarterly* 9(2):129-141, 9(3):225-237.

Leventhal, H. and Cameron, L. 1987. "Behavioral theories and the problem of compliance." *Patient Education and Counseling* 10:117-138.

Maiman, L. A., Becker, M. H., and Katlic, A. W. 1985. "How mothers treat their children's physical symptoms." *Journal of Community Health* 10:136-155.

Maiman, L. A., Becker, M. H., and Katlic, A. W. 1986. "Correlates of mothers' use of medications for their children." *Social Science and Medicine* 22:41-51.

National Council on Patient Information and Education. 1989. *Children and America's Other Drug Problem: Guidelines for Improving Prescription Medicine Use among Children and Teenagers*. Washington, DC: NCPIE.

Obeidallah, D. A., Turner, P. L., Iannotti, R. J., O'Brien, R. W., Haynie, D., and Galper, D.I. 1993. "Investigating children's knowledge and understanding of AIDS." *Journal of School Health* 63:125-129.

Pantell, R. H., Stewart, T. J., Dias, J. K., Wells, P., and Ross, A. W. 1982. "Physician communication with children and parents." *Pediatrics* 70: 396-402.

Piaget, J. 1932. *The Moral Judgement of the Child*, translated by M. Gabain, NY: Harcourt, Brace and World.

Chapter 14

Self-Medication Among Families with Children in Jyväskylä, Finland

Riitta Ahonen
Olli Kalpio
Tuula Vaskilampi
Outi Hallia

Self-care is the most common way people handle acute symptoms (Tibblin 1984; Lilja 1988). Self-care can be defined as an intentional behavior that a layperson takes on his or her own behalf or on behalf of family, friends, or community, to promote health or to treat illness (Levin, Katz, and Holst 1976; Levin and Idler 1983). Families treat most of the minor medical complaints and illnesses of their children that last only a few days at home by means of self-care without seeking professional help (Dahlqvist et al. 1987). People may also pursue self-care after consultation with a physician. Thus self-care is supplementary to, not necessarily compensatory for, professional health care.

Self-medication forms a part of self-care. There are several definitions for the concept of self-medication (c.f., Fryklöf and Westerling 1984). In this chapter, we use the concept self-medication as synonymous with the use of nonprescribed drugs, i.e., those sold "over-the-counter" (OTC) without a doctor's prescription.

There are about 3,700 pharmaceutical products on the market in Finland; about one-fifth are OTC drugs. When a new pharmaceutical product obtains its sales license, the Finnish National Agency for Medicines decides whether the drug will be a prescription only

(Rx) or an OTC drug. This decision can be changed afterwards if the medicine is regarded safe enough to be used for self-medication.

In Finland, pharmaceutical products (OTC or Rx) can only be bought from pharmacies and Rx drugs are impossible to obtain without a doctor's prescription. Public pharmacies are staffed by qualified personnel (with three- or five-year university degrees), who have the sole right to sell and dispense medicines. Finnish pharmacies are strictly professional, with over 90 percent of the turnover represented by licensed medicines.

Due to the strict control of pharmaceuticals exercised by the state, health officials can easily regulate the health behavior of the population, including self-medication, through government policy. The official health policy in Finland during the 1970s and early 1980s tended to guide people toward use of professional health care services. This was a result of the Primary Health Care Act introduced in 1972, which provided all citizens with free access to health services. This act also resulted in a rapid increase in the resources allocated to primary health care. At the same time, new medical faculties were established to train more physicians for health centers established all over the country. The primary health care services, including visits to health center physicians, have been free of charge since 1993, when a small fee was introduced. As a result of these changes, the use of health services (especially visits to physicians) increased during the late 1970s (Kalimo et al. 1982).

These changes in the Finnish health policy were also reflected in the use of medicines. According to the nationwide surveys conducted by the Finnish Social Insurance Institution, the proportion of adult users of prescription drugs was 44 percent in 1968, 45 percent in 1976, and 61 percent in 1987 (Klaukka, Martikainen, and Kalimo 1990). This increase in the use of prescription drugs coincided with a decrease in OTC drug use. In 1968, the proportion of users of OTC medicines during the two days prior to interview was 30 percent but fell to 24 percent in 1976 and then rose again to 35 percent in 1987. The increase in the proportion of OTC drug users in the late 1980s was accounted for by a growth in the use of vitamins and mineral supplements, with the use of other OTC medicines remaining at the same level from 1976 to 1987. Among children under 15 years of age, the growth in prescription drug use was faster than among adults and the proportion of users in 1987 (12 percent) was three times greater than in 1964 (4 percent).

During the late 1980s and early 1990s, the public health policy changed due to the economic recession experienced in Finland. Furthermore, there was great political pressure to reduce the costs of health care. The public was encouraged to assume more responsibility for its own health, with great emphasis being placed on self-care. These attempts to reduce costs also led to changes in drug policy and drug use, reflected in the last four years by a tendency to switch medicines from prescription only to OTC status. For instance, ibuprofen, ketoprofen, several cough remedies (pholcodine, bromhexine, dextromethorphan), and decongestants (xylometazoline, oxymetatzoline), which could earlier only be obtained on prescription, are now available from pharmacies as OTC medicines. Most of these medicines also include indications for children.

The public marketing by mass media of these "former prescription drugs" has been aggressive. "Now without a prescription . . ." has been one of the leading slogans in advertisements. Sales statistics show that the consumption of ibuprofen, for instance, increased twelvefold since becoming available as an OTC drug (Ahonen et al. 1991; FSM 1993). There are, however, no studies on the use of these former prescription drugs; neither do we know how the attitudes and beliefs of the public changed in response to the change in status of these drugs.

In this chapter we describe the kinds of medicines kept available at home by families with children. We also analyze the perceptions and attitudes that the parents have about self-medication for some common symptoms concerning their children and themselves. Special attention is paid to those OTC drugs that have formerly been available on prescription only.

MATERIALS AND METHODS

The study formed a part of the COMAC Childhood and Medicines Project,[1] and thus the methodology and the selection criteria for the study sample were guided by the international study group (see Chapter 2). In Finland, the study was carried out in Jyväskylä, a town with 71,200 inhabitants in central Finland. Two neighborhood schools, Halssila and Kypärämäki were chosen on the basis of their demographic structure (middle-class families) and the availability of statistical data. Seventy children were interviewed at school in the first stage of the study. In the second stage of the study, 51 children and 46 parents were interviewed at home. The selection of the children and the methodology of the Finnish study is represented in more detail elsewhere (Vaskilampi et al. 1994; see also Chapter 2, this volume).

During the interview with parents, a questionnaire, the Medicine Cabinet Inventory (MCI) was left to obtain quantitative data about medicines kept in the households. The parents were asked to list by brand names all of the medicines they had in their homes. In addition, questions concerning the use of medicines (e.g., who used it and when, where stored, when purchased) were included (see Chapter 5, this volume). The brand names were later coded according to therapeutic categories also described in Chapter 5.

The parents returned the medicine inventory questionnaire by mail to the researchers. Of 46 households receiving the questionnaire, 40 families returned it, thus representing information on 197 family members (Table 14.1).

The main caretaker of each child was interviewed at home. In most families this was said to be the mother (38/46), and in the remainder of cases, the father (8/46). In four interviews, both parents were present during the interview, although only one of them answered most of the questions.

The interview was conducted as an open theme discussion. Although the interview focused on the child, it was also used for gathering background information on the family. Questions were asked concerning the socioeconomic background, the medical history of the family, and the use of various treatments. Themes focusing on self-medication and OTC drugs were also discussed.

RESULTS

Medicines at Home

Of the 40 households that returned the MCI questionnaire, two indicated they had not a single medicine at home; 13 indicated only

TABLE 14.1. Household Members by Gender and Age Group

Age in Years	Female	Male	Total
≥ 3	1	2	3
3 - 14	42	40	82
15 - 24	10	13	23
25 - 44	36	33	69
45 - 64	10	10	20
≥ 65	0	0	0
Total	99	98	197

OTC medicines, two only Rx medicines, and the remaining 25 households indicated medicines from both of these drug categories. OTCs constituted 59 percent of all 320 medicine packages stored at home and these represented 190 different brand names; Rx medicines represented 38 percent, and 2.5 percent were not categorized.

The average number of medicines was about eight per household. For OTC medicines, the average number/household was 4.8 (± 3.0 S.D.) and for Rx medicines 3.1 (± 3.4 S.D.). Altogether, 312 medicines were later coded according to the therapeutic groupings presented in Chapter 5. Analgesics and antipyretics, including NSAIDs, were the most often kept OTC drugs in homes, followed by topical products and vitamin and mineral supplements (Table 14.2). These three drug groups constituted 63 percent of all OTCs. As can be seen in Table 14.2, the order according to therapeutic grouping of medicines was somewhat different from that for prescribed medicines.

The three most popular medicines stored in homes were all OTCS: Panadol® (in 17 households), Disperin® (in 13 households), Burana® (in 10 households). All these are analgesics: paracetamol, acetylsalicylic acid (ASA), and ibuprofen respectively. Other typical medicines available at home were cough/cold remedies, topical products for skin problems, (e.g., corticosteroids), antihistamines, and tablets for diarrhea. An example of the typical content of a household's medicine cabinet can be seen in Table 14.3.

TABLE 14.2. Medicines in the Household by Therapeutic Category

Therapeutic Category	OTC		RX		All[1]	
	%	n	%	n	%	n
Analgesic/antipyretic (incl.NSAID)	33.2	63	10.6	13	24.3	76
Vitamin/mineral	13.7	26	0.8	1	8.7	27
Topical (mainly for skin)	15.8	30	23.0	28	18.6	58
Gastrointestinal[2]	11.1	21	0.8	1	7.1	22
Eye/nose/ear	6.3	12	24.6	30	13.5	42
Cough/cold[3]	12.6	24	11.5	14	12.2	38
Antiinfective	0	0	0	0	0	0
Antihistamine	3.1	6	8.2	10	5.1	16
Antiasthmatic	0	0	6.6	12	3.8	12
Psychotropic	0	0	9.8	8	2.6	8
Other	4.2	8	4.1	5	4.1	13
Total	100.0	190	100.0	122	100.0	312

[1] eight medicines indeterminate.
[2] includes antidiarrheal, antacid, laxative, and other stomach medicines.
[3] includes decongestants, sore throat medicines, antitussives/expectorants, combinations.

Families with only one child had more prescribed medicines at home than those with two or more children (Table 14.4). However, no such relationship was found with the number of OTC drugs. Also, no correlation was found between the number of medicines stored at home and family income.

About 44 percent of all OTC medicines kept at home were used by female and 34 percent by male family members; 15 percent of

TABLE 14.3. Typical Medicines in a Jyväskylä Household

Brand Name	Generic Name	Purpose Last Use	Who Used It
Burana®	ibuprofen	headache	mother
Panadol®	paracetamol	fever	female child
Disperin®	ASA[1]	headache	father
Coldrex®	ASA with vit. C	headache	mother
Fortus®	combination	cough	female child
Betnovate®	betamethasone topical	unknown	female child
Strepsils®	dichlorbenzyl-alcohol	sore throat	mother
Tavegyl®	clemastine	itching/chicken pox	mother
Hydrocortisone	hydrocortisone topical	skin problems	female child

[1]ASA: aspirin (acetylsalicylic acid).

the medicines had multiple users (Table 14.5). Male children were found to use more Rx medicines than female children but slightly fewer OTCs.

Self-Medication Reported by Parents

Although the families had OTC medicines at home, many of the parents doubted their effectiveness compared to prescribed ones. Some of the parents had, however, positive experiences with OTC medicines (e.g., analgesics). Those OTC medicines that had earlier been prescription-only status were regarded as especially powerful. Some of the parents thought that "they have taken away some of the most active substances from (OTCs compared with Rxs)."

A child's sickness was usually first treated with nonpharmacological remedies such as rest and hot or cold drinks. OTC medicines were also used, but these were not the drugs of first choice; instead they usually formed only part of the treatment. Many parents

TABLE 14.4. Average Number of Medicines in the Household According to Family Size

Number of Family Members	OTC		Rx*	
	Mean	Std Dev ±	Mean	Std Dev ±
3	4.62	4.03	4.75	5.31
4	4.73	2.68	2.93	2.76
5	5.00	3.01	2.28	2.70
6	4.00	3.00	2.66	3.05
Total	4.75	3.01	3.05	3.39

* OTC: over the counter; Rx: prescription only.

emphasized that they did not give medicines to a child unless it was absolutely necessary. Most of the parents reported that they first needed to "analyze the situation" and asked the child to rest. Symptoms and changes in the state of the child were observed for a time before further actions were taken, e.g., give a medicine or seek professional care. If the illness continued or the symptoms become more serious, the parents then decided to contact a doctor. This was often reported to be done in order to obtain a more effective medicine (i.e., prescription medicine). If the parents themselves became sick or showed minor symptoms (e.g., headache), they often used OTC medicines more readily than they had done with their children.

Treating Coughs

For cough, nonmedical treatments (e.g., hot drinks, rest, garlic with warm milk) were mentioned as the treatment of first choice. The most common opinion about the treatment of cough was that "cough goes away by coughing." Most of the parents, however, said they use cough medicines themselves and also for their children if "the cough gets bad" or if it disturbs sleep during the night. They used both OTC and prescribed cough remedies, although most of the parents shared the opinion that "cough remedies don't really cure the cough, they just make you feel a little bit better." Most of

TABLE 14.5. Number and Percentage of Household Medicines by User's Age and Sex

User	OTC		Rx		Both*	
	%	n	%	n	%	n
Males						
≤ 3 years	1.8	3	0.8	1	1.4	4
3 - 14 years	13.4	22	30.0	36	20.5	58
15 - 24 years	3.0	5	5.1	6	3.8	11
25 - 44 years	14.0	23	11.7	14	13.0	37
45- 64 years	1.8	3	7.5	9	4.2	12
Females						
≤ 3 years	-	-	-	-	-	-
3 - 14 years	15.4	25	17.6	21	16.2	46
15 - 24 years	2.4	4	-	-	1.4	4
25 - 44 years	23.9	39	20.1	24	22.2	63
45 - 64 years	1.8	3	3.0	4	2.5	7
Multiple children < 15 years	4.3	7	-	-	2.5	7
Multiple adults ≥ 15 years	3.0	5	1.7	2	2.5	7
Multiple children and adults	7.3	12	-	-	4.2	12
Unknown	7.9	13	2.5	3	5.6	16
Total	100.0	164	100.0	120	100.0	284

* 16 medicines unknown.

the parents regarded prescribed cough medicines to be more effective than the OTCs, however, some parents reported that there are no real differences between them. Some parents admitted that when some of the family members get a cough, a prescription cough medicine is used even though the medicine was prescribed earlier for another person.

The parents knew that there are two kinds of cough remedies: expectorants and antitussives. They also said that the choice between the two categories of cough medicines depends on the type of cough; for an irritating cough they used an antitussive and for bringing up mucous they used expectorants. Surprisingly few brand names were mentioned in the interview (e.g., Silomat,® Vicks Formula 44®), although questionnaires revealed that many of the families had cough medicines at home.

Only a few parents talked about those OTC cough medicines that had previously been only available on prescription. One mother (a nurse) commented that, "One good cough medicine has now been switched from prescription to OTC . . . it's a good choice for prescription-only medicines, but I have not bought it myself. It's Silomat® (clobutinol) and has been on prescription before. One little substance is missing compared with the same prescription drug. But nowadays you can buy better medicines from pharmacies than about three years ago. The Social Insurance System doesn't take responsibility for these things nowadays for economic reasons, thus we have better opportunities for treating symptoms with OTCs so that you do not need to see a doctor for every reason . . . ."

Treating the Common Cold and Fever

In addition to medicines, other treatments for the common cold were first mentioned. These included hot drinks, sleeping, breathing hot steam, and onion juice. The parents reported that they usually did not give medicines to the children for the common cold. If the child had a fever, then antipyretics were given. The most commonly used medicine for fever was Panadol® (paracetamol) for children and Disperin® (ASA combined with antacid) or Aspirin® for adults. Some of the parents also reported giving aspirin to their children in dosages of half a tablet. Other cold remedies used included Burana® (ibuprofen), Coldrex®, Fortal-C 200®, Posivil® (fixed combinations of ASA, caffeine, and vitamin C), although these fixed combinations were seen as medicines more especially intended for treatment of the common cold than the single ingredient products, which were also used for pain and aches. This is a reflection of the drug advertisements; fixed combinations of ASA and vitamin C are marketed as "common cold medicines," whereas single ingredient products are claimed to be effective for both common colds and pains and aches.

The use of vitamin C as a preventive measure, but also as a treatment for the common cold, was mentioned by several parents. One of them commented that "if you take vitamin C daily, you don't get a cold during the whole winter." If a family member had a cold, many families took large doses (one gram twice a day) of vitamin C, e.g., effervescent tablets with large doses of vitamin C. One negative aspect of these tablets commented on by parents was the good taste of the bubbly orange or lemon flavored drink, which tempted the children to drink too much of it ("like soft drinks").

Two medicines, which were previously on prescription-only status, were also mentioned for the treatment of common colds and fevers. These were Burana® (ibuprofen) and Nasolin® (a nasal decongestant containing xylometazoline). The same mother mentioned Silomat® and talked about Nasolin®:

> This nose spray was before on prescription only; it is now an OTC. We have used it when the nose is so stuffed up that you can't sleep. It really helps you to breathe better. I got these dosage regimens (and the prescription, too) from an ear specialist when the children were smaller and have used it when needed. It's Nasolin® nose spray, which takes away the inflammation from the nose and really helps you to breathe. You can use it for both adults and children.

Treating Pains and Aches

Analgesics (including nonsteroidal antiinflammatories [NSAIDs]) were the most frequently mentioned drugs in interviews with the parents. The general opinion (with some exceptions mentioned later) was that "you should not take a painkiller immediately yourself and especially not give them to children at the first opportunity." One comment of a mother is very descriptive in this respect:

> I myself have a headache when I have a lot of stress and then I feel guilty if I take Panadol®, but I do it after some serious consideration. If the headache is not over by late afternoon, then I have to turn to medicine for relief . . . Then, if you have a lot to think about and you do not feel able to concentrate,

then you have to take it (tablet) . . . But this happens very seldom . . . usually it is rest that helps . . . .

There was an exception to this "general cautiousness" in treating pains with medicines. The three nurses (mothers) in the study stated that children should not need to suffer from, for instance, headache, when effective medicines are available.

The parents pointed out that children rarely have pains, although headache was the most frequently mentioned. For headache, Panadol® (paracetamol) was the drug of first choice for children and ASA (Disperin,® Aspierin®) and ibuprofen (Burana®) for the parents. Some parents reported that they gave half a tablet of aspirin to their children for headache. Growing pains were also mentioned by several parents, for which massage of the legs, hot baths, and warm or cold dressings were the nonpharmacological treatments most frequently used. The medicines that were used for growing pains were the same as for headache. In addition to these, vitamin B was also used.

It was interesting that many of the parents talked about the strengths of analgesics, e.g., 200 milligrams, 400 milligrams, 500 milligrams. They felt that the more milligrams contained in a tablet, the more effective the medicine would be. One father, however, compared aspirin and ibuprofen in this respect:

"I don't get pain relief from Disperin® even though I take 500 milligrams twice, but one 400-milligram Burana® helps me quickly . . . " One slogan in the marketing campaign of Burana® has been, "Now twice the strength of before . . . Burana® 400 milligrams." This is because when ibuprofen was switched from Rx status to OTC status in 1986 it was initially only available as 200 milligram (mg.) strength and it was not until two years later that 400 mg. tablets also became available OTC.

Inappropriate use of analgesics was not found with the exception of two parents who reported that they would use analgesics (Burana®) for stomachache. On the other hand, another two parents pointed out that analgesics can cause gastrointestinal disorders. These two parents also mentioned that it is possible to abuse analgesics and become dependent on them. Other side effects of analgesics were not mentioned in the interviews with the parents.

Treating Stomach Problems

Parents reported that their children have several kinds of stomach problems but they usually are harmless, e.g., stomachache due to stress or tension, diarrhea or vomiting caused by viral infections, and do not need to be treated with medicines. Diet, rest, and special drinks or food were the nonpharmacolocigal treatments most commonly mentioned. Although the parents talked considerably about the stomach problems of their children, they rarely spoke of such problems as affecting themselves.

For diarrhea, soft drinks (yellow Jaffa) and dietary changes were the most common forms of treatment. Lactophilus powder (acidophilus bacteria) was mentioned by several parents as well as Tannopon® tablets (opium extract), which were used with children, despite the warning on the package that the tablets are to be used "for children under 12 years only according to doctor's prescription." The parents, however, stressed that they give only half a tablet of Tannopon®. In addition, Carbo® tablets were reportedly used as well as liquid mineral supplements (Osmosal®). One parent remarked that diarrhea caused by the rota virus could be fatal and for this reason Osmosal® should be used with children "to avoid dehydration." Both her children had had diarrhea caused by this virus and the children were very ill and had to be hospitalized.

Two parents mentioned Imodium® (loperamide), which was switched two years ago from prescription to OTC. Both of them regarded Imodium® to be a good and effective medicine.

As previously mentioned, stomachache caused by tension, stress, or unsuitable food were usually not treated with medicines. Laxatives were mentioned by only a few parents. The most common treatments for constipation both for children and parents were plums, licorice, and "just waiting until the intestines begin to work . . . ." One mother told about her son's prolonged constipation:

> The boy has had some problems with constipation. It was Metade (Metalax®?) or something, those suppositories, . . . something without a prescription. There were five suppositories in the package; it was not in any case meant for prolonged use. It was really bad this constipation, such that he was afraid when he had to void . . . you could see how painful it was.

Then he just tried to avoid voiding and got stopped up, so we had to relax it with suppositories. He was about three years old then. Then we tried to pay attention to the food he ate, to avoid eggs and cheese and to add vegetables, fibrous bread, etc.

Treating Other Symptoms

The parents talked very little about vitamins and mineral supplements, although they constituted the second largest OTC drug group stored in homes. Several parents mentioned, however, fixed combinations of vitamins and minerals such as Multitabs® and RaMaVit®. They reported that they use them for themselves and sometimes also for their children to avoid fatigue during the dark seasons (i.e., autumn, winter, and early spring) or as stimulants. Preparations containing iron and cod-liver oil were used for poor appetite with the children of some families, and vitamin C to prevent or treat the common cold as mentioned earlier.

In Finland, fluoride tablets are recommended to be given to children daily. It is surprising that the parents did not mention them, nor were they listed on the medicine cabinet questionnaire. This finding may implicate poor compliance in this respect or that the parents did not regard fluoride tablets as medicines.

Several other nonprescription drugs were mentioned during the parents' interviews, e.g., antihistamines (for allergy and for itching after insect bites), drugs for allergy, topical products for skin problems and for cuts. One mother talked much about herbs that could be used for self-medication. Some other natural medicines were also mentioned.

DISCUSSION

In this chapter some features of self-medication among families with children in Jyväskylä have been described. The participants were a group of middle-class families from two neighborhoods. Most of the families had two or three children. All the families chosen for inclusion in the study group did not participate and it may be that those parents who were more health conscious were more likely to participate.

Self-medication with OTCs was not the "treatment of first choice" for minor symptoms or sicknesses in children. The parents tried to treat minor symptoms first with other home remedies such as rest, sleep, hot, or cold drinks. The same was revealed in the interviews with the children; drugs were not spontaneously mentioned by them (Vaskilampi et al. 1994). It was also obvious that the parents themselves used OTCs more readily than they did with their children.

The parents were suspicious about the effectiveness of OTCs compared with the Rx medicines, although they also had positive experiences with OTCs. Especially those OTCs that had formerly been available by prescription only were generally seen to be more effective than the "old OTCs." Two medicines were particularly notable in this context: Burana® (ibuprofen) and Nasolin® (nasal decongestant).

Most of the medicines stored at home were nonprescription drugs, with over one-third analgesics (including NSAIDs). This result supports earlier findings that pains and aches are the most commonly self-medicated symptoms among people both in Finland (Klaukka et al. 1990) and in other countries (Bush and Rabin 1976; Dunnell and Cartwright 1972; Hansen 1984). Most brand names mentioned by the parents during the interview were also analgesics. Analgesics were the most frequently stored drugs not only in this Finnish sample, but also in other European locations and the USA (see Chapter 5, this volume).

The order according to therapeutic grouping for Rx medicines was different from the order for OTCs, reflecting the difference between self-medication and prescribed medication. Eye/nose/ear drops, topical products, analgesics, and cough/cold medicines, respectively, were the major Rx drug groups in descending order of occurrence at home. This order is different from that found in the whole Finnish population where drugs for cardiovascular diseases account for the largest share (Klaukka et al. 1990). In our data, only one family had cardiovascular drugs at home. This difference is explained by the age structure of the families; the families were nuclear families without grandparents living in the household.

Our study found no connection between family income and the number of medicines stored in the home. In contrast earlier studies examining the relationship between use of medicines and the socioeconomic class of the users have yielded mixed results (Dunnell and Cartwright 1972; Ambert 1982; Johnson and Pope 1983). The families in our study formed a very homogenous group of middle-class people, and thus the variation of family income was rather low, which may also explain this result.

An interesting finding in this study was that families with only one child had on average more prescribed medicines than those with two or more children. In the case of OTCs, no difference was discerned between these two groups. One explanation for this might be that the parents with only one child were more prone to seek advice from the doctor because of inexperience and resulting anxiety.

The absence of natural medicines in our MCI data may be one reason for finding that the number of medicines per household was lower than that of the other European locations and the USA (see Chapter 5, this volume). This does not mean that such remedies are not kept in Finnish households, since the interviews showed that both some parents as well as children spoke of them. The lack of natural medicines in the MCI data can be attributed to the laymen's definition of the concept of medicine. The parents were asked to list all the medicines they kept at home and thus may have defined the term medicine as only those licensed pharmaceutical products available from a pharmacy. Finns usually buy their natural medicines elsewhere than from a pharmacy (Airaksinen, Ahonen, and Enlund 1994). Thus, it appears that the parents defined the concept of medicines in the same way as the health professionals and health authorities, or their definition of the term might have reflected social desirability.

Inappropriate drug use (e.g., using a medicine for a wrong indication or symptom) was not found by the MCI questionnaire. This does not mean that all the medicine use among the families was rational. Most likely the result may be explained by the methodology of the study; the parents wrote the names of the medicines themselves on the MCI questionnaire and may have read the labels as well as the indications on the packages. In the interview, inappropriate drug use was noted. Two parents said that they would give aspirin or Burana® (ibuprofen) to their children for stomachache. As we know, these analgesics are most unsuitable for such symptoms; moreover, they can cause gastrointestinal disorders.

Many parents had also given children OTCs that, according to the labeling, should only be given to children under 12 years of age after a consultation with a doctor. Although the parents knew this, they believed they could still give half a tablet to children. Thus, they made the decision by themselves that, if they decreased the dosage, they could also use these drugs with children. This indicates the parents think it is the dosage that makes the drug dangerous to children, not the special chemical substance itself. Moreover, some parents reported that they could use aspirin for fever, which based on the present knowledge is not suitable, due to the possible connection between aspirin use and Reye's syndrome.

The dosages and especially the strengths of tablets also came up when the parents talked about other drugs, especially analgesics. This may reflect the present drug marketing strategy in Finland in which the strength of a tablet (e.g., 400 milligrams) is emphasized as in the advertisements of Burana® (ibuprofen), one of the most popular OTC drugs in the whole country. Thus, it can be argued that the parents thought that the more milligrams contained in one dose the more effective the drug.

It was interesting to compare the parents' interviews with the information from the MCI data, as they partially contradicted each other. In the interview, most of the parents reported that they do not very readily use OTC medicines themselves and especially do not give them to their children. However, the MCI data indicate that the same parents had frequently given OTCs to their children. It seems likely that the parents tried to report behavior that they thought would be more socially acceptable and would demonstrate their adequacy as parents (see Baruch 1981).

Finland is characterized by Calvinistic values, reflected in the attitude toward pain; it is more virtuous to suffer than to readily treat and alleviate discomfort. This was evident when the parents talked about pains and aches, as these were not treated with OTCs immediately. Klerman (1970) has called this type of behavior "pharmacolocigal Calvinism."

Risks connected with the use of OTC medicines in children were not spontaneously discussed by the parents, although they came up indirectly in the general cautiousness of self-medication with children. Some side effects of OTC drugs were, however, mentioned;

these included gastrointestinal disorders and possible drug dependency related to analgesic use.

Self-medication with OTC drugs has its own specific and limited role in home health care. The decision to use OTCs depends on the seriousness and the etiology of the symptom or illness; when the symptom is regarded to be serious or prolonged, the families are prone to seek professional advice. Often the decision to seek professional care was seen as a means of obtaining a more effective remedy in the form of a prescribed medicine. Thus, the parents could be seen to make a clear distinction between the effectiveness of the two drug categories.

NOTE

1. The COMAC Childhood and Medicines Project was funded through a European Economic Community (EEC) *Comité d'Action Concerté* (COMAC) contract, COMAC/HSR MR4*-CT90-0319, awarded to The Institute on Child Health, Athens, Greece, with Deanna J. Trakas as the Project Leader. The official title of the Contract was "Medicine Use, Behaviour and Children's Perceptions of Medicines and Health Care." In Finland, additional support was received from The Academy of Finland.

REFERENCES

Ahonen, R., Enlund, H., Klaukka, T., and Martikainen, J. 1991. "Consumption of analgesics and anti-inflammatory drugs in the Nordic countries between 1978-1988." *European Journal of Clinical Pharmacology* 41:37-42.

Airaksinen, M., Ahonen, R., and Enlund, H. 1994. "Pharmacy in the health food product market-consumer experiences from Finland." *Journal of Pharmaceutical Marketing and Management* 8(1):207-221.

Ambert, A. M. 1982. "Drug use in separated/divorced persons–gender, parental status and socio-economic status." *Social Science and Medicine* 16:971-976.

Baruch, G. 1981. "Moral tales: Parents' stories of encounters with the health professions." *Sociology of Health and Illness* 3(3):275-295.

Bush, P. J. and Rabin, D. L. 1976. "Who's using nonprescribed medicines?" *Medical Care* 14 (12):1014-1023.

Dahlqvist, G., Sterky, G., Ivarsson, J. I., Tengvald, K., Wall, S. 1987. "Health problems and care in young families–load of illness and patterns of illness behaviour." *Scandinavian Journal of Primary Health Care* 5:79-86.

Dunnell, K. and Cartwright, A. 1972. *Medicine Takers, Prescribers and Hoarders.* Routledge & Kegan Paul, London.

Fryklöf, L. E. and Westerling, R. 1984. "Self-medication. Proceedings from an international symposium." Stockholm, November 9-11, 1983. Swedish Pharmaceutical Press, Stockholm.

FSM 1993. Finnish Statistics on Medicines 1992. The Finnish Committee on Drug Information and Statistics, Helsinki.

Hansen, E. H. 1984. Self-medication in Scandinavia. A review of studies with special reference to methodological aspects. *Self-Medication* edited by L. E. Fryklöf and R. Westerling. Stockholm, Swedish Pharmaceutical Press, pgs. 15-18.

Johnson, R. and Pope, C. 1983. "Health status and social factors in nonprescribed drug use." *Medical Care* 21:225-233.

Kalimo, E., Nyman, K., Klaukka, T., Tuomikoski, H., and Savolainen, E. 1982. "Need, use and expenses of health services in Finland 1964-1976." Publication of the Social Insurance Institution A:18. Helsinki.

Klaukka, T., Martikainen, J., and Kalimo, E. 1990. "Drug utilization in Finland 1964-1967." Publications of the Social Insurance Institution M: 71. Helsinki.

Klerman, G. K. 1970. "Drugs and social values." *The International Journal of the Addictions* 5(2):313 -319.

Levin, L. S. and Idler, E. L. 1983. "Self-care in health." *Annual Review of Public Health* 4:181.

Levin, A. H., Katz, H. E., and Holst E. 1976. *Self-care: Lay Initiatives in Health.* New York: Prodist.

Lilja, J. 1988. "Theoretical social pharmacy: The drug sector from a social science perspective." Publications of the University of Kuopio. Statistics and Reviews 2. Kuopio, pgs. 231-246.

Tibblin, G. 1984. "The role of self-care in medical treatment." *Self-Medication* edited by L. E. Fryklöf and R. Westerling. Stockholm, Swedish Pharmaceutical Press, pgs. 15-18.

Vaskilampi, T., Kalpio, O., Ahonen, R., and Hallia, O. 1995. "Finnish study on medicine use, health behavior, and perceptions of medicines and health care." *Childhood and Medicine Use in Cross-Cultural Perspective: A European Concerted Action*, edited by D. J. Trakas and E. Sanz. Luxembourg: Office for Official Publications of the European Community, (EURO Report), pgs. 191-220.

Chapter 15

From Catching a Cold to Eating Junk Food: Conceptualization of Illness Among Finnish Children

Tuula Vaskilampi
Olli Kalpio
Outi Hallia

Pain, disease, and feelings of ill health are embodied in cultural explanations and behavioral regulations. Every individual and community deals with these experiences within its specific sociocultural context.

Cultural definitions of illness situations explain symptoms, diseases, treatments, and outcomes by providing the structural framework for the constant creation and interchange of ideas and signs related to well-being and illness. In other words, in different communities there exists a collective discourse that provides meaningful explanations of biological misfortune. Moreover, professional and lay discourses can be distinguished as well as other discourses according to different subgroups in Western industrial societies (see e.g., Sigerist 1951; Vaskilampi 1982; Herzlich and Pierret 1985).

It can be argued that the notions on causality of illness and health are crucial in the belief system of any society. We observe and theorize in order to understand the origin of human history and causal thinking (Herzlich and Pierret 1986; Riese 1950).

Children as their own subgroup have emerged as independent study subjects only recently. They are observed in meaningful social interactions (Prout and James 1990). Their viewpoints and notions on health matters have become a matter of inquiry relative to whether they represent directly the views of their parents and wider national culture or whether they arise independently. Various studies involving interviews of children have shown a systematic structure to their health perceptions and behaviors (Gochman 1977; Gochman and Saucier 1982; Bush and Iannotti 1990). Bush and Iannotti (1988, 1990) applied a comprehensive Children's Health Belief Model encompassing children's and primary caretaker's health perceptions, beliefs, and use of health services to predict children's expectations to take medicines for common health problems.

In Finland there have been large follow-up studies on the health behavior of teenagers (12-18 years of age). The rationale for this research emerged from the needs of health education for information on smoking, sexual behavior, and subjective health status, which have been the main problems studied (Rimpelä et al. 1983, 1987). Also performed have been large surveys on the health status and the use of health services among Finnish children. However, these quantitative data were collected from the mothers of the children and not the children themselves (Kalimo et al. 1989, 1992).

In the Finnish health studies, the use of qualitative methods, in which the children are seen as autonomous study subjects able to form opinions and to interpret the opinions of others, has been quite unknown. Nor has information been gathered from preadolescents. Thus very little is known about the health and illness related life styles and cultural meanings of health among younger schoolchildren in Finland.

Home has been the primary health care domain of these Finnish children (cf., Mayall 1993). The beliefs and attitudes of the family are manifested there in daily activities and knowledge gathered from various sources adapted to everyday life situations. In most cases, both parents work outside of the home and before school age the children have been in private or public day care. If they live in tranquil suburbs (as did the children in the study described in this chapter), the children can play out in the neighborhood with their friends after school without adult supervision. This represents another important social domain where friendships and age-group interaction are promoted.

The children have been exposed to health care from the public sector since birth (and before that). They have all gone through the program of Maternity and Child Health Care by which prevention, health checkups, and health education have been the main strategies to maximize health status. This reflects the aims of the Nordic Welfare State model in Finland.

Regular health checkups continue throughout the school years. Almost all the children in Finland go to primary schools which have similar curricula that includes health education. The dual role of a primary schoolteacher as a caregiver and as a teacher as observed by Mayall (1993) is important during the first school years.

Besides the official health "socialization agents," there exist private economic markets with their advertisements and the mass media. Especially the TV is a source of information on health-related issues for children.

Finnish society has quite recently gone through an exceptionally rapid modernization process. Urbanization and industrialization came later than in the other European countries (Senghaas 1985). When comprehensive social institutions of religion and family have broken, a new type of individualism and different integrative strategies have emerged. It can be argued that under these social circumstances health has become one of the basic values and a source of behavioral regulation, while at the same time, health care as a social institution has widened its power (Crawford 1980). This medicalization of everyday life and health ideology (healthism) seems to be visible and widely accepted in Finnish society. For instance, one of the first large scale community-based intervention programs in the world, the North Karelia Project, which aimed to decrease cardiovascular diseases by changing individuals' eating and smoking habits, was launched in the beginning of the 1970s. Since that time, public health education programs have aimed to change individuals' behavior toward professionally accepted health beliefs (Vaskilampi 1981).

All these factors have created a shared sociocultural context for the children who participated in our study. As Cornwell (1986) concluded, social and personal experience are important sources of ideas and theories about the causes of illness, but there are others. There are "common stocks" of information and ideas in different social milieus; there are information and ideas specific to particular families and informal social networks, and there are "external" and "official" sources of information about health matters, i.e., the formal health care system and the media.

This chapter focuses on the cultural and social construction of illness among the Finnish children. When undertaking the research, plans were made to seek answers to the following questions: How do the schoolchildren in our study see illness? How have they experienced illness? What does health and illness mean for them?

METHODS AND MATERIALS

This study was a part of the COMAC Childhood and Medicines Project[1] and was performed as a case study in the Finnish town of Jyväskylä. In accord with the study protocol, the participating children were from the first grade (seven to eight years of age) and third grade (nine to ten years of age) of two comprehensive schools in a middle-class area.

The data were collected by semistructured interviews in two stages. The first interview at school was based on the drawings made by the children about their own illness episodes. In the second interview, which was conducted at a child's home whenever possible, the themes of the first interview were revised and broader themes about health and illness were introduced. This chapter is based mainly on the children's descriptions of their illness episodes and their discussions about what they liked and disliked in being ill, what they regarded as serious and mild diseases, and how they characterized a sick and a healthy individual.

There were 29 boys and 41 girls who participated in the drawing interview and 26 boys and 25 girls in the second interview. All of the children were from middle-class families. The methodology is described in more detail in Chapter 2 and in a study report (Vaski-lampi et al. 1995).

RESULTS

Etiological Concepts in the Children's Narratives

The causality of diseases can be expressed in several dimensions and levels of rationality. In lay explanations, a mutually exclusive classification does not necessarily exist, but instead several notions might coexist. The scientific explanation of illness is based on the chronological and observable cause and effect relationship. This disease etiology has dominated scientific medicine since the discovery of bacteriology (cf., Whitbeck 1977). However, in recent years, a multifactorial model has arisen within the domain of etiological explanation.

Although scientific explanations have acquired legitimacy (cf., Freidson 1970), there still exist lay belief systems in modern Western societies. Throughout the whole history of modern medicine, there has been constant interchange of ideas between the scientific and lay belief system (see, e.g., Helman 1978, 1982).

In lay health cultures, a search for causes of illness includes a search for meanings as well. And as Herzlich and Pierret (1986) said, people have been trying to relate illness to the order of the world and to the social order by explaining illness with religious, ideological, and physical terms, for instance regarding illness as God's will or fate or as an effect of natural law. Thus the lay explanation of illness extends beyond the biological level. But at the same time individuals explain illness by their daily observations and perceptions. All individuals think, observe, and respond to evidence at a sensory level. It can be concluded that scientific and lay conceptualizations of etiology operate partly in the same, and partly in different dimensions, and provide answers to different questions.

The Finnish children in our study named several causes for illness and by this gave meaningful explanations. However, some of the children did not verbally express any explanations for illness saying that they did not know. For some children illness just happened and seemed to be very natural phenomena of everyday life that did not require any explanation.

Transmission of Diseases

Contagion was a cause of illness that was known to all the children. A disease had been caught from another person, who was often mentioned along with the situation where it was suspected to have been transmitted. However, knowledge about the mechanism of contagion varied considerably. Especially when talking about chicken pox, the children often used the expression "it was going round" or "it" was going "from one person to another."

Q. Where does that chicken pox come from?
A. I don't know. It just came. It was going round a lot at that time.
Q. Do you know how an infection happens?
A. Yes, it is like for example when [in the neighborhood] there is a stomach disease going round and then it always goes round and then it comes.
Q. How does it go round?
A. I can't explain that.
A. I haven't had much else, but when our neighbors had a stomach disease, the whole family had it. It may have been transmitted from them to me somehow. Later my mother told me.

The situation in which the disease is transmitted appears in an interesting way in the children's reasoning.

Q. Where does such a thing like a chicken pox come from?
A. When I was visiting [a class mate] they had chicken pox some time ago. It is for some three, two weeks that it germinates. I think I got it from there.
Q. How was it transmitted?
A. I didn't even notice it myself.

According to some children the duration of time one spends with a sick person also determines if one will be infected.

A. They had flu some time ago and then I spent only a little time with them.
A. If another person is too long near that sick person it [the disease] can spread.

In addition to the duration of the contact, the distance was emphasized in the narratives. Usually it was thought that being near a sick person is enough to become infected.

Q. What makes the chicken pox spread then?
A. If you are quite near and you should not be near at all, if you are in the same room then it can spread easily. But not all diseases spread so very easily.
Q. Do the adults get it, too?
A. Well they can get it but mother isn't always so near except when eating; at the dinner table she is quite near but she has not been infected yet, at least not so far.

The explanations were specified by saying that something concrete was moving from one person to another, for example when sneezing.

Q. It doesn't matter at all, even if you had a fever?
A. No, I don't think so, if you just don't go very near.
Q. Why can't you go near?
A. Well, if you are coughing and sneezing–sneezing by accident toward another person–it can spread very well.
Q. What is it in the sneeze that makes the disease spread?
A. I don't know.
Q. How do you think a disease spreads?
A. Well somehow, when you are coughing at someone; I don't really know.

Contagion and spreading of a disease were related to microbes. These were called bacteria, bacilli, viruses, or by a popular term "bugs" ("pöpö") which were used synonymously. The bugs were said to be small and either invisible or visible only with a microscope. One boy said that when he had been smaller he had imagined them as "furry little beasts," another described them as "little bugaboos."

The penetration of microbes into a human being was described as usually happening through the mouth as drops, e.g., when sneezing, from hands or in breathing air, but also through other orifices in the body or "under the skin" through a wound. The microbes were also said to "jump from a person to another." They were known to be found in dirty places and in birds. To some children the microbes were also related to pollution and poisons.

When describing how microbes act in a person's body the children used expressions "causing a disease" or "causing damage inside a person." Microbes were said to cause pain, too. Bacteria could "carry the disease" and a virus "hit." Microbes could also try to "kill a person." One child said they cause "injuries to blood."

For most children microbes were something that penetrate into people from outside and cause a disease. A few children also said that the microbes exist in "both ends" of a person especially if one is dirty. In one exceptional description the bacteria were divided into good and bad ones. This description illustrates very well how the children constructed systems from different kinds of knowledge.

Q. Do you know where that fever comes from?
A. Well, or I don't really know where it comes from.
Q. What do you suppose, where it comes from?
A. Yes, but from the temperature of the body.
Q. Well, how does it, what will the temperature of the body be like?
A. Well such overheated.
Q. Why is it so . . . what is causing it?
A. Bacteria.
Q. Ahh. What are the bacteria like?
A. They are such little things that we, we people do not see as they are too small, and there are good ones and bad ones.
Q. What kind of ones are bad?
A. Such ones that they do all, well, all pains and lots of, they make diseases.
Q. What about the good ones?
A. Well they are here in the stomach and they do . . . well they receive the food and melt it there.
Q. Where have you learned that from, of the bacteria?
A. My father has told me.
Q. Does your father know it well?
A. Yes, as he is that, a psychologist, or was that.

Since the discovery of microbes and the elaboration of Pasteur's model of specific etiology, people have become familiar with the contagion concept. The Finnish schoolchildren expressed the germ theory as explaining the cause as do nowadays most of the adults in

Western societies (cf., Helman 1982; Herzlich and Pierret 1986; Pill and Stott 1986).

Generally, the children did not relate germ theory to the concept of vulnerability or resistance. An exception was one child who said that if you once had chicken pox you will not have it again.

It seemed that for most of the children, germs represented learned metaphor or hypothesis–something that cannot be observed at the sensory level and also something that is exterior, outside the individual. In scientific understanding, germ theory is neutral, objective, and unable to carry emotions and signs. However, the children constructed it in their own belief system wherein germs could be seen as independent entities with personal qualities that were also associated with individual behavior and responsibility.

Life-Style as a Cause of Illness

The concept of life-style integrates various factors from the physical environment, social relationships, and personal habits in a model to explain causality. Unlike germ theory, life-style theory is multifactorial; microbiological factors are only one explanation within it. Lay understanding and scientific medical theories (especially epidemiology) interact in life-style theory. Whereas germ theory has been effective in explaining infectious diseases with disease-specific causality, it has not explained most degenerative diseases.

The children expressed some behavioral causes for their getting ill. Often these were associated with food. Food that was contaminated, spoiled, or unhealthy, or of which too much was eaten, was seen as causing illness.

> A. I had a bit of a bellyache in the evening. We were at my cousins, the youngest one of them had vomited, and then it had transmitted, [and] I had bellyache in the evening. First I thought that I had got it from the sweets as I had eaten a lot of sweets, but it wasn't. I vomited in the night.
>
> Q. Do you get bellyache from sweets?
>
> A. Oh yes, like Annina had vomited from sweets.

The etiological concepts of the children, as we see later, also included other notions of dietary risks. In their narratives, the chil-

dren associated their own illnesses with food and eating and sometimes with clothing they wore (or did not wear). Exercise was
mentioned only in the general conceptualization but not in the children's narratives of their own experience. This is discussed in more
detail later.

With food and eating, as well as with clothing, expressions were
in terms of "right" or "proper" qualities and also quantities, i.e.,
"too much" or "too little." Thus, ethical issues were pointed out
that touched on the notion of personal responsibility in the illness
process.

Climate, Weather, and Natural Conditions as Illness Cause

Natural conditions such as climate, weather, air, and cosmology
have been historical explanations for illness. They still exist very
persistently in lay concepts of illness causation.

For the causes of fever, the explanations were almost invariably
of physical origin like the weather, climate, or seasons. Bad weather
(cold, wet, rainy, wet snow), getting wet (usually wetting one's feet)
and then feeling cold were the main reasons for getting fever.

Nevertheless, it seemed to be clear for the children that these
external circumstances would not cause the illness alone but also
one's own behavior contributes to it. "Wearing too few clothes,"
"not remembering to at once go in when one has got wet," or
"staying too long out in the cold" describe the way children took a
part of the blame for their illness.

> A. Well I try, that I do not go out bareheaded so that I won't
>   catch a cold.

According to the children, getting a fever could be prevented by
acting "in the right way." Wearing a (knitted) cap and clothes that
are warm enough can prevent one's getting ill.

The fact that the children know how they ought to behave does not
mean that they would always do so. Playing and other outdoor activities, regardless of the weather, were nice, important things, whereas
caution and proper dressing were dull, secondary ones. Due to this,
the children did not seem to feel guilty for their behavior.

A. At least [one could] stay away from all those puddles and such where we usually play.
Q. Where did you get fever, then?
A. Well, from the puddles usually, where we splash water on each other.

In the same way that being properly clothed is a way of being prepared against external circumstances it is also a way of maintaining the internal balance and order in its relationship with the external. A lack of control of one's own behavior may cause illness.

Q. Where does fever come from?
A. Well it can come from having had too little clothes on and wetting your feet and then playing too wild. If you are very wild then it can come from that, too.

A change of temperature risks illness. Hot and cold is one theme on which the children speculated.

Q. How does [a fever] come from that?
A. You get hot and when you go somewhere where it is a little colder, then when you have had very cold, hot and then cold, then you get so that you start to feel cold and when it has been hot then you can get fever.
Q. What made you get fever, then?
A. I can't remember, something it was . . . I might have had too little clothes outside, or I'm not quite sure.

A disease developing from another disease as a chain of chronological cause and effect was a characteristic way for some children to explain why they became ill.

Q. What did cause it? Where did such a thing come from?
A. Well it came in such a way that I had a bit of a cold, then I started coughing and sniffing, then I got fever. For some time I had a cough and a runny nose. After a couple of weeks I got fever.
Q. Where do you think fever comes from?
A. If you have a runny nose then you can get fever.

Q. Why is it so?
A. What?
Q. That you can get fever from a runny nose?
A. Well if it could go up into your head, or I don't know . . . .

Another explanation for illness was that it comes from the ground: from sand, mud, water, or snow. These elements, in the urban environment where the children live, were related to uncleanliness and dirt. When talking about dirt the children mentioned "bugs," bacteria, bacilli, and viruses.

All the causes for illness described here are connected to the idea that an illness is something that comes to a human being from outside. Internal causes for illness such as heredity or congenital disabilities and diseases appeared only fragmentally. The children did not give any psychological explanations for illnesses. When a concept of an external cause is so strong, questions of one's own responsibility follow: could the illness have been avoided (Pill and Stott 1986)?

Categorizing Illness

A consideration of what is serious, dangerous, or frightening is a part of the illness concept. When the children described their own experiences, the illnesses were in most cases acute and mild. Nearly all the episodes had been treated at home and medicines had not played an important role in the treatment. Most illnesses appeared in the narratives as relatively usual episodes in the everyday life of the children, without big dramatic details. The children reported when and where ill health was recognized. "I was visiting my godmother in Helsinki," "We had guests in the evening . . . ," "I was playing outside."

The degree of seriousness was defined according to whether the disease could not be treated at home or whether it was painful. Diseases that required visiting a doctor or a hospital were regarded as serious. In these cases effective medication was needed or it was not known what was wrong. A few children related seriousness also to the risk of secondary diseases, e.g., a pneumonia developing from bronchitis. At a more general level seriousness was related to death.

Cancer was identified as a disease leading to death. The experiences and knowledge the children had about it had come from family members and relatives. Also mass media were a source of knowledge.

The children mentioned various cancers (cancer of the lungs or breast) and changes in the appearance of a cancer patient (losing weight), also some treatments (operations, radiotherapy, medicines). One child told of the pains suffered by a relative before dying of cancer.

The etiology of cancer included smoking, fats, and unhealthful food, but also environmental risks were mentioned. Radioactive pollutants like ones from the Chernobyl nuclear power plant disaster were said to be one cause of cancer.

Q. Why is cancer a serious disease?
A. I don't know really. It is a serious disease anyway, and I've heard somewhere that if it gets really bad then you can die from that cancer.
Q. Where does a cancer like that come from?
A. At least if you don't eat lots of vegetables . . . if you eat really fatty food.
Q. Are there any other causes?
A. If you do not exercise a lot.
Q. Is it infectious?
A. No, I don't think so.

Another disease regarded as serious was AIDS. Those few children who mentioned it gave a distant and dim picture of it. It was known to be infectious and the themes of AIDS education came out in the children's narratives.

Q. Where does AIDS come from, then?
A. Well either if there are dirty needles, like there seldom are, or if there are too little, if one makes sex without being protected.
Q. Where does it come from?
A. AIDS? It comes from some person who has got AIDS, it can be transmitted.
Q. How is it transmitted?

A. Well, for example in such a way that another person has a
   wound, a person that has AIDS, and I have a wound and
   when we shake hands for a long time and rub those hands,
   then it should come.

Also heart problems, epilepsy, diabetes, and tonsillitis were
thought to be serious. Some other diseases mentioned in this category were rather rare and exotic: hemophilia, jaundice, dysentery, lep-
rosy, scurvy, or spotted fever. A reason for remembering these diseases may be the concreteness and impressiveness of their Finnish
names, such as "bleeding disease," "yellow disease," or "red disease."

The children classified the diseases they had themselves experienced as both mild and typical for children. Children's diseases
were thought to include especially cough, fever, and a runny nose
which were all considered to be mild. Also chicken pox and ear
infections were regarded as normal childhood ailments. An opinion
that serious diseases are a problem particularly belonging to adulthood was clearly visible in the interviews.

A large group of common diseases was classified as possible for
both children and adults. The experiences of the children and their
families were reflected in this categorization.

Illness as a Social Experience

From the children's point of view, being ill is an interruption of
normal life, causing limitations in their social relationships.

A sick child is "ordered" to go to bed for rest, to stay inside, and
to stay away from school. Inside the family the child moves to a
kind of a social core, to a passive role where the others act for
him/her and arrange special privileges–an act representing the classical Parsonsian sick role with its rights and obligations (Parsons
1951). However, there are also differences, for the children do not
need to justify the sick role by emphasizing their symptoms; the
decision as to whether the child is really ill is made by the parents.

Illness in general was found as a negative experience. What was
notable is that the symptoms or the disease in itself were not always
the greatest disadvantage. Most annoying things for the children
were isolation, staying inside, separation from friends, getting bored,

and lack of activities. Even though the children had not been separated from the other members of the family, their friends and classmates were not usually allowed to visit the child except for briefly bringing homework. According to the parents this was not so much for the risk of infection as for the child's need of peace and rest.

When the children were asked whether they found any good things in being ill, however, only a few did not find any. Some of the children viewed the rest and especially the possibility to sleep late in the morning as pleasant. One boy said that sometimes "it is nice to stay at home longer than for two days." In these responses the children described illness as a "break" from the rapid pace of everyday life. Some statements reflected enjoyment of being "in peace" or alone at home.

For many children an illness gave a possibility for playing, listening to music, and watching videos. The parents also tried to find entertainment for their children so that they would not get bored. A sick child feels he/she is getting special attention and care during the illness. Rented videos and books and tapes from the library were mentioned as a part of it. The children also said they were given their favorite food and drinks, sometimes also sweets.

Even though all these things were considered to be extra attention, the children also found illness to mean being closer to the parents than usual. When ill, the children were allowed to sleep in the parents' bed or on the sofa in a bed made for them. They found their position as ill to be different than at other times. The children said they also received more than their usual amount of attention:

Q. In what kind of way more [attention]?
A. In such a way that when I am not ill then almost all the time they are with my little brother but then they are not.

Some narratives of the children conveyed coziness in being ill, a situation also observed by Sachs (1990) and discussed in Chapter 9 (this volume). Some children felt they had been pampered. An interesting detail was that of these "pampered" children, the boys slightly more than the girls said that being ill is cozy and that the negative sides of an illness are getting bored and suffering from the symptoms. This might hint at different kinds of relationships between mothers and children of different genders: mothers as the primary caretakers responding to their son's needs in a different way than to the needs of their daughters, or a son's illness being a rare possibility when a school-aged son allows a mother to show affection.

When the children deliberated the advantages (rights) and disadvantages (obligations) of being ill the school was a central theme. The children saw their relationship with school as dichotomous: the school being both work and a social environment. Those children who thought staying at home was an advantage found the extra spare time a pleasure. Some saw this as a disadvantage because of getting more homework and having a fear of "being behind" the others. On the other hand the sick child also missed what the classmates do and experience during the day at school; especially the girls emphasized missing their good friends (cf. Prout 1989).

General Concepts of Illness and Health

The children were also capable of speaking about and defining illness and health in general and abstract terms. Most of the children gave their own definitions when they were asked and only a few could (or would) not give any.

The children dichotomized health and illness (Figure 15.1). These were seen as the opposite end of the same dimension and were often expressed as opposite qualities: health with positive characteristics and illness lacking those qualities. However, at the same time, the children could also see them in different dimensions. Often illness was seen as physiological phenomena and health more in psychological and mental terms.

The children defined illness and health by using qualitative and behavioral dimensions (Figure 15.1). They gave general prototypes with some exceptions of specific symptoms and disease. Health was defined in a negative way as a lack of disease and symptoms, but also often in a positive way to mean something more or different from mere shortage of illness. The children gave comprehensive concepts on health which included physiological, psychological, and social aspects. Their conceptualizations cameclose to the famous World Health Organization definition of health (WHO 1946).

Health included positive behavior–obeying the social norms. Healthy people were thought to be nice and fit; also activity, energy,

FIGURE 15.1. The children's definitions of health and illness

Health		Illness	
Qualities		**Qualities**	
Healthy Not Feeling Sick Not Seriously Ill No Cold No Cough	Somatic and psychosomatic qualities	unhealthy ill health pains sick cough cold	Somatic and psychosomatic qualities
Active Energetic Vital Not Tired		tired fatigue weak not active	Personal and mental qualities
Nice Happy Glad Normal	Personal and mental qualities	abnormal mentally ill lunatic dull stupid not nice	
Good-Looking	Visible qualities	bad-looking pale red crippled	Visible qualities
Behavior		**Behavior**	
Walking briskly Being outside all the time Can go to school Can go anywhere Exercising Not sleeping all the time	Activities	Walking with a limp Being passive Cannot go to school Cannot go anywhere Sleeping all the time Things have been done to him by the others	Activities
Eating properly Not smoking Not watching TV all the time	Life style	Doing wrong things Not acting as one should Eating improperly Smoking, drinking Watching TV all the time	Life style

and vitality were often emphasized. The children gave a picture of an ideal type of person who follows professional health instructions and leads a successful life (cf. Crawford 1980). The boys more often than the girls expressed health in a negative way and the girls more often than the boys related health to happiness and activity.

It was interesting to notice that mental and emotional dimensions were emphasized in the children's definitions whereas these aspects were not taken into account by the children in their etiological perceptions. Illness was seen as a negative phenomenon which integrated the negative characteristics of people, their unhealthful behavior, and physical symptoms. It can be seen to represent degeneration. Illness was seen as an intentional phenomenon which people had obtained by their own behavior.

Figure 15.2 represents a semantic map drawn from the children's health and illness definitions. The map can be distinguished from the definition of health and illness as shown in Figure 15.1 as illustrating, on the one hand, qualities that might be physical or mental (psychological) abilities, and on the other hand, various behaviors. Among the different abilities are psychosomatic status and physical as well as mental outlook.

In their perceptions on health promotion, the children found health to be obtained by their own efforts. Health was something that is under control and for which individuals are accountable. It was emphasized that with special health behaviors health can be attained: right (proper) diets, e.g., fat free, lots of vegetables and fruits, no junk food, not too many sweets. Exercise and sports were stressed, too.

Also, watching too much TV was considered bad for your health. Smoking and alcohol were mentioned by only a few children. Hygienic health habits were mentioned very rarely.

In their general opinions, the children seemed to be quite firm and absolutist. However, they did not express guilt or shame about their own health behavior. Their notions on health behavior reflected Finnish health education programs.

DISCUSSION

The children in the study came from middle-class families, and during the selection process, health-conscious parents were prob-

FIGURE 15.2. The semantic map of the children's health and illness definitions

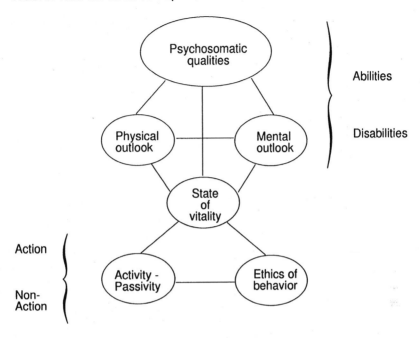

ably more likely to volunteer to participate. The data were collected via semistructured interviews. Thus, those children who were the most verbally talented and socially active provided more opinions.

The children described the main disease etiological classifications: contagion, climate, and life-style. Transmitted diseases with bacteriological explanations were described most often, and most completely with varied expressions.

The children, consistent with the adults in the Finnish Welfare State, generally indicated that they had adopted a microbiological etiological model (Helman 1982; Pill and Stott 1986). This model is perceived as neutral and objective, as setting the cause outside the individual and his/her responsibility. However, the children expressed in their narratives behavioral factors in the process of falling ill, indicating that one can avoid illness by one's own behavior. Although health promotion and illness prevention were seen to be the responsibility of the individual, the children did not seem to feel guilt or shame in association with their own illness episodes.

The most modern etiological concepts of the relationship between lifestyle and illness were well known among the Finnish children. They were familiar with health risks, especially dietary.

The children saw the causes of diseases to be exterior, i.e., outside individuals but relating to their own behaviors. There were few expressions about possible interior causes: hereditary or psychological.

Also the children did not attribute, nor did they express any need to attribute, illness to ideological, religious, or supernatural causes. It seemed to be satisfactory for illness to be explained at an observable sensory level or with the help of professional explanations.

Illness meant almost entirely acute minor health problems for the children, as also has been shown to be the case for adults (cf. Field 1976). Chronic and serious diseases are known, however, and especially by the children whose family members or friends have them. Also, the mass media have brought AIDS and environmental catastrophes into the children's world. However, serious diseases are generally associated with others.

A child's illness episode appears socially and culturally structured. A child has special rights (privileges) and obligations (limitations with regular everyday routines). Structurally this can be described as a Parsonian sickness role (Parsons 1951). However, at the same time, according to the children's experiences, illness was perceived to be quite natural and a normal part of children's lives. Illness is, above all, experienced. Children are ill and the performance of illness is within temporal and spatial conditions (cf. Christensen 1994; Frankenberg 1986).

Their own illness episodes provide children a chance to find a new "secret world" and become exempt from the routine of everyday life. There the child has more attention from the parents and time to think and do things (cf. Herzlich 1973). At the same time, however, the child suffers from loneliness due to social isolation. The illness creates the fear that the child will be cut out of associating with friends and schoolmates. The second fear is falling behind in school work.

Health and illness were perceived as the opposite end of the same dimension to the children. Whereas health was seen in the children's definitions as a positive phenomenon, illness was the opposite, representing the negative characteristics. Health has, however, a much wider definition than mere lack of disease and it was associated with qualities covering the right way to behave and personal and mental abilities (cf. Crawford 1980; Vaskilampi 1982, 1983; Zola 1972, 1975).

From the children's health and illness definitions, we can interpret their image of body and self. They expressed a biological outer body which can be observed and also a socially and culturally constructed body, which is the image of a self that is controlled by social regulations and norms (cf. Scheper-Hughes and Lock 1987). The ethical core of postmodern society can be seen reflected in these definitions.

The children and their parents have been raised within the Finnish Welfare State in which health education has played an important role. Their health and illness concepts and experiences represent the modern society. Activity and work are appreciated and illness is related to behaviors that are under one's own control. The sickness role is, in this respect, losing the characteristic of unintentionality (cf. Parsons) and is becoming more intentional. Health has moved into the individual's own domain of responsibility. The breaking down of many social institutions has generated a demand for new social control agents and new sources of norms. Health and health promotion are fulfilling some of this demand. Health has entered the marketplace of postmodern society. The Finnish children's perceptions and experiences of health and illness are well within this emerged mainstream (Vaskilampi 1995).

NOTE

1. The COMAC Childhood and Medicines Project was funded through a European Economic Community (EEC) *Comité d'Action Concerté* (COMAC) contract, COMAC/HSR MR4*-CT90-0319, awarded to The Institute on Child Health, Athens, Greece, with Deanna J. Trakas as the Project Leader. The official title of the Contract was "Medicine Use, Behaviour and Children's Perceptions of Medicines and Health Care." Additional funding for the study was provided by The Academy of Finland.

REFERENCES

Bush, P. J. and Iannotti, R. J. 1988. "Origins and stability of children's health beliefs relative to medicine use." *Social Science and Medicine* 27:345-352.

Bush, P. J. and Iannotti, R. J. 1990. "A children's health belief model." *Medical Care* 28:69-86.

Christensen, P. H. 1994. "Vulnerable bodies: Cultural meanings of child, body, and illness." Presented meeting Royal Anthropological Institute. Pauling Center for Human Sciences, Oxford.

Cornwell, J. 1986. "Health beliefs in old age: The theoretical grounds for conceptualizing older people as a group." *Working Together for Health: Older People and Their Careers*, edited by F. Glendenning. Stoke-on-Trent, Beth Johnson Foundation, pgs. 9-25.

Crawford, R. 1980. "Healthism and the medicalization of everyday life." *International Journal of Health Services* 10 (3):365-388.

Field, D. 1976. "The social definition of illness." *Introduction to Medical Sociology*, edited by D. Tuckett. London: Tavistock, pgs. 334-366.

Frankenberg, R. 1986. "Sickness as cultural performance: Drama, trajectory and pilgrimage. Root metaphors in the making social of disease." *International Journal of Health Services* 16(4):603-626.

Freidson, E. 1970. *Profession of Medicine. A Study of the Sociology of Applied Knowledge.* New York: Dodd, Mead.

Gochman, D. S. 1977. "Perceived vulnerability and its psychosocial context." *Social Science and Medicine* 11:115-120.

Gochman, D. S. and Saucier, J. 1982. "Consistency in children's perceptions of vulnerability to health problems." *Health Services Reports* 86:247-252.

Helman, C. 1978. " 'Feed a cold starve a fever': Folk models of infection in an English suburban community and their relation to medical treatment." *Culture, Medicine and Psychiatry* 2:107-137.

Helman, C. 1982. *Culture, Health and Illness.* Bristol: Wright. Herzlich, C. 1973. *Health and Illness.* London, NY: Academic Press.

Herzlich, C. and Pierret, J. 1985. "The social construction of the patient: Patients and illnesses in other ages." *Social Science and Medicine* 20 (2):145-151.

Herzlich, C. and Pierret, J. 1986. "Illness: From causes to meaning." *Concepts of Health, Illness and Disease*, edited by C. Currer and M. Stacey. Leamington Spa: Berg, pgs. 73-96.

Kalimo, E., Häkkinen, U., Klaukka, T., Lehtonen, R., and Nyman, K. 1989. Tietoja suomalaisten terveysturvasta. Kelan julkaisuja M:67, Helsinki. (with English Summary: Data about the health security of the Finns. Health status, use of health services, health related life-style and health care costs to families by population group in 1987.)

Kalimo, E., Klaukka, T., Lehtonen, R., and Nyman, K. 1992. Suomalaisten terveysturva ja sen kehitystarpeet. Kelan julkaisuja M:81, Helsinki (with English Summary: Health security in Finland and needs for development).

Mayall, B. 1993. "Keeping healthy at home and school: 'It's my body, so it's my job'." *Sociology of Health and Illness* 15 (4):464-487.

Parsons, T. 1951. *The Social System*. Glencoe: Free Press.

Pill, R. and Stott, N. 1986. "Concepts of illness causation and responsibility: Some preliminary data from a sample of working- class mothers." *Concepts of Health, Illness and Disease*, edited by C. Currer and M. Stacey. Leamington Spa: Berg, pgs. 259-277.

Prout, A. 1989. "Sickness as a dominant symbol in life course transitions: An illustrated theoretical framework." *Sociology of Health and Illness* 11 (4):336-359.

Prout, A. and James, A. 1990. "A new paradigm for the sociology of childhood?" *Constructing and Reconstructing Childhood: Contemporary Issues in the Sociological Study of Childhood*, edited by A. James and A. Prout. London, New York, Philadelphia: The Falmer Press, pgs. 7-34.

Riese, W. 1950. *La Pensée Causale en Médicine*. Paris: PUF.

Rimpelä, M., Rimpelä, A., Ahlström, S., Honkala, E., Kannas, L., Laakso, L., Paronen, O., Rajala, M., and Telama, R. 1983. Nuorten terveystavat Suomessa. Nuorten terveystapatutkimus 1977-79. Lääkintöhallituksen julkaisuja, sarja Tutkimukset 4/1983, Helsinki.

Rimpelä, M., Rimpelä, A., Karvonen, S., Siivola, M., Rahkonen, O., and Kontula, O. 1987. Nuorten terveystottumusten muutokset 1977-1987. Lääkintöhallituksen julkaisuja, sarja Tutkimukset 7/1987, Helsinki.

Sachs, L. 1990. "The symbolic role of drugs in the socialization of illness behaviour among Swedish children." *Pharmaceutisch Weekblad Scientific Edition* 12:107-111.

Scheper-Hughes, M., and Lock M. 1987. "The mindful body." *Medical Anthropology Quarterly* (New Series) 1(1):6-41.

Senghaas, D. 1985. *The European Experience. A Historical Critique of Development Theory*. Leamington Spa: Berg.

Sigerist, H. E. 1951. *A History of Medicine*. New York: Oxford University Press.

Vaskilampi, T. 1981. "Sociological aspects of community based health intervention programs." The North Karelia project as an example. *Revue d'Epidémiologie et Santé Publique* 29(2):187-197.

Vaskilampi, T. 1982. "Culture and Folk Medicine." *Folk Medicine and Health Culture: Role of Folk Medicine in Modern Health Care*, edited by T. Vaskilampi and C. P. MacCormack. Publications of the University of Kuopio. Social Sciences 1/1982. pgs. 2-16.

Vaskilampi, T. 1983. "Health as a Goal of Eternal Life or Ability to Survive." Proceedings 12th World Congress on Health Education Dublin 1993. pgs. 1250-1251.

Vaskilampi, T., Kalpio, O., Ahonen, R., and Hallia, O. 1995. "Finnish study on medicine use, health behavior, and perceptions of medicines and health care." *Childhood and Medicine Use in Cross-Cultural Perspective: A European Concerted Action*, edited by D. J. Trakas and E. Sanz. Luxembourg: Office for

Official Publications of the European Community, (EURO Report), pgs. 191-220.

Whitbeck, C. 1977. "Causation in medicine. The disease entity model." *Philosophy of Science* 44:619-638.

WHO 1946. Constitution of the World Health Organization. Geneva.

Zola, I. M. 1972. "Medicine as an institution of social control." *Sociological Review* 4:487-504.

Zola I. M. 1975. "In the name of health and illness: On some socio-political consequences of medical influence." *Social Science and Medicine* 9:83-87.

Chapter 16

Children's Knowledge of Medicines in Trieste, Italy: Situations and Perspectives

Giampaolo Canciani
Patrizia Romito

The Italian part of the COMAC Childhood and Medicines Project[1] was carried out in Trieste, a seaport with approximately 250,000 inhabitants. Its main area of employment is in the tertiary sector and it has a high percentage of elderly people. Its birth and perinatal mortality rates are lower than the national average. Pediatric care is provided on a more widespread basis than in the rest of Italy for the following reasons:

1. a high number of Day-Clinic pediatricians (who are self-employed and paid by the National Health Service) with respect to the number of children resident;
2. the presence of a local Pediatric Hospital which is also a National Research Institute with specialist pediatric departments and an emergency department open round the clock;
3. the existence of a medical faculty and School of Specialization in Pediatrics situated at the Pediatric Hospital whose Directors have established excellent working and training relationships with Day-Clinic pediatricians throughout the region.

In addition emphasis has been placed for nearly 20 years on "demedicalization" and "dehospitalization" (the current average hospital stay is 1.8 days).

Some more general comments are in order. Health care in Italy is free of charge for hospital admissions (funded out of tax contributions) and almost completely free of charge for clinic services, tests, and treatment. As yet, there is no system for calculating costs, and therefore no rigid protocol of diagnostic/therapeutic interventions such as that existing in the United States of America, where private health insurance schemes predominate.

On the one hand, this makes it impossible to control health expenditure (as the amount of debt of the Italian Health Service shows). On the other hand, the pediatrician is not obliged to work within strict diagnostic/therapeutic protocols in order to avoid the risk of administrative, legal, and financial sanctions. Prescribed therapy is more likely to be based on purely clinical motives.

METHODOLOGY

The comments in the section following are based on an analysis of the data emerging from the Drawing Interview done with the children and from the Medicine Cabinet Inventory (MCI) of the families interviewed (see Chapters 2 and 5 for a description of these methods). The instruments for gathering these data were designed in the preparatory phase of the project and were common to all participating centers.

Sixty-four children were interviewed and 35 families agreed to the home visit. The socioeconomic level of 48 families was determined (including the 35 who had the MCI). Of a total of 96 parents, 52 had attended school until age 14, while 44 had a high school certificate or a university degree.

RESULTS AND COMMENTS

The wide availability of health services might lead one to expect that they would be used more frequently and that there would consequently be greater recourse to medicines, resulting in bigger stocks at home. Indeed, the everyday working experience of one of the authors (G. C. in the emergency department of the Pediatric

Hospital) is that people often consult the pediatrician not only with often trivial medical problems but also with problems unrelated to health. Instead the results were very different from what was expected. The interviews with the children showed that the Hospital and the family doctor were rarely used and that the latter made few home visits (Table 16.1).

The family doctor was usually a well-liked figure, with whom the child had a trusting relationship and sometimes almost a friendship. All the children had some experience of medicines apart from the most common remedies. The most familiar ones, both in terms of their names and their purpose, were the antipyretics. The others were recalled more imprecisely. The names of antibiotics and how often they were administered was often recalled incorrectly. Other products were mentioned because of their purpose (cough medicine or throat pastilles without more detail being given [Table 16.2]).

TABLE 16.1. Use of Medical Services as Referred by the Drawing Interview

TYPE OF SERVICE	TYPE OF EPISODE	
	MEDICAL	**TRAUMATOLOGICAL**
FAMILY PEDIATRIC		
- phone	1	
- at home	5	
- consulting room	11	
- didn't come	1	
HOSPITAL		
- examination	3	2
-admission	2	6
NOT MENTIONED	30	
MENTIONED BUT NOT USED	3	
TOTAL	**56**	**8**

TABLE 16.2. Medicines and Remedies as Recorded by the Drawing Interview

MEDICINE CATEGORY	NUMBER OF CITATIONS
General Remedies	30
Analgesic/Antipyretic (name remembered)	25
Analgesic/Antipyretic (name not remembered)	2
Vitamin	1
Other stomach	3
Topical	1
Eye/ear/nose	2
Antibiotic (name remembered)	5
Antibiotic (name not remembered)	7
Antiasthmatic/bronchodilator	3
Combination cough/cold	28
Sore throat lozenges	4
Orthopaedical/Surgical medication	5
Other	4
Undetermined	59

The MCI carried out with the parents showed that good use was made of medicines overall. In our opinion, the number of medicines in each household was reasonably low (Table 16.3). Most families had no more than 15 medicines which seemed acceptable considering an average household size of three to four members. With regard to expiration date and storage, 21 families out of 35 (60 percent) had no expired medicines, and with the exception of one family with 69 products, half of which had expired, only two out of 452 products overall (4.4 percent) had expired (Table 16.4).

TABLE 16.3. Modal Distribution of Medicines in the Households

NUMBER OF MEDICINES	NUMBER OF FAMILIES
From 0 to 5 (min. 3)	4
From 6 to 10	8
From 11 to 15	12
From 16 to 20	5
From 21 to 25	2
From 26 to 30	3
Over 30 (69 drugs)	1

TABLE 16.4. Number and Percentage of Expired Medicines in the Households

EXPIRATION STATUS	N	%
yes	52	10.0
no	470	90.0
Total	522	100.0

Note: One family showed 69 medicines, 31 of which (44.9%) had expired. The other 34 families showed a mean of 4.4% expired medicines. Twenty-one out of 35 families (60.0%) did not have any expired medicine at home.

In most cases (three families out of 35), all of the medicines were stored in the same place thus making it easier to check their state of preservation, expiry dates, reserve stocks, and consumption rates (including checking the child's "autonomous" consumption whether accidental or purposeful).

The medicines for adults and children were stored with the same amount of care for all household members regardless of age. Moreover, there was little difference in knowledge about how the medicines for adults and children worked.

Knowledge of the medicines' effects and the purposes for which they were last used was almost always correct (86.4 percent of the total of 521 medicines). (See Table 16.5 for incorrect knowledge.) This would seem to indicate that the prescription was clear and the instructions were read carefully.

The adults used a greater variety of medicines. There were 98 different brand names among the products for adults, as compared with 26 brand names among the products for children.

Medicines observed during the MCI corresponded to the information provided by the children in their interviews. In fact, the most common children's medicines were the antipyretics followed by products for the eyes/ears/nose, remedies for "colds and coughs," antibiotics, and "mucolytic/expectorants" (Table 16.6). Because the most common illness in this age-group is upper airway infection of a viral origin, the medicines inventoried showed a certain degree of consistency between the most prevalent problems and the most appropriate treatment.

When these MCI data were compared with those from the interviews with the children, it was found that the medicines the children recalled the best were the antipyretics (medicines taken frequently that are useful but that only treat symptoms). Other medicines were recalled vaguely or not at all, despite being used to treat the same kind of problem. Other products were hardly mentioned at all, even when the children were asked which medicines were used in other situations, and despite their presence in the home as revealed by the MCI (e.g., externally applied creams or "topicals"). Similarly, no reference was made to the "nonclassifiable" items though they also

TABLE 16.5. Parents' Incorrect Knowledge of the Effect and the Purpose of the Last Time Medicines Were Used

	EFFECT vs PURPOSE*	EFFECT AND PURPOSE UNKNOWN**	TOTAL
PEDIATRIC	16	7	23
ADULT	17	21	38
TOTAL	**33**	**28**	**61**

* Different referred effect and last use purpose.
** Effect and purpose not recalled or unknown.

TABLE 16.6. Medicines by Therapeutic and Age Category (Number and Percentage)

MEDICINE CATEGORY	N FOR PEDIATRIC USE	N FOR ADULTS' USE	TOTAL (%)
Analgesic/antipyretic	45	37	82 (15.7)
Topical	30	44	74 (14.2)
Indeterminate/other	25	45	70 (13.4)
NSAID	3	36	39 (7.5)
Eye/ear/nose	28	7	35 (6.7)
Antibiotic/antiviral	19	16	35 (6.7)
Mucolytic/Expectorant	17	15	32 (6.1)
Combination cough/cold	18	10	28 (5.4)
Vitamin/mineral	6	14	20 (3.8)
Antiacid/Other stomach	3	14	17 (3.3)
Antihistamine	5	8	13 (2.5)
Laxative	3	9	12 (2.3)
Decongestant	6	4	10 (1.9)
Sore throat lozenges	7	2	9 (1.7)
Antidiarrheal	3	5	8 (1.5)
Antiasthmatic/bronchodilator	6	1	7 (1.3)
Homeopathic remedy	4	3	7 (1.3)
Tranquilizer/sedative/hypnotic	3	4	7 (1.3)
Antihypertensive/diuretic	/	6	6 (1.1)
Antiemetic	2	3	5 (0.9)
Hormonal supplements	/	2	2 (0.4)
Heart (angina/other)	/	1	1 (0.2)
Oral contraceptive	/	1	1 (0.2)
Steroid oral	1	/	1 (0.2)
TOTAL	234	287	521

were well represented at home. Evidently, the children make a clear distinction between a bout of illness and the transitory, trivial "upset," probably because the latter has little or no effect on their daily routine. In addition, during an illness, the children make a distinction between the "important" medicines, those used continually, and the "unimportant" ones, used occasionally. A high temperature clearly represents a problem, although it is only a symptom from a clinical point of view and rarely worries the doctor; antipyretics are therefore employed frequently and methodically. Other products, whether used correctly in the course of bouts of illness or used on other occasions, were not recalled and would therefore seem not to be used so frequently and methodically.

A comparison between the children's medicines and those for adults showed a big difference in the number of nonsteroid anti-inflammatory drugs (NSAIDs) and some other groups, with a large number of "vitamins/minerals" and "topicals" for adults. The surprisingly low number of contraceptives was probably due to failure to declare them. The larger number of NSAIDs and "stomach" medicines for adults is not surprising. What is interesting is the number of "vitamins/minerals," "topicals," and "other" products. Because no real therapeutic efficacy can be attributed to the first of product, their main usefulness must be as placebos. The second group consists of useful drugs, but it would seem that they are being used more than necessary; adults are not particularly susceptible to skin disorders. Perhaps the visible nature of skin problems leads to a prompt visit to the doctor and hence to an immediate prescription.

GENERAL CONSIDERATIONS AND DISCUSSION

Many studies have been performed on the doctor-patient relationship from the patient's perspective (e.g., Sachs 1992). Here, in contrast, we provide a simple evaluation of our results from the doctor's perspective. From a purely technical point of view, a physician is trained to work within the following mechanistic scheme:

explanation of problem -> analysis of problem ->
identification of solutions -> prescription of solutions ->
application of solutions -> disappearance of problem

The scheme is a simple one, and undoubtedly effective when applied to a simple system. It becomes inadequate, however, when applied to a complicated system such as the individual. The complexity of biological phenomena is in itself enough to make it inadequate. If we then consider the individual's social interactions, certain stages in our scheme clearly appear over-simplistic. In addition, there is the relatively limited sphere of action of the medicines available, compared to the vast number of problems the individual brings to the physician. The kinds of problems emerging are discussed below.

If the data collected in Trieste are interpreted using the perspective of the mechanistic scheme outlined above, they appear to be quite satisfying. The children recalled the essential medicines, did not take them autonomously, and recalled their effects and purposes fairly well. The parents kept a reasonably low number of products at home, knew their effects and purposes and were careful about conditions of storage. The variety of brand names was fairly limited indicating a well-aimed choice of products. The situation seemed to be extremely positive and it suggested that the abundance of health facilities present in the area has produced a high level of knowledge about use of medicines. Because no planned health education programs have been implemented in this sector, the results suggested that this level of knowledge may have been attained from frequenting health facilities and that their personnel conveyed consistent messages.

However, whereas from a technical point of view there may be good reason to be satisfied with the concrete application of the scheme proposed and with the degree of adherence to existing diagnostic and therapeutic protocols, some other points need to be discussed. First, there is the question of the nature of the problems presented to the physician. Two levels should be distinguished. The most important, in clinical terms, represents those serious disorders that jeopardize a person's life or health. For these problems, the place of treatment is the hospital; the type of medicine is highly specific, and the management protocols are clearly defined. The second level consists of those problems that are less threatening to life and health or of longer (chronic) duration. The place of treatment is outside the hospital; management protocols are less important and more flexible, and the way they are implemented varies. The latter is the most frequent context; there sociocultural factors play an extremely important role and the hypothesized scheme is no longer enough from the very outset, i.e., from the problem presented by the patient.

Obviously the data were collected within the context of the second level and indicated an excellent level of technical management of medicines, for the most part for symptomatic relief. After all, a high temperature is an individual's defense mechanism; vitamins do not greatly alter the course of an illness, except in specific disorders. The use of topical creams on the other hand would be worth investigating further.

Our sample consisted of young parents with very few clinical problems of a chronic nature; the main health problems seemed to be connected to "quality of life." Remedies were sought for problems that interrupted the daily routine. In this perspective, the issue of "noncompliance" is unimportant, because failing to take medicine in the situations reported would probably make no difference from a clinical point of view. It would be different in the case of a chronic illness in which a correct methodical compliance with the therapeutic regime should guarantee certain results (from a statistical point of view) (Wirsing and Sommerfeld 1992).

But in both cases, the basic problem is how to provide the "patient" (who may not always be ill) with the correct information regarding the functional model of illness/disorder in every individual. A clear understanding on the part of the individual of the reasons for his or her own malaise may make it easier to decide whether the problem can be solved by the physician and, if so, may make the description of the problem clearer, thus giving the best possible start to the functional scheme proposed earlier. This would produce the correct "technical" expectation with regard to the medicine's effect, and acting indirectly through the patient, it would be possible to modify the motives which induce the physician to make the prescription. In this way, "self-medication" could be reduced to "physiological" levels.

Until now, we have remained in a purely rational dimension, in which our original scheme still seems relevant. But this leaves a series of questions unanswered. The physician may be a "cure" in her/himself. Recourse to a physician expresses a need on the part of the patient and the physician's actions are usually trusted; certain expectations are created. Perhaps the physician of today, accustomed to dealing with every problem mechanically, is no longer aware of the semiological aspect of the physician role. The patient's expectations are disappointed and the problem, which might have been solved without recourse to medicines, remains. The result may be a pointless prescription, a failed "application of the solution" (to return to our original scheme) and a consequent (and justified) "noncompliance." Is it possible to change the physician's "scheme of functioning?"

We have investigated stable situations of young families with small children. But what is the situation of adolescents who are in the self-identification phase, who need to present a strong image of themselves, free of problems, both physical and social?

In conclusion, what is the correct educational message for the use of medicines? Of course we must continue to provide the basic technical information as it is is vital to keep risks and errors to a minimum. But we must not lose sight of the many psychological and sociocultural aspects that turn a medicine or a cure or a physician into a "placebo" but which may still be highly effective in enhancing the quality of people's lives. Such decisions clearly depend on the basic approach adopted at the level of primary health care (Haiijer-Ruskamp 1992).

If the trend for the future is toward a health system requiring itemized accounting of all interventions, those problems that are not of a strictly clinical nature will have to be delegated to others who will deal with them for what they are, without turning them into "*problems*" of a medical (or nonmedical) kind. Or perhaps we should already be looking for ways to handle them in their true light within the present system. These considerations go beyond the functional scheme of the physician's daily work and enter the sphere of social interaction. Here, besides the culture of the individual and group, those economic and political factors that are involved play a crucial role.

We are unable to provide any clear solutions to these problems. We hope simply to have provided some starting points for future discussions.

NOTE

1. The COMAC Childhood and Medicines Project was funded through a European Economic Community (EEC) *Comité d'Action Concerté* (COMAC) contract, COMAC/HSR MR4*-CT90-0319, awarded to The Institute on Child Health, Athens, Greece, with Deanna J. Trakas as the Project Leader. The official title of the Contract was "Medicine Use, Behaviour and Children's Perceptions of Medicines and Health Care."

REFERENCES

Haaijer-Ruskamp, F. M. 1992. "Medicine Use as a Social Phenomenon." *Studying Childhood and Medicine Use*, edited by D. J. Trakas and E. J. Sanz. Athens: ZHTA Medical Publications, pgs. 33-55.

Sachs, L. 1992. "Health and Illness: Theoretical Perspectives: Some Concepts within the Anthropology of Medicine." *Studying Childhood and Medicine Use*, edited by D.J. Trakas and E. J. Sanz. Athens: ZHTA Medical Publications, pgs. 7-15.

Wirsing, R. and Sommerfeld, J. 1992. "Compliance–A Medical Anthropological Reappraisal." *Studying Childhood and Medicine Use*, edited by D. J. Trakas and E. J. Sanz. Athens: ZHTA Medical Publications. Athens: ZHTA Medical Publications, pgs. 17-30.

SECTION IV:
VIEWPOINTS

Chapter 17

Implications for the Health Care Provider: Viewpoint of a Pediatrician

Eleni Valassi-Adam

I spent a whole summer reading the contributions for this volume, and all along, while mentally debating with the authors and enjoying every page of it, I worried, querying its accessibility, its readability, and its effectiveness to the people who should use the knowledge it contains–the health care providers. The work presented in this book could, and should, have important implications for medical practice. The approach of the authors, many of their points, and some of their conclusions are, in general, greatly needed in health care. To be used, this knowledge, or the recognition of its lack, must reach and be appreciated by the health care givers. Under present circumstances, I doubt if it will.

Once again, the long existing difficulties in communication between scientists of different disciplines are demonstrated. To physicians, anthropologists seem to work with a view to enriching their own science. They communicate their new knowledge to their own colleagues. The implications that this knowledge might have for the health of children appear to be of low priority. Pediatricians have not yet learned to appreciate this knowledge. Naturally, each scientist publishes in books or in specialist journals, rarely attracting the attention of other disciplines. Thus, one of the values of this work is the multidisciplinary teamwork on which it is based.

Members from different disciplines have tried to bridge the communication gap by pooling their knowledge from the start, and their search for common methodology, viewpoints, and conclusions has obviously led to the discovery of a common communication path. It should not be forgotten though, that this is an achievement limited to their group. To the reader, the path may still be unclear, leaving ample room for confusion and misunderstanding. In many passages, although the terminology is familiar, I felt that the author meant something different from what I as a pediatrician understood. Words such as autonomy, dependence, locus of control, are known to physicians but not necessarily with same meaning as to social scientists. Readers with a biomedical background might come to conclusions that are far from representing the authors' view. I felt much more secure in chapters with a dominant biomedical authorship. I would consider it a major contribution of anthropology to health care if researchers would use the expertise acquired through this interdisciplinary work to ensure that their knowledge be transcripted into a "physician compatible language."

Medical anthropology is a rather new discipline. Like any new drug or other product, its use by the consumer depends largely not only on its quality but on appropriate promotion as well! The anthropological approach, methodology, and concepts are to a large extent unknown to pediatricians and commonly considered irrelevant to medical practice. The average physician would tend to have a negative reaction (sometimes ironic, sometimes querying, quite often defensive) to any other professional's involvement in his/her own cherished territory of children's health. Some even have difficulties in accepting the involvement of patients with their own health! However, the request for a minimum understanding of child health for any scientist interested in the field, is neither irrational nor solely due to professional exclusiveness. Some of the authors appear to assume an understanding which might render them unreliable to the health care giver. They seem to perceive terms such as fever, diarrhea, and vomiting as quantitatively and qualitatively stable variables when they are not necessarily so. For example, the variable "fever" might differ according to age, duration, and etiology. In studying the concept of "diarrhea" in children (who had too much ice cream or acute viral gastroenteritis or cholera) one should be very cautious in attributing variance to cultural differences!

Even the most sensitized physician would not easily invest the time required to read this book. The new, stimulating knowledge it offers will be lost unless presented in an attractive, concise, easily digestible form. Much consideration should be given to which form would meet the scientific standards required by both authors and health care givers: raw data? analyzed and processed findings and conclusions? simplified condensed summing up by a high-powered expert? This is a challenge for both social and biomedical scientists!

The most important point made by this book, which would have significant implications in health care, is the concept that the child is a person and should be approached as such by the physician. In most applied medical models the child is not approached directly but through the parents. The questions put to him/her are seldom seeking information. They are merely used to put the child at ease. The medical history is elicited from the adult caregiver who is erroneously thought to be more reliable: How does she feel? How did he fall? (even when the adult was not present at the accident!) What did she have for breakfast? (in case of a discrepancy the adult's reliability is taken for granted). Where does it hurt? (Yes, the question is often addressed to the adult escort in outpatient clinics!) The finding that four-year-olds already have structured concepts on disease and the use of medicines should give physicians cause for reflection.

Intercountry differences are observed and given varying interpretations according to the authors. This made me realize that my own understanding and interpretation of the findings, which I believed to be based on scientific knowledge, are greatly influenced by my personal attitudes and my childhood experiences. I identified more with the children of the sample than with their unseen health care givers! This was an impressively effective intervention of the researchers and it should be acknowledged with admiration!

In my childhood, and in the childhood of half of the contemporary prescribing physicians and medical teachers, cough medicines had a bitter taste and the daily spoonful of sticky foul-smelling cod-liver oil left a revolting memory. The popular children's comics showed how the naughty boy managed to pour the foul medicine down the sink, water the house plant with it, or feed it to the cat! It is not surprising then that today's generation of parents was nurtured in the opposite philosophy. They were encouraged to take their super-tasty, extra-sweet, wonderful medicines which would make them healthy in no time, help them grow, give them energy, ensure success in sports, help them concentrate, help them sleep, keep away their troubles, control stress and melancholy, make the future look brighter . . . . The potential dangers of this attitude seem to have been noted by the population in Germany and by the health authorities in Finland. German parents are reported to go to extremes, totally rejecting conventional medicines. They turn to "Anthroposophica." The term would be enchanting to anthropologists and Greeks and the movement would be highly desirable for the health of the population if what it implies was actually applied. The literal interpretation of the term would be "means of the wisdom of man." The study in Germany describes a misconception: It seems anthroposophica simply substitute for conventional medicines which are ostracized with almost medieval fanaticism. Data in Finland and Trieste give much more encouraging information: "The wisdom of man," which is common sense, and the skill to make informed decisions on the use of medicines and health services, seem to have reached the children.

There is much discussion on whether contraceptives, vitamins, and fluoride supplements are perceived by people as medicines. The authors tried to find some explanation as to why contraceptives were not mentioned by parents in any of the study sites. I was a little disappointed to see much reasoning on medicines not mentioned by the children and no analysis of the concept of "doctor" who is very often mentioned in the interviews. Is not the doctor considered part of the local culture? Did the children refer to "a doctor," "the doctor," "a specialist," "my doctor?" In most chapters I felt the authors related doctors only to disease and not to prevention or health promotion. But what about the children? Perception of the doctor by some of the authors seemed rather negative! What about the children?

In most countries represented in the study, doctors and parents are reported to perceive side effects, accidental overdosage, and poisoning as the major dangers of medicines. Awareness of the risks of irrational use, of ineffective or outdated preparations and of addiction to common medicines such as analgesics, antibiotics, or vitamins is observed in rather few sites. Only in Finland did parents express the concern that children are tempted to use bubbly orange flavored vitamin C preparation as a "soft drink." In all study sites some parents caution children against side effects but in a rather negative paternalistic way. There seems to be virtually no organized attempt at positive health education on how to use medicines and health services.

The findings and conclusions of the study would deter the foreign-educated doctor from approaching his/her patient with techniques acquired in another country or with data collected from another population. In some sites the doctor is expected to use the thermometer himself, in others to prescribe an antibiotic or an antipyretic. Even the doctor with much experience in the local concepts and behavior should be aware that there are intergroup differences and variations. It is irrational to think in terms of Greek children, Finnish parents, American four-year-olds, the Spanish concept of fever. There are only individuals whose concepts and beliefs might change with age, circumstances, or education. Health care providers are advised to get to know their patients and their parents, to understand the basis of their concepts and beliefs, and to adapt their therapeutic and health-promoting approach accordingly.

Any differences observed among countries seem to relate more to contemporary local medical policies or practice than to traditional habits and beliefs. This is most encouraging. People's health behavior seems to be ready to change within a period of time much shorter than in previous generations. Any change in doctors' philosophy and practice can be expected to have some effect.

The messages I got from this work as a health care giver are very clear:

- Do not simply prescribe medicines; teach their rational use. Prescribe self-help, minimal intervention, appropriateness, measure.

- Don't limit your history taking to biological variables, try to include concepts, habits, phobias, expectations.
- Do not think in terms of age, social class, ethnic, sex groups. There are individual variations.
- Do not think in terms of compliance only. Try to influence concepts and beliefs. It is in your power to direct patients according to contemporary scientific knowledge and help them to become immune to misinformation.
- Do not believe you always know best. Anthropologists may know something valuable. It is about time they are welcomed in the health care team!

Chapter 18

Grasping the Children's Point of View?
An Anthropological Reflection

Sjaak van der Geest

... children as people to be studied in their own right, and not just as receptacles of adult teaching.

Charlotte Hardman 1973:87

How interesting are the chapters of this book for cultural anthropologists and, more specifically for medical anthropologists, especially those who study people's perception and use of pharmaceuticals?[1] Do the various contributions on children, medicines, and culture enrich our theoretical insights, our methodological skills and our ethnographic understanding? Conversely, what critical comments need to be made about these contributions from the viewpoint of cultural and medical anthopology? To me, cultural anthropology is first and foremost the art of understanding others in the context of their culture. Malinowski's admonition of more than 70 years ago still inspires the present generation of anthropologists.

> [T]he final goal, of which an Ethnographer should never lose sight . . . is, briefly, to grasp the native's point of view, his relation to life, to realise *his* vision of *his* world. We have to study man, and we must study what concerns him most intimately, that is the hold which life has on him. In each culture, the values are slightly different; people aspire after different aims, follow different impulses, yearn after different forms of happiness. (Malinowski 1961:25)

That art of understanding is a melange of surprise and familiarity. At first sight, the "otherness" is most conspicuous. Anthropologists are fond of describing–and, in a sense, defending–other ways of acting and thinking. According to some critics, they practice exoticism. At second sight, however, anthropologists rather portray the other as familiar to us. By describing the other people's way of life as logical, meaningful, and practical within the context of their own culture, as Evans-Pritchard did for witchcraft beliefs among the Azande, we come to realize that "we" and "they" have common grounds, or, to say it with a paradox, that we are the others. Evans-Pritchard's study, for example, helped Polanyi (1958:286-294) to discover striking parallels between belief in witchcraft and scientific thought. In second instance, therefore, anthropologists contribute to the awareness of pan-humanity in the diversity of cultures (cf. Jackson 1989). In his introduction to a trendsetting anthropological publication Clifford (1986:23) puts it thus:

> Ethnography in the service of anthropology once looked out at clearly defined others, defined as primitive, or tribal, or non-Western, or preliterate, or nonhistorical. . . . Now ethnography encounters others in relation to itself, while seeing itself as other.

Before that awareness of commonness is reached, however, the ethnographer needs to delve deeply into the lives of those he wants to describe and understand. Anthropological research includes cerebral as well as emotional involvement.

> To study the institutions, customs, and codes or to study the behaviour and mentality without the subjective desire of feeling by what these people live, of realising the substance of their happiness–is, in my opinion, to miss the greatest award which we can hope to obtain from the study of man. (Malinowski 1961:25)

Medical anthropology is a test case of this ambition because it wants to approach and understand the other in his most lonely and inaccessible situation, during sickness and depression.

If understanding "the other" is so fundamental in my concept of anthropology, it will come as no surprise that I was fascinated by the choice of the "others" in this collection of studies: children. Children have been a widely neglected "tribe" in the work of anthropologists and sociologists (cf. Goodman 1957, Erikson 1965, Hardman 1973, James and Prout 1990, Christensen 1994). Of course, we do have studies *about* children, for example about child-rearing practices in various cultures but ethnographic work which attempts to grasp the child's point of view is extremely rare.

All critiques which in recent years have been launched against the anthropological treatment of "others" (cf. Clifford and Marcus 1986, Dwyer 1987), suit the treatment of children particularly well. The subjects of anthropological research have been objectified, silenced, and reconstructed; their statements have been twisted and alienated. They were regarded as primitives whose words and actions–which usually had been distorted and misunderstood–were perhaps interesting for the collector of *curiosa*, but did not contain much worth to be taken seriously. It is significant that "those primitives" were often likened to children with their preliterate, mistaken and immature concepts. Children provide the proverbial metaphor to characterize the "primitive other" encountered in anthropological fieldwork. Early theories of child psychology lent support to evolutionist views on "primitive people":

> Just as the child . . . is ignorant of the course of things and therefore believes in fiction as readily as fact, so the savage, similarly without classified knowledge, feels no incongruity between absurd falsehood and established truth. (Spencer, cited in Hardman 1973: 86)

When Edwin Ardener (1975a, 1975b) described the place of women in ethnographic work as "muted," he borrowed a term from an article about children (Hardman 1973). In a world where adults set the tone, children seem inarticulate and are not listened to.

> "What is it that makes a group muted?" We then become aware that it is muted simply because it does not form part of the dominant communicative system of the society. . . .

Why have children been so maltreated by anthropologists? One reason, of course, is that their views are–almost by definition–

regarded as incomplete, not deserving serious attention. Children may take a central value in a culture (in fact, they do in many cultures), not as human beings, but as future human beings. They are near-objects, extremely precious, but mute. Their position is not much different from that of cows in a Nuer village, canoes among Trobriand men, or marbles in a group of Dutch children: cherished, omnipresent, and without words (cf. Ardener 1975a:4).

Another reason is perhaps that the ideas of children do not rouse the interest of adults. The latter may think they know those ideas already since they have been children themselves. Viewing children as incomplete versions of themselves is the ultimate form of "ethnocentrism" and renders any ethnographic attempt meaningless beforehand. Moreover, it is ahistorical; it denies the social and cultural changes which have taken place in the meantime and reduces the lives of children and adults to mere phases in an ever-identical biological cycle.

If a "mature" anthropology of children is indeed so full of pitfalls, it will surprise no one that this book on "Children, Medicines and Culture" roused my interest. It seemed an almost heroic enterprise to give voice to the ideas and experiences of children with respect to feeling sick and taking medicines. I soon discovered that my expectations were misplaced. The book hardly touches upon the views of children. Some authors of the book hastened to explain to me that it had never been their intention to describe the children's world of illness and medicine. As a matter of fact, the funders of the research project preferred that its emphasis would be on quantitative data that could be used to improve the quality of medicine use by children. The anthropological fascination with what children think about medicines, what medicines mean to them, was not shared by those who had to pay the bills. My lamenting about "missed chances" and lack of anthropological empathy should therefore not so much be taken as criticism of those who carried out the research but rather as a complaint about the general low appreciation for the qualitative approach in circles of pharmaceutical research funding. By pointing out what—to my taste—is missing from this collection of articles, I hope to provide an outline of a medical anthropology of children and to elicit interest in such an undertaking.

Ninety percent of the book is a continuation of the tradition of "adultism" or adult-centrism: it contains information *about* children by nonchildren such as parents, particularly mothers, and by teachers, caregivers, and social scientists themselves; it presents the adult perspective of children. Only the chapter by Prout and Christensen is a modest attempt to grasp the children's point of view. Quotations from children have been taken out of context and are counted without much concern about their meanings from the children's perspective. The quantitative treatment of this extremely qualitative material deprives the children from what they had wanted to say. One would have wished more attempts had been made by the writers of this book to become, as it were, child with the children and allowing the reader to enter the world of children–of sick children, to be more precise. The researchers have opted for an easier approach–in the eyes of many a more appropriate one: they discussed the children's practices with the adults.

At the initial stage of the research an interesting approach was suggested: asking children to make a drawing of themselves being sick, and talking with them about that drawing. It looked a promising approach, but its results have not reached the pages of this book. The reason is not given.

Even if the emphasis were quantitative, qualitative data of this kind would have been enlightening, providing context and meaning to the counting of children's practices. Why did the researchers not add a qualitative dimension to their work? Were they unable to grasp the children's views? Did they find the children inarticulate, incoherent, unsuitable, or unreliable informants? Or did the researchers realize that they were unable to become acceptable and "natural" conversation partners for children? Personally I do not think that participant observation with children of one's own culture is more difficult than with adults in another culture.[2]

Do anthropologists–and other social scientists–miss the imagination which is required for an intelligible and empathic description of the children's world? Is it only literary writers who succeed in putting themselves in the situation of children and producing a convincing story, true from the children's point of view?

Or, finally, is the topic of this book, pharmaceuticals, unsuitable for a serious treatment of children's views? After all, pharmaceuticals are overwhelmingly regarded as things to be kept out of the reach of children, like matches. Was the choice of children in this case too farfetched? The fact that in some societies children seem to be rather free in handling certain medicines, as is shown in this book, does not change the general feeling, that medicines are forbidden territory for children.

Let me pick out four examples of children's views which are mentioned in this book and which seem to me worth of a more elaborate anthropological discussion. The first is the observation by Trakas and Botsi (Chapter 9) that children's taste of medicines reflects their feeling during illness. For Swedish and Dutch children, being sick means being pampered and getting special attention. It is a "cozy" period for them. Those positive feelings are reflected in the "sweet taste" of the medicines they take. Conversely, Greek children say they are bored and lonely during sickness and refer to their medicines as "bitter." The medicines thus become metaphors for the entire experience of being ill.

Prout and Christensen (Chapter 3) noticed that children usually did not mention the use of pharmaceuticals when they spoke about their illness. For them, another aspect was much more important—the fact that during that period they enjoyed special care and attention. Illness was first and foremost described in social terms. In an article coauthored by Whyte (Van der Geest and Whyte 1989), I have suggested that pharmaceuticals are means by which sick people liberate themselves from the control by powerful others. Medicines often replace the people who impose themselves upon the patient as healers or counsellors. Escape from that imposition may prove the greatest benefit of pharmaceuticals. If the observation by Prout and Christensen presents a more general trend in the experience of children, this would prove a sharp difference with the experience of adults. In that case, children would rather use the illness as an opportunity which allows them more social dependence and care than they are entitled to in ordinary life. The medicines are not alternatives for that care but rather part of it. That is why they taste sweet.

In the same chapter, Prout and Christensen remark that pharmaceuticals communicate to children the power that adults hold over them. As objects used by adults, forbidden to children, medicines represent the boundary between child and grown-up. Taking a medicine for the first time, without the interference of an adult, is like crossing that boundary, an act of ritual importance. Christensen, in a personal letter, gave me a vivid example: A seven-year-old boy with a cold was allowed by his mother to apply a nasal spray. His reaction was that he was now as big as his ten-year-old brother. That brother often used an inhaler to treat his asthma.

The fourth observation worthy of more anthropological attention is the role of the thermometer marking the boundary between health and illness. The instrument assumes an air of strict objectivity. The cultural construction of that objectivity passes unnoticed. Its truth is simple and clear because it is able to reduce a complex whole of bodily and emotional sensations to a straightforward figure, in which both adult and child firmly believe. That the thermometer can also be used to cheat is not mentioned. Did the children not tell the researchers?

For children, medicines become symbols of power and adulthood and markers of the transition from childhood to adolescence. Medicines are the child's concretization of feelings experienced during sickness. These may be fascinating insights to the anthropologist interested in symbolic meaning, but they do not seem very relevant to the scientist–social, medical, or pharmaceutical–who is after solutions to practical problems in medicine use. The latter's lack of interest in the symbolic meaning of pharmaceuticals is regrettably misplaced, however. Understanding how children perceive and experience pharmaceuticals can be of immense value for the improvement of medicine use by children.

Undoubtedly, the various studies in this book have enlarged our knowledge about children as consumers of medicines. My criticism has been that this knowledge is predominantly from the perspective of the adult outsider. The children themselves hardly raise their voice and are never given the chance to tell their whole story.

My complaint should be taken as a positive suggestion to put more effort into grasping the children's point of view. Following a good tradition of entering the world of "others" and giving voice to their muted views, anthropologists could make a significant contribution to the social and cultural understanding of pharmaceuticals by studying children in their own right, not as receptacles of adult teaching.

The rare anthropological studies of children's views and practices suggest that children have an autonomous world which is, however, not entirely incomprehensible to adults (Hardman 1973:95). Children perform without inhibition and with great virtuosity what adults do clumsily and furtively: they follow their imagination. In their games, children do not let themselves be confined to the physical entity of objects and environment. They have a remarkable competence for changing the function of things in their surroundings and subjecting them to the purpose of their games. A carpet becomes a ship, a planet, a boxing ring, or a forest; a table changes into a castle, an airplane, or an island.

> The environment has no idiosyncratic meaning at the level of play; the objects, including their own bodies, are at the mercy of the realm of their imagination. (Hardman 1973:95)

In the hands and minds of children, objects are used as playthings, but their function in the play is not based on what they are in themselves, but on the meaning given to them by the child, which could be almost anything. One may assume that medicines in the children's world are subjected to a similar transformation.

Studying the creative, "magical" handling of medicines by children does not confront us with a totally different world, however. Adults too attach meanings to pharmaceuticals which manufacturers, physicians, and pharmacists have never dreamt of. In the spontaneity of the playing child we are likely to discover some of the more hidden and surreptitious practices and concepts of adults. One sometimes learns most about adults by listening to children. The proverbial saying that children (and crazy or drunken people) speak the truth occurs in every language with which I am familiar.

NOTES

1. The invitation to write this reflection on anthropology and children reached me while I was preparing for fieldwork among old people in an African community. It seems to me that old and young have some striking similarities. Both are being marginalized and silenced. During my fieldwork I heard many adults refer

to the old as "children." Having completed this reflection I feel I have gained understanding of the old. I thank Pia Christensen, Anita Hardon, and Patricia Bush for their critical comments on an earlier version of this text.

2. Christensen (1993: 490) has the following to say about the delicate role of ethnographer among children:

> My aim . . . was not to assume the status of a "child," which from the point of view of children (or other adults), might have been perceived as patronising and insincere. Thus the study was conducted as a constant balancing act between being recognised as an "adult" and avoiding the preconceived ideas, practices and connotations associated with "adulthood." This status as an "other" was inevitably negotiated and renegotiated with both children and adults during the entire process of the study.

In a personal communication she gave me an example. During a holiday camp the children were to choose their mates for a game of soccer. Although the adults (teachers) were excluded from the selection, one team chose her. Apparently she belonged to another category.

REFERENCES

Ardener, E. 1975a. "Belief and the problem of women." *Perceiving Women*, edited by S. Ardener. London: Aldine, pgs. 1-17.

Ardener, E. 1975b. "The 'problem' revisited." *Perceiving Women*, edited by S. Ardener. London: Aldine, pgs. 19-27.

Christensen, P. H. 1993. "The social construction of health among Danish children." *Sociology of Health and Illness* 15 (4):488-502.

Christensen, P. H. 1994. "Children as the cultural other: The discovery of children in the social cultural sciences." *Kea Zeitschrift für Kulturwissenschaften* 6: 1-16.

Clifford, J. 1986. "Introduction: Partial truths." *Writing Culture: The Poetics and Politics of Ethnography*, edited by J. Clifford and G.E. Marcus. Berkeley: University of California Press, pgs. 1-26.

Clifford, J. and Marcus, G. M. (editors). 1986. *Writing Culture: The Poetics and Politics of Ethnography*. Berkeley: University of California Press.

Dwyer, K. 1987. *Moroccan Dialogues: Anthropology in Question*. Prospect Heights: Waveland Press.

Erikson, E. H. 1965. *Childhood and Society*. Harmondsworth: Penguin (first published 1950).

Goodman, M. 1957. "Values, attitudes and social concepts of Japanese and American children." *American Anthropologist* 59:979-999.

Hardman, C. 1973. "Can there be an anthropology of children?" *Journal of the Anthropology Society Oxford* 4 (1):85-99.

Jackson, M. 1989. *Paths Toward a Clearing. Radical Empiricism and Ethnographic Enquiry*. Bloomington: Indiana University Press.

James, A. and Prout, A. (editors). 1990. *Constructing and Reconstructing Childhood: Contemporary Issues in the Sociological Study of Childhood.* London: Falmer Press.

Malinowski, B. 1961. *Argonauts of the Western Pacific.* New York: Dutton (first published 1922).

Polanyi, M. 1958. *Personal Knowledge.* Chicago: University of Chicago Press.

Van der Geest, S. and Whyte, S. R. 1989. "The charm of medicines: Metaphors and metonyms." *Medical Anthropological Quarterly* 3 (4):345-367.

Chapter 19

Implications for Health Educators

Concha Colomer

In relation to the economic crisis of the 1970s, a series of studies and publications was produced that began to question the prevailing paradigm on the health-illness process and interventions for its promotion-prevention. Cochrane (1972), Illich (1976), and McKeown (1971) developed hypotheses which questioned the positive role of medicine on the state of the population's health. McKeown suggested that the improvement in the health of the inhabitants of England and Wales from the eighteenth century onward, is owed more to the effects of improved environmental factors (nutrition and hygiene) and to changes in certain types of behavior (e.g., fall in birth rate) than to the contributions of scientific medicine.

At that time, which also coincided with a change in the illness pattern as shown by an increase in chronic and psychosomatic diseases, the Canadian Health Minister, Lalonde, proposed a framework strategy for health promotion and illness prevention among Canadians. The Lalonde (1974) report has been—and still is—one of the most influential governmental documents on health policy ever published in the modern world. Its importance emerges basically from the recognition—in which it makes clear—that the determinants of health are numerous and diverse (Health Field Concept). Apart from the importance of the organization and the quality of medical care, hereditary factors (human biology), life-styles, and environmental factors play important roles in the making and promoting of health.

Also at that time, the World Health Organization (WHO) gave a show of support for a new health strategy, developing that of

"Health for All by the Year 2000," which has been spread, adopted, and adapted in the majority of countries across the world. Within this strategy, a health promotion program has been developed which is based on the social concept of health. Now health is defined in more operational terms instead of the classic WHO (1977) definition of "complete physical, mental, and social well-being." Health is now treated as, "the capacity by which the individual or group is able to realize his aspirations or satisfy his needs, and at the same time is also capable of changing or coping with the environment in which he lives." The focal point is on health rather than illness and also on health as a resource for everyday life, not as an ultimate goal to attain. Health is a social idea with psychological, cultural, economic, political, and biological elements. This concept of health is not new, neither does it emerge from the health service sector. The popular view of health is fundamentally and naturally holistic and seeks improvements in the very community resources which are characterized by their lack of paternalism, their respect for popular knowledge, and their strengthening of individual or group capabilities on a pragmatic level (WHO 1978). There are many examples of attempts on the part of the population to win control over its health (e.g., feminists, ecologists).

Health promotion has been defined as "the process of enabling individuals and communities to increase control over health determinants and, thereby, improve their health" (WHO 1977). This process employs various complementary approaches such as health education, facilitation, and regulation. Its focus is on advocacy, enabling, and mediation of health; building healthy public policy; creation of supportive environments; strengthening community action; developing personal skills; reorienting health services (WHO 1986). Worth noting in this approach of the last decades is the importance for health of life-styles—understood to mean ways of living or life patterns—in an interrelationship with the sociocultural contexts in which they are developed. This contrasts with other approaches which interpret life styles as a set of behaviors, generally negative for health, and supposedly independent of their sociocultural contexts.

Life styles signify a bridge between culture and individual behavior; therefore, their study is complex and should bear in mind the different components that interact and address them with different methodologies. The different chapters of this book are a good example of this approach; they represent one aspect of life style but they show that different methodologies were applied to the problem. This is what is currently recommended, once the inefficiency of previous approaches is ruled out (*Lancet* 1994).

Life styles have three main components: one individual or self-help component, another social and personal relationships component, and finally a component considered environmental or referring to the availability of services (WHO 1986). The complexity of the components and mechanisms of life styles is such that both research and interventions for life style modification should bear in mind this complexity and be approached in the same dimensions. This requires use of an extensive and varied combination of approaches, ranging from individual to community actions, from health education to healthful public policies.

Self-care and self-help are understood to be activities organized in an informal way that involve decision making. When the decisions are related to health, they include self-medication, self-treatment, and first aid in the normal social context of everyday life. It is in this context where the use of medication is fundamentally manifest as a specific aspect of life styles and as the object of health education. But we should not forget that the social component is important, and that attitudes of others, especially of the family, influence the attitudes of children and, finally, their decision making. On the other hand, the facilities that the environment provides with regard to access to services—in this case to sales of medication— also marks a difference in use, as is reflected in some of the studies in this book.

In recent years, there have been, without doubt, great developments in health education which have been implemented in schools in all countries to a greater or lesser extent. Also, all governments, national and regional, have been sensitive to the need for reporting the health status of children and for understanding how children's health can be improved and maintained.

The results of all these programs and activities for health education in schools have been highly contradictory, have given rise to a methods crisis, and even have deceived those, who at first, defended these innovative initiatives. The analysis which should be conducted on health education programs and activities should take into account the aims of health education which are to transmit information and, in any case, create favorable attitudes toward certain healthful behaviors. These aims are within reach of school health education. The problems and the deceptions have arisen when aims to modify behavior, or even create life styles, were based exclusively on didactic methods. This has resulted from a lack of knowledge of factors that intervene in the establishment of life styles. Individual values have been maximized; forgotten have been the effects of environmental and political aspects on life style. Obviously these factors do not alter with health education approaches toward children, but they require specific multisectoral action (Nutbeam and Catford 1987).

At the same time, the older didactic approaches have lacked a fundamental element for their effectiveness, which is the participation of those involved in their definition and execution. It has been shown that the impact of school health education programs is greater when the children themselves are the ones to define the priorities, aims, and methods of the programs (Arborelius and Bremberg 1988; Conell, Turner, and Mason 1985).

Another fundamental element for the success of promoting healthful life styles is to avoid tackling the different aspects which compose it separately, (e.g., sexuality, nutrition, exercise, medicine use), as if they were divisible parts of everyday life. Given the falsity of this separation, the danger for the results is apparent. The strategy should be empowerment of individual values and capabilities, strengthening people so that they are capable of facing up to situations and of freely deciding their best options. Decisions made in real life are almost never independent; they are interrelated; they involve assessment of what may appear to be a partial element, but in fact, are influenced by the personal and social factors of the individual's environment (*Social Science and Medicine* 1993; Hunt 1988).

In conclusion we may say that, if we want to promote rational use of medication by children, we should not forget that this is a behavior that is integrated with other components in children's life styles, their families, and society as a whole. For this reason, actions should consider all these aspects in order to be effective. Also, the different actors involved should develop, not only didactic skills, but also intersectoral work skills to introduce healthful modifications into the environments of children and into the related public policies.

Neither should we forget that the end objective of this process is to improve the health and the quality of life of children. The basis for doing so is to facilitate their empowerment, in order for them to be capable of making healthful decisions in the context of their daily lives in an informed, responsible, and self-confident way.

REFERENCES

Arborelius, E. and Bremberg, S. 1988. "It is your decision!" Behavioral effects of a student-centered health education model at school for adolescents. *Journal of Adolescence* 11(4):287-297.

Cochrane, A. L. 1972. *Effectiveness and Efficiency*. Nuffield Provincial Hospitals Trust.

Conell, D. B., Turner, R. R., and Mason, E. F. 1985. "Summary of findings of the school health education evaluation: Health promotion effectiveness, implementation, and costs." *Journal of School Health* 55:316-321.

Editorial. 1993. *Social Science and Medicine* 37:vii-viii.

Editorial. 1994. "Population health looking upstream." *Lancet* 343:429-430.

Hunt, S. M. 1988. "Health related behavioral change–A test of a New Model." *Psychology and Health* 2:209-230.

Illich, I. 1976. *Limits to Medicine: Medical Nemesis, the Expropriation of Health*. London: Marion Boars.

Lalonde, M. 1974. *A Perspective on the Health of Canadians*. Ottawa: Department of National Health and Welfare.

McKeown, T. 1971. *The Role of Medicine: Dream, Mirage or Nemesis*. London: Nuffield Provincial Hospital Trust.

Nutbeam, D. and Catford, J. 1987. "Welsh heart program evaluation strategy: Progress, plans and possibilities." *Health Promotion* 2:5-18.

WHO. "Lifestyles and Health." 1986. *Social Science and Medicine*. 22:117-124.

WHO. 1977. "Health for all by the year 2000." World Health Assembly Resolution 30.43. Geneva.

WHO. 1986. Health Promotion: Concept and Principles in Action–A Policy Framework. Copenhagen.

WHO. 1978. *Primary Health Care. Health for All. Alma-Ata 1978*. Series No. 1. Geneva.

Chapter 20

Implications for Health Policy

Abraham G. Hartzema

Use of medicines in children has attracted little scientific research (as noted in Chapter 15). While clinicians and pharmacoepidemiologists have been busy implementing clinical trials in the middle aged, and sociologists and health educators have directed considerable energies in understanding and changing health behaviors of the aged, the process of the socialization of our children in health care has been left relatively unexplored. However, its significance cannot be overestimated. Appropriate health behaviors are important for leading a complete and fulfilled life. Teaching children correct health behaviors could significantly reduce health care costs by reducing adverse health behaviors and providing the basis for efficient health care utilization.

The policy recommendations provided in this analysis are largely based on the research, emerging findings, and discussion provided in the preceding chapters. The focus of the analysis is on *the family* as a source of variation in medicine use, and as an explanation for this variation. Only few outside reference materials were involved or were consulted. For a more detailed description of the pharmaceutical distribution system, the nation-to-nation differences in legislation and regulation impacting on the distribution system, and the resulting variation in medicine use, the reader is referred to Chapter 4.

GENERAL BACKGROUND

In their formative years, children go through different phases in knowledge acquisition. In each of these phases, different needs for information arise. Providing an environment that serves as a model for good health behaviors and supporting that environment with tailored and targeted educational strategies should greatly contribute to appropriate health behaviors later in life. Providing a policy framework that contributes to such an environment and that fosters good health behaviors in society is of paramount importance.

Before we discuss such a policy framework, its characteristics as well as the structures, the processes, and the outcomes relevant to policy development should be identified. What have we learned of the project, medicine use in childhood, that may guide us in policy development? What are the elements in individual health behaviors that should be reinforced, augmented, or modified? What are the age-specific characteristics, the cultural sensitivities? What is the contribution of the parents, the influence of the environment? How do illness episodes modify these behaviors, and what is the role of the health care system? Why is medicine use rarely included as a topic in schoolchildren's health education curricula as observed by Bush and Hardon (1990), whereas most children's medicine use is not instigated by health care professionals but rather by children or families?

What are the resources available for treatment in the family and the environment? How are these resources being used? Can we optimize the use of these resources to provide a more efficient and cost-effective approach to health care? How are physicians being used? Do children and parents have access to over-the-counter (OTC) medicines so they can self-medicate? How are diseases diagnosed and treated in the family? What is the availability of different treatment modalities? Each of these considerations has consequences for policy development.

Understanding the principles involved in reducing the risk of attracting disease to oneself by avoiding disease-inducing exposures and behaviors, as well as actively adopting the behaviors that may reduce disease, is important in disease prevention. Recognizing illness symptoms and the ability to distinguish between self-limiting diseases and those needing medical attention and intervention, and understanding the importance of properly following a recommended plan of treatment, contribute to an effective use of health care resources.

Fundamental to proper health behaviors is a knowledge base with a supporting vocabulary and a set of attitudes and values that support these behaviors. This complex of attitudes, values, and knowledge can be acquired in several ways, but an appropriate combination needs to exist in all instances of appropriate health behavior. A combination of parental role modeling and formal information transferred by parents, information filtered through the peer network, knowledge obtained through the media, and formal educational processes in the school system all contribute to a cognitive system of knowledge. Some of these information sources may augment each other, others may be conflicting and thus left for the child to sort out the correct information.

INTERACTION OF HEALTH KNOWLEDGE, VALUES, AND ATTITUDES WITH DEVELOPMENTAL STAGES

Cognitive Development Theory (CDT) as proposed by Piaget (Inhelder and Piaget 1958), emphasizes stages for children's cognitive development of causal thinking from the preoperational through concrete operational to formal operational. It suggests that stages of development, although influenced by personal experience, are not formed as the direct response to parents, peers, or the child's own behavior, but result from the child's cognitive processes as they develop and operate within their environment. After infancy, children go through three different stages in their development. These developmental stages are: (1) the preoperational stage, (2) the concrete operational stage, and (3) the formal operational stage. In the preoperational stage (two to seven years of age) the children's understanding centers around observable events and whether or not there is a direct relation between the observable event and the health event. In the concrete-operational stage (seven to ten years of age), children's thinking becomes logical and systematic. Their understanding of health and illness now incorporates internal physiological characteristics.

The formal operational stage, approximately age range 11 years to adult, shows individuals who are capable of logical and systematic speculation about processes and consequences. Children's health-related beliefs and behaviors are relatively stable by the time they are in third and fourth grade (eight to 10 year olds), and the changes that take place when they are moving to into adolescence are relatively small (Bush and Iannotti 1988). A better understanding of health-related processes and the coordination of internal systems and external factors becomes apparent during this period. Individuals do not reach this level fully until late in adolescence and the skills associated with this level are not always applied to all content areas.

Analysis of the cognitive development stages in 119 classifiable cases of the 150 children observed in Novi Sad, Yugoslavia, (see Chapter 13) indicated the distribution of cases over developmental stages as shown in Table 20.1.

Apparently of the four-year-olds who should be in the middle of the prelogical (preoperational) stage according to strict Piagetian age ranges, 11 percent were already in the concrete logical (operational) phase. Whereas the age of seven marks the transition from prelogical to concrete logical, 41 percent of the seven-year-olds had not made this transition; of the 11-year-olds, only 23 percent had made the transition to the formal logical phase. Thus, the development of health concepts may trail the children's cognitive development in other life science areas, although this may not be the case for Finnish children who are exposed to a formal health education program (see Chapter 15).

Bandura (1986) put forward the Social Cognitive Theory to explain the interaction of the person, the environment, and behaviors. Behaviors are acquired through the process of attention, retention, production, and motivation. These processes operate in three domains: the personal, the behavioral, and the environmental domain.

TABLE 20.1. Development Stages of the Study Sample is Novi Sad*

Stage	4 years old	7 years old	11 years old
Prelogical	34 (89%)	19 (41%)	0 (0%)
Concrete logical	4 (11%)	27 (59%)	30 (77%)
Formal logical	0 (0%)	0 (0%)	9 (23%)

* 119 classifiable of 150 children (Chapter 13).

Personal factors include the child's own value system; expectations are derived from observation and experience; behavioral factors include skills in performing behaviors; environmental include peers, family members, and media which both model and influence through expressed opinions (Chapter 7). Illness episodes, dealt with in the family, are important contributors to forming the cognitive structure and lay the basis for subsequent health behaviors and attitudes.

FINDINGS RELEVANT TO POLICY DEVELOPMENT

The Family as Source of Variation: Fever as a Model

Chapter 3 defines illness episodes as "broad cultural events through which children experience the structure of their world and the social relations within it." During illness the children learn, *inter alia*, fundamental aspects of the social processes that occur between children and adults in their specific social and cultural contexts and experience child-adult hierarchies, relations of power, and the distribution of knowledge. Fever is used in this study to frame the sociopsychological processes that occur during an illness episode.

In Chapter 6, fever is defined as a socially and culturally constructed health problem. Although medical consensus holds that temperatures below 38°C (100.4°F) are normal, temperatures between 38 and 41°C (100.4 and 105.8°F) warrant monitoring and treatment by parents, and only temperatures over 41°C (105°F) need attention by a physician, a large variation in the interpretation by parents of these range delimiters was found. This variation in interpretation of the fever temperature results in a large variation of physician contacts.

Higher fevers might be more to likely cause a physician contact; also symptoms differing from those normally accompanying fever episodes, such as headache and belly ache, and in particular cough with vomiting, increase the likelihood of a physician contact (Chapter 11). Middle-ear infection and measles are also seen as serious diseases (Chapter 12). German parents appeared well informed about the meaning of temperature: 37 to 38°C (98.6 to 100.4°F) was considered raised, 38 to 39°C (100.4 to 102.2°F) was fever not needing physician attention if the duration is shorter than two days; 39 to 40°C (102.2 to 104°F) was defined as high fever. Uncertainty about the meaning of the temperature may result in an earlier physician contact; knowledge about the meaning of the temperature reading may result in symptom containment by an OTC medicine.

The number of physician contacts for fever episodes ranged from a high of 70 percent in Athens and Madrid, to 50 percent in Chapel Hill, to a low of 30 percent in Finland; physician contacts were often initiated after a "wait and see" period. In Germany, a physician contact was more likely than in other study locations to be followed up by a visit to a naturopath or homeopath. If the first visit was to a naturopath, then if the disease worsened, a visit to an allopath would follow. Parents from higher socioeconomic status were more likely to use a naturopath or homeopath (Chapter 12). Differences in type of provider contact may emerge from differences in the uncertainty about the underlying cause of the fever. Parents do not like to take risks with their children; thus, in cases of rising or high fevers, allopaths are consulted.

The presence of fever was usually first reported by the child, then assessed using sensory means (feeling the skin temperature with the hand) by the mother, followed by an assessment with the thermometer. Children learn to recognize the symptoms by experience; they know the symptoms and can judge if they have fever even though their experience is rather small because most children do not experience many illness episodes. In Chapter 13 it was shown that 93 percent of the children were aware they had fallen ill before recognition or confirmation of the illness by the parents. The confirmation that the child is sick was made in the following order: (1) the child him/herself, (2) the mother, (3) the doctor. More children in Chapel Hill self-diagnosed their disease than in other locations. School health education programs can play a role in bringing children in tune with their body by discussing fever-related symptoms.

Mothers are the main caregivers, but a greater availability of the mother may likely be a contributing factor (see Chapter 14 and others). When children's fever episodes began in the evening or weekend, fathers played a larger role. In the two Spanish locations (see Chapter 8) the main caregiver was more likely to receive help from relatives and others such as friends and neighbors; the extended family or lay network is more involved. On average, caregivers lose two workdays. Current labor laws permit sick leave days only for the wage earner. Where both parents are wage earners and the parents have to take unpaid sick leave, it becomes more likely that the child may be left on his or her own. In those cultures with extended families, which include, for example, grandparents, often child care responsibilities are shared by family members.

Children characterized their illness primarily in terms of change in their social relations and not in bodily symptoms. The experience of a fever episode was expressed by children in terms of isolation, restrictions, and privileges. Parents differed with children on their view of the imposition of isolation. An analysis of the illness experience as expressed in the children's drawings in Novi Sad (Chapter 13) showed that 42 percent of the children portrayed themselves alone in bed, 39 percent with the mother present, 14 percent with a "fearful medical instrument or equipment," and 5.3 percent with either the father or grandparent. The four-year-olds were more likely to draw themselves with the father. An illness episode was not seen as a pleasant experience. In contrast, the Finnish children considered being sick as a period of rest with the possibility of playing, and the warmth and coziness of more attention from the parents (Chapter 15). Illness meant also an absence from school with two implications, relief from school pressures but also the lack of social interactions. Older children more often reported to be alone or isolated, with being alone considered a negative experience. It is likely that older children were more likely to be left alone at home; the Finnish response reflects the more liberal sick leave provisions in the labor laws benefitting the child. Also, countries with low labor market participation can rely on the mother or the extended family to take on child care responsibilities. Current sick leave provisions in most countries only cover sick leave by the wage earner. They should not discriminate between parents and they should base sick leave time on the number of children in the family.

Mothers and their children differed greatly in the explanation of the cause of the child's illness. While mothers attributed the cause to viral infections, children attributed the cause to their own actions, such as going outside without a coat, essentially reiterating the maternal warnings received on those cold days. In the Finnish sample, most children recognized the concept of contagion but the actual processes involved were still unclear. Illness episodes were largely attributed to contagion, climate, and lifestyle. Concepts of internal causes of diseases were unknown with diseases considered to be caused by something entering the body from the outside (Chapter 15). Whereas younger children may perceive an illness as external to the body, older children will localize the illness in the body (See Chapter 13). Finnish children defined illness and health as two opposite concepts: illness was considered a physiological concept, whereas health was considered a psychological concept. Children were also more likely than the parents to think that they could prevent fever.

The cognitive development of children, aged seven to 11, can be characterized by the use of logical reasoning in solving problems. Concurrent to this developmental stage, the presentation of disease models may be most interesting. Children start also to include internal physiological characteristics in their descriptions of illness causation and effects of medicine. Older children describe contagion in terms such as bacteria and bugs, younger children in terms of transmission routes. Older children use brand or generic names in referring to medicines; younger children more often describe medicines by color and taste. Older children believe that the ability to recover is vested in their own body; younger children believe in external sources that lead to recovery. In the German sample (Chapter 12) few children differentiated between "natural" or "plant-based" or "chemical" medicines. The homeopathy or naturopathic products were heavily used in this sample and were considered harmless. Medicine shape, color, and taste appeared to be important; tastes bitter, sour, and alcoholic were least preferred. Parent perceptions about the danger of medicines may lead to stopping antibiotic cures when the child appears to recover (Chapter 12). In the Finnish sample, little evidence of the use of natural products was found; the investigators attributed this to the fact that natural remedies are not referred to in the Finnish culture as medicines.

Vocabulary and references to illness processes change according to developmental stage. Children have only limited experience with illnesses, because they do not encounter many illness episodes.

Parents see illness episodes and resulting experiences as a part of growing up. School-based health education can play an important role in developing children's vocabulary, processes, and concepts used in explaining health-related events, preventive or curative, in accordance with their cognitive developmental stage. Such a program should parallel the natural history of childhood illnesses and concentrate on those that are most likely to be acquired by children in the age group addressed. Diseases such as cancer and AIDS evoke strong associations by children but are of lesser importance in this age group.

A conclusion in Chapter 3 is that children see the nonpharmaceutical therapeutic actions of their caregivers as the most important aspect of their recovery. Nonpharmacological treatments used in the illness episode are resting, special diets, and beverages. In Finland the first line of treatment for a child's fever episode is a nonpharmacological course of action; the second line is a prescription medicine. Finnish parents indicated they were more likely to use OTC medicines in their own illness episodes than for their children (Chapter 14). Parents often expressed a suspicion about the effectiveness of OTC products as compared with prescription medicines.

In the "wait and see" period, most of the medicine use was initiated by the mother, followed by the doctor upon medical attention to the illness episode. Parents in the three samples, Madrid, Tenerife, and Chapel Hill did not realize that children perceive themselves as decision makers and active participants in the process (Chapter 8). When asked which decisions they were most likely to be involved in, the children responded: (1) bringing fever symptoms to the attention of the parents; (2) reminding parents about the right time to take the medicines; (3) telling parents that they were feeling well enough to go back to school. In many situations (including medicine taking) children did not have much room for independent action, although the autonomy of children in medicine use is greater than most adults assume.

In Chapel Hill, children are more active partners in decision making regarding treatment choices than in Madrid and Tenerife as recognized by both parents and children. Spanish children showed more autonomy in taking medicines and purchasing medicines. In the German sample (Chapter 12), older children had the autonomy to take the medicine themselves but under parental supervision. Understanding the structure of decision making in the family, and understanding when and under which conditions the transfer of authority takes place will help tailor planned health education efforts and determine the information need.

In the "wait and see" period, parents in the German sample were more likely to use medicines that were already available in the household (Chapter 12). Fifty percent of the medicines used were those already stored in the Dutch sample homes (Chapter 11). Chapter 5 refers to the "medicine cabinet" as an indicator of the "pharmaco-medicalization" of families. The number of medicines available in the typical household ranged from eight (Jyväskylä, Finland) to 24 (Chapel Hill, USA) with up to 70 different medicines identified in some households. Of these medicines, 40 percent had OTC status and 60 percent prescription (Rx) status. In descending order, the most frequent present were: topicals, cough/cold products, analgesics, antipyretics, and nonsteroidal antiinflammatory agents. In Finland, families with one child had more prescription medicines stored per person than families with two or more children (Chapter 14). The expiration date had passed for 10 to 30 percent of the medicines. Often the expiration date could not be identified; for example, on tubes with the expiration stamped on the bottom, after use and rolling up of the tube, the expiration date disappeared. Also, an erroneous indication was sometimes provided by the family when asked. Prescription medicines are stored because they represent the total of opportunity cost, visit cost, and medicine cost, and thus represent significantly more than the cost of the medicine alone.

Medicine use differed significantly among countries with 50 percent in Finland, 78 percent in Spain, and a high of 96 percent of families in the USA indicating medicine use for the treatment of a fever episode. Paracetamol and aspirin were the most commonly used medicines, while also antibiotics were mentioned. In Chapel Hill, 90 percent of the parents used paracetamol, in Madrid and Tenerife 32 percent, and in Jyväskylä, 30 percent. Antibiotics and other medicines were most frequently used in Athens, 39 percent. The leading norm in parent-initiated medicine prescribing was: "only when really needed, I may give a tablet to my child, preferably a *half* one." Children offered a lower opinion of the effectiveness of medicines than the parents.

The storage place was predominately the kitchen or the bathroom; the medicines were rarely locked up and were usually accessible to children. Seventy to eighty-five percent of the children said that medicines are accessible to them. Some medicines were given to children under 12 years, even when the label stated that the medicine should be given to children under 12 only after consultation with the physician. The parents would not consult the physician but would provide the child with a half dose. The parents apparently saw danger in the dose and not in the chemical structure.

Children commonly made references to restrictions and regulations concerning pharmaceuticals. Many children understood that the doctor prescribes medicine and that an adult in the household (usually the mother) distributes it. Chapter 13 reported that 40.6 percent of the children mentioned that the doctor decides which medicine to take; for 35.0 percent the mother makes the decision. In asking what contributes most to their recovery four-year-olds most often mentioned their mother together with medicines, seven-year-olds the mother and the doctor, and for 11-year-olds the most potent force in their recovery was viewed as their doctor and the medicines. Some children pointed to their own role as one in cooperating in taking medicine (Chapter 3). The degree of control children have differed by location. In the USA sample (Almarsdottir and Bush 1995), it was found that children may take medicines independently of parental approval; in other samples, such as ones in Great Britain and Denmark, the level of autonomy appeared less. In this concept, children are seen as independent actors, interrelating with their larger environment.

Only a few children ten years and under in any study location had ever bought medicines, whereas most children have physical access to the medicines and know where they are stored. More children in Chapel Hill than in Madrid or Tenerife said that they had treated themselves for a headache without parental involvement. In general, children identified their medicines as curative and not as preventive; only a little understanding of adverse medicine reactions was present and this was only in relationship to overdosing. Healthy children rarely had a concept of preventive medicines or chronic diseases (Chapter 10). Medicines were rarely identified to inter-viewers according to their pharmacological action but descriptors such as color, size, and taste were often used.

The parent's choice of medicine was found to be based on experi-ence and information acquired over time. None of the caregivers ac-tively looked for information; information acquisition appeared to be quite truncated (Chapter 11). From the information sources available, the mass media were mentioned as an important source of information on health and illness. Television programs were mentioned most often, followed by women's magazines, medical handbooks, and brochures. The presence of a chronic disease precipitated an active search for information (Chapter 11). Acute, short-term illnesses generally did not cause an information search. In the Spanish sample, children's knowl-edge and attitudes relating to health, sickness, and medicine use were developed almost exclusively through personal experience and family influence; little health education is available (Chapter 8).

Several issues relevant for policy development arise from the synthesis of the research findings presented above. Cultural differ-ences, as presented in the characteristics of the family structure, the interpretation of symptoms, the expression of the fever experience, treatment choices, and the amount of autonomy delegated to the child in the management of fever, are important considerations in developing health education programs and in strengthening protec-tive mechanisms. Health education programs need to be sensitive to cultural differences in society while providing a rational approach to health behaviors.

Also, strengthening the protective structure which surrounds child health and disease management needs to be considered. Fiscal measures are needed to promote medicine development for child-hood diseases, medicine testing specifically for the younger age groups, and medicine formulation, packaging, and promotion to foster appropriate medicine-taking behaviors. Other important areas for consideration in this domain are child care provisions and the extension of sick leave benefits. Governments play increasingly a greater role in information provision and regulation. Policy implica-tions emerging from the research findings are discussed in greater detail below.

Policy Implications

Earlier studies in medicine use conducted under the auspices of the World Health Organization led to the conclusion that major differences in medicine use are prevalent among the European countries, but also among countries outside Europe (Chapter 4). Such differences are due in part to the regulatory environment, the organization of health care resources, and the payment mechanism, but a large variation in medicine consumption remains. This variation cannot be explained with morbidity models alone, thus other factors must be responsible for these differences. These factors are strongly cultural and can only be explained in an anthropological and sociological context. As observed in Chapter 3, there are "cultural patterns in the meanings associated with medicine use and these patterns, learned in childhood, may be used to explain variations in pharmaceutical use enacted in adult life."

Moreover, the health care system can be considered to be composed of three interrelated sectors: a professional, a popular, and a folk sector. The professional sector is defined by the professional diagnostic, treatment, and care procedures. The popular sector contains the approaches used in lay management of diseases. The folk sector includes traditional healing methods, including homeopathy, herbalism, and other folk practices that are endogenous. Different cultures place different values and beliefs in each of these sectors; economically more advanced communities show a higher affinity for professional approaches, while economical disadvantaged countries rely more on the folk practices. The German observations in which higher income families were involved in the use of naturopathy may be due to payment mechanisms where use of a naturopath requires an out-of-pocket payment.

Also, pharmaceuticals may express some form of hierarchy in health care at different levels, at the macro social level through the restrictions surrounding the approval and marketing of medicines, and at the intermediate level through restrictions in the prescriptions necessary to purchase medicines (Chapter 3). At the micro (family) level, the relationship between the child and the adult hierarchy emerges from the oversight and gate-keeping position of the parent.

Study findings show how medicines communicate messages about hierarchy, authority, and power in the family.

Health policy facilitating good health practices in children—health practices that may benefit them in adulthood—should be based on research and development into the strategies and practices that may facilitate these practices. Policy needs to be developed along three broad lines: (1) strengthen the protective environment; (2) assist the cognitive development of health behaviors and practices through child and adulthood; and (3) stimulate qualitative and quantitative research in health behaviors and practices and the culture surrounding these behaviors and practices.

Policy Framework for a Protective Environment

Medicine Development

Little is known about the effectiveness and safety of a medicine product when admitted to the market. Clinical trials often enroll middle-age volunteers; the extremes in the population age distribution, the young and the old, are underrepresented in such trials. Thus clinical information on prescription medicines, including toxicity and kinetic information for new medicines for pediatric populations, is inadequate. This lack of good medicine information makes it difficult to extrapolate the therapeutic schemes from adults to children. Medicine evaluation mechanisms should be extended to include children, so that kinetic and safety data become available for those products that have potential value in the treatment of childhood diseases.

Most illnesses are self-limiting; the literature suggests that maybe 80 percent of all illness episodes are self-limiting and do not need the attention of the physician. Thus, it becomes important that an arsenal of childhood-specific products becomes available that alleviate symptoms and allow children as well as parents to cope with self-limiting illness episodes. In the USA, OTC medicines currently are sold in two different dosages: a dosage size for the adult, and a dosage size for children six to 12 years of age. These latter packages include a warning not to use the medicines for children younger than six years of age. The question remains, what does one do for a child less than six years of age? Clearly, there is a need for medicines specific for childhood illness in the very young or doses adapted to their needs.

That no such medicines, dosage forms, and packaging, currently are available may be related to market conditions. This market segment involves more risk and a lesser return than the adult or the elder market. How can we entice the pharmaceutical industry to provide for this market segment? One could think about the orphan medicine act as an example, providing additional incentives to develop new chemical entities for childhood diseases and facilitate the formulation of OTC products for the very young. In the USA, a new set of initiatives by the National Institute of Health (NIH) may stimulate medicine development for the young and very young.

Medicine Approval

Kogan et al. (1994) studied the prevalence of OTC medicine use in 8,145 children whose mothers were interviewed for the 1991 Longitudinal Follow-up to the National Maternal and Infant Health Survey. In the 30-day recall period, 53.7 percent of three-year-old children in the sample had used an OTC product, 40 percent of the children received two OTC medicines, and 5 percent received three or more medicines. The medicine most commonly used was Tylenol® (66.7 percent) and cough and cold medicine (66.7 percent). The use of OTC products for three-year-olds was more prevalent in white, higher socioeconomic families, and in families without health insurance. From these findings, the authors concluded that OTC medicines play an important role in the treatment of illness episodes in preschool-age children, while little scientific evidence about their efficacy and safety in this population is known.

According to NIH sources, of the approximately 80 medicines used in children, only five have Food and Drug Administration (FDA) approved label indications for pediatric use. In response to these findings, the NIH recently initiated a network, referred to as the Pediatric Pharmacology Research Unit (PPRU) Network and sponsored by the Center for Research for Mothers and Children of the National Institute of Child Health and Human Development. The purpose of the network is to stimulate investigator-initiated studies on the pharmacodynamics and pharmacokinetics of medicines in children; conduct pre- and post-marketing clinical trials, provide pediatricians and others with experience in pediatric clinical pharmacology, and establish a network for multicenter clinical trials. Six centers are participating in the network (NIH 1994).

Efficacy and safety of natural products for children also need to be assessed (Chapter 12). Differences in countries can be observed in the availability and use of natural and homeopathic products. From the observations made in these studies in selected countries, homeopathic and naturopathic products are frequently used in childhood diseases because they are thought to be safe and healthful. Little efficacy data support the use of these products and safety profiles supporting their use in children is not available. It appears rational to hold these products to the same efficacy and safety standards as are set for allopathic medicines.

Medicine Marketing

The role of the government in providing public information has increased over the last few years; examples are legal requirements for warning labels on smoking articles, alcoholic beverages, and other consumer products. The FDA revised requirements for food labeling which now requires extensive nutritional information. Although currently not addressed, there appears to be a need for medicine information distinct from the information contained in the current mandated package inserts. Product information, both for prescription and OTC medicines, needs to be made available to the consumer.

Rx to OTC Switch

A trend can be observed in society to switch prescription (Rx) medicines to OTC status. Three reasons are indicated for this transfer, (1) increased self-care with individuals demanding a wider range of treatment options without having to consult a physician; (2) the pharmaceutical industry, upon patent expiration of prescription medicines, favors a switch to OTC status to retain or expand market share, and (3) some governments with extensive medicine insurance programs support shifts from Rx to OTC status to remove expensive medicines that are reimbursable. Bringing a prescription medicine to OTC status means that individuals can buy the product for self-medication purposes without a prescription from a physician.

For medicines switched from Rx to OTC status, there is a need for public education to introduce the new treatment in the self-care domain. The introduction of a new OTC product based on a previously unavailable chemical class, is a product innovation in the public domain. Directed information programs identifying the place of such a treatment in the marketplace are of paramount importance to assure proper use of a new class of OTC products. Although OTC advertising by manufacturers plays a role in increasing the awareness of the product innovation, the government may play a role in further educating the public about the appropriate use of the self-treatment with the new OTC product.

In addition, when medicines are transferred from Rx status to OTC status, the switch often does not generate sufficient revenue for the company to provide separate data supporting efficacy and safety claims in younger populations. Thus, most medicines are poorly researched in younger populations. The NIH, recognizing this problem, organized a network of investigators with access to pediatric populations. The purpose of this network is to evaluate medicines for pediatric use, a policy decision that can significantly influence the availability of OTC medicines for childhood illnesses.

Medicine Formulation

Two sets of observations become important in the formulation of pediatric medicines. First, children have strong feelings about the shape, color, and taste of medicines. These strong feelings are positive if medicines are formulated as candies and negative if medicines are formulated as medicines, i.e., large in shape, white in color, and alcoholic or bitter in taste. Despite the special formulations available, in which the taste of the medicine is disguised, it appeared from interviews in Greece that mothers, even for those medicines brought to the market as child formulations, further sweeten the medicine to make it more palatable and easier to swallow (Chapter 9).

Medicines for pediatric use should be formulated so that errors of accidental use of the medicine as candy are avoided. Pediatric formulations should not disguise the taste of the medicine or make them look like candies, the benefit being that children early in their cognitive development process acquire an understanding that medicines are different in both form and purpose. Presenting children with medicines in the form of medicines may help children move from the preoperational to the concrete operational phase in their cognitive development to understand that the purpose and mode of action of medicines are greatly different from that of candies.

Medicine Packaging

Encapsulating study findings in policy implications, the following conclusions can be drawn. In a review of the medicine cabinets as observed in Chapters 5, 11, 12, and 14, it appeared that a large number of medicines are not completely finished. Parents may stop giving the child the medicine as soon as the symptoms disappear, behavior also common among adults. Expired medicines were identified for both Rx and OTC medicines.

Several policy issues emerge from these behaviors. The completion of therapies is necessary to achieve the intended effect, especially for antibiotics. Medicines have a limited shelf life, in particular under conditions that are adverse to the chemical integrity of the medicine such as often prevail in kitchens and bathrooms. In these places where the medicines are stored under adverse conditions, warmth and humidity accelerate the decomposition of medicines. Then the expiration date of medicines becomes more important. Expiration dates should be identifiable even when the outside package is disposed of, and only the blister pack is left. Also the identification of medicines that are kept for later use may be difficult, for example, containers may be damaged, instructions may be unreadable, or medicines may be repackaged. Some of the parents interviewed could not give the appropriate indication for the medicines stored. Then there is the question of how to dispose of medicines in an environmentally acceptable way.

These observed manifestations of patient behaviors, largely induced by lack of information, confusing information, conflicting information, and information not available should be addressed. Clarity in labeling and packaging of the products can solve many of these problems. The following are conditions and requirements that can resolve the medicine-use problems observed in the Childhood and Medicines Project.

An emphasis should be placed on unit-of-use packaging to reflect differences in children's ages in the package design and length of therapy. Packaging designs should clearly distinguish the medicine from candy, and establish within the child's frame of reference a disease/health connotation. Then, it appears that the unit-of-use packaging should be adapted for the normal course of an illness episode. For influenza, which runs its course over a six- to seven-day period, the package should provide therapy for such a period of time; antibiotics for a ten- to 12-day period. Unit-of-use packaging should reduce the number of expired medicines lingering in the medicine cabinet.

Expected outcomes of the medicine treatment should be clearly identified on the package and on the unit of packaging. If the last pill is taken and the symptoms remain, clearly a follow-up strategy, almost always implying a physician visit, should be indicated. Information presented on the packaging in a decision tree or algorithmic format may be helpful. OTC medicines are relatively inexpensive, so inexpensive that the cost-effectiveness ratio of keeping a medicine stored versus discarding it, and if necessary purchasing a new product, is negative. The expiration date coupled with the unit of packaging should largely reduce medicine storage. A barrier to discarding medicines may be the ambiguity and public concern regarding the disposal of chemicals. Clearly, identified approaches to the disposal of the medicine may also reduce the number of unnecessary medicines kept in storage at the home. Moreover, such an approach would reduce the chance for accidental poisonings.

Stricter guidelines for developing pediatric packaging and information provided on the package is strongly recommended. Such information should provide an algorithmic approach to therapeutic decision making including: indication for start of the therapy, expected outcome of therapy, follow-up on therapy, and disposal of medicines. Labeling may be required to clearly state the indication for the drug and the interpretation of the symptoms related to that indication, resolving in part the confusion caused by combination products. An index of the therapeutic value of the medicine–its ranking as compared to other products on the market–may benefit the consumer. Such a therapeutic value could be modeled after the energy consumption rating on refrigerators or after food labeling as currently implemented in the USA. Production of a basic list of drugs to be kept in the household for self-medication by family members–in analogy to home first aid kits–should be fostered.

Policy Framework for Health Education Programming

The basic viewpoint of health policy on medicine use is to enhance rational medicine therapy. From this viewpoint emerges how adequate health education for children can be made available, and what regulations should be implemented as part of a protective structure to guide the development of a cognitive structure precipitating rational medicine-use behaviors.

Children are a high risk group for the inappropriate use of medicines. Among the multiple factors defining risk are: immaturity of knowledge about medicines; mistaking medicine for candy or food; disagreement between children's perceived autonomy in the use of medicines and the autonomy perceived by parents, and the availability and accessibility of medicines stored at home (Chapter 10).

Children's behaviors as related to health and medicines are developed early in life, and these behaviors reflect their culture as well as their stage of internal cognitive development. Children have beliefs, attitudes, values, and behaviors toward treatment that are possibly distinct for each child, but are formed by the surrounding culture (Chapter 8). Behaviors are acquired through the process of attention, retention, production, and motivation (Bandura 1986). Therefore, differences in knowledge, behavior, and attitudes regarding treatment and use of medicines during childhood illness should be expected across cultures.

The socialization of children in their early stages of development as described by Piaget has been found important. Most socialization of children takes place through parents who serve as role models. Mothers have a strong influence on their children's health behaviors, which become relatively stable at school age. Only in later stages in development do media become important. Schools could play a more important role in providing health education since most of the child's knowledge acquisition takes place in the school. Health education provided at an earlier age may be more effective than education provided at a later age. Such education could parallel the development of the different childhood diseases which are a part of growing up.

It is possible to start educating about medicines as early as second grade. Children think about medicines and have already discovered the Western paradigm of the role of medicines in the repair of the body's malfunctions. Having medicines available in pediatric packaging and adapted formulations but resembling medicines may help start the socialization process in medicine use. Whether knowledge acquisition by children is purely a function of development, or whether there are important social factors at work, we do not know. We also do not know when children are knowledgeable enough and behaviors are developed enough to take responsibility for their medicine taking.

Advertising may be an important factor in enhancing children's perceptions that medicines are beneficial, but may not increase actual knowledge about medicines. Knowledge acquisition is facilitated by other resources such as value systems and parental background (Chapter 7). The influence of children's books, and the role of doctors pictured in children's books should be explored, as well as how medical encounters are reviewed in children's literature.

POLICY FRAMEWORK FOR FUTURE RESEARCH

In conclusion, the study increases the recognition that variations in medicine use, controlling for differences in legislative environment and morbidity, are socially and culturally determined. Second, the study provides significant information about developing educational strategies and illustrates the importance of providing an environment that fosters good medicine taking. Third, the project employed a triangulation of qualitative and quantitative methods for cross-cultural comparisons of childhood medicine use, an approach significantly adding detail and depth to the data presented. Fourth, the project brought researchers together who overcame three main cultural barriers to achieve the collaboration.

The three barriers, which have some degree of operational overlap, reflect differences in research culture. Research culture differences refer to (1) differences in research approach, activity, and productivity; (2) differences in professional prerogatives as exemplified in health care providers working together with anthropologists, sociologists, and epidemiologists; and (3) the research schism between the qualitative and the quantitative scientists which needed to be overcome. This dimensionality, which provided the project with a culturally rich environment, translated into a kaleidoscope of important results. Certainly, the contrasts in findings, flowing from the amalgam of qualitative and quantitative studies, contributed to a rich vein of knowledge. This newly opened vein deserves all efforts at further exploration.

REFERENCES

Almarsdottir, A. B. and Bush, P. J. 1995. "Children's experience with illness in Chapel Hill, North Carolina, USA." *Childhood and Medicine Use in Cross-Cultural Perspective: A European Concerted Action*, edited by D. J. Trakas and E. Sanz. Luxembourg: Office for Official Publications of the European Community, (EURO Report), pgs. (in press).

Bandura A. 1986. *Social Foundations of Thought and Action*. Englewood Cliffs, NJ: Prentice-Hall.

Bush, P. J. and Iannotti, R. J. 1988. "Origins and stability of children's health beliefs relative to medicine use." *Social Science and Medicine* 27(4):345-352.

Bush, P. J. and Hardon, A. P. 1990. "Toward rational medicine use: Is there a role for children?" *Social Science and Medicine* 31(9):1043-1050.

Inhelder B. and Piaget, J. 1958. *The Growth of Logical Thinking from Childhood to Adolescence*. New York: Basic Books.

Kogan, M. D., Pappas, G., Yu, S. M., and Kotelchuck, M. 1994. "Over-the-counter medicine use among US preschool-age children." *Journal American Medical Association* 272:1025-1030.

NIH. 1994. "NIH funds network of centers for pediatric medicine research." *American Journal Hospital Pharmacy* 51:2546.

Chapter 21

Pharmacoepidemiology and Children

Göran Tomson

In recent decades, medicine has been blessed with pharmaceutical tools that are much more powerful than before. Although this provided opportunities for treating global major public health problems such as malaria, pneumonia, and tuberculosis in a much better way, it also resulted in the ability to do much greater harm. The history of drug regulation, in fact, parallels the history of major adverse drug reaction disasters. Pharmacoepidemiology is the study of the use of, and effects of, drugs in large numbers of people (Strom 1994). The discipline has become increasingly important for regulatory agencies and public health.

NEED FOR PHARMACOEPIDEMIOLOGY AMONG CHILDREN

Children, newborns, and fetuses often have been the victims of major drug safety catastrophes. The infamous "thalidomide disaster" in the early 1960s (McBride 1961; Lenz 1966) in which children exposed to thalidomide in utero were born with phocomelia, i.e., with flippers instead of limbs, greatly stimulated interest both in drug regulation and pharmacoepidemiology. The "grey syndrome," wherein premature newborns reacted with circulatory collapse to chloramphenicol, is another example of a drug safety catastrophe. In the 1970s, clear cell adenocarcinoma of the cervix and vagina and other genital malformations were found to have been caused by in utero exposure to diethylstilbestrol two decades earlier (Herbst, Ulfelder, and Poskanzer 1971). Reye's syndrome, a serious disease characterized by coma and hepatic dysfunction, was demonstrated in a case-control study to occur in children following use of salicylate during febrile illnesses (Hurwitz et al. 1987). Obviously children have been at risk and the need for drug safety mechanisms, pharmacoepidemiology being one, is clear.

A recent review of the epidemiology of drug use in children (Bonati 1994) concluded that studies monitoring drug prescriptions and their rationality in this age group appear to be a rarity more than a routine. The few studies published (Adams 1991; Bush, Iannotti, and Davidson 1985; Hardon 1987; Ray, Federspiel, and Schaffner 1967; Ray, Federspiel, and Schaffner 1977; Rylance 1987; Rylance et al. 1988; Sanz, Bergman, and Dahlstrom 1989; Schaffner et al. 1983; Tomson, Diwan, and Angunawela 1990) showed that antibiotics for upper respiratory infections and antipyretics were the most common classes of drugs for children. Paracetamol was generally preferred to salicylates (e.g., aspirin) for safety reasons, whereas the antibiotic profiles varied among countries without obvious explanatory factors.

Given that children, especially young children, constitute a population that has been shown to be vulnerable to the toxicity aspects, as well as representing a large proportion of consumption of specific classes of drugs, e.g., antibiotics and antipyretics, it is surprising that more systematic approaches have not been developed. This situation holds true both for industrialized and developing countries. In the latter, children under fifteen years of age represent about half of the population (World Bank 1993) and suffer from communicable diseases treatable with drugs at the primary health care level.

PHARMACOEPIDEMIOLOGY

History

Drug Utilization Research was conceived in northern Europe in the late 1960s. The comparative studies conducted were mostly of a descriptive nature showing major unexplained differences in drug use between and also within countries (Engels and Siderius 1968).

Numerous factors, as shown in Figure 21.1, influence prescribing including technological achievements, the health care system, national drug policies with regulations, drug and therapeutic committees, marketing, and sociocultural determinants including professional and public preferences and information efforts (Sterky et al. 1991). Comparative research should have a multidisciplinary approach (Sachs, Sterky, and Tomson 1988), but only recently have social and behavioral scientists become more involved, enabling more analytical, "why" research. This perspective was thus very much welcomed when the multidisciplinary "COMAC Childhood and Medicines Project" was initiated in 1989 supported by the commission of European Communities. It had by then become obvious to professionals, administrators, politicians, and the informed public that something had to be done to achieve higher quality of drug use in all segments of the population in industrialized and developing countries alike.

Whereas pharmacoepidemiology is a relatively new discipline (Strom 1994), one might say that epidemiology is as old as medicine itself (McBride 1961). In the fifth century B.C., Hippocrates, the "father" of modern medicine, first suggested that the development of human disease might be related to the external as well as personal environment of an individual. The word "epidemiology" is semantically composed of the Greek "epi" = among, "demos" = people, and "logos" = science, i.e., it is concerned with what happens with the population. Pharmacology is the study of the effects of drugs.

Epidemiology is based on two assumptions: first, that human disease does not occur at random, and second, that there are causal and preventive factors associated with human disease, that can be identified by systematically investigating different populations (or subgroups of individuals within a population) in different places or at different times. This leads to the definition of epidemiology as "the study of the distribution and determinants of disease frequency" in human populations. These three closely interrelated components—distribution, determinants, and frequency—encompass all epidemiologic principles and methods. The field of pharmacoepidemiology has primarily concerned itself with the study of adverse drug effects (Cluff, Thornton, and Seidl 1964; Farquhar et al. 1977; McEwen

FIGURE 21.1. Factors Influencing Prescribing

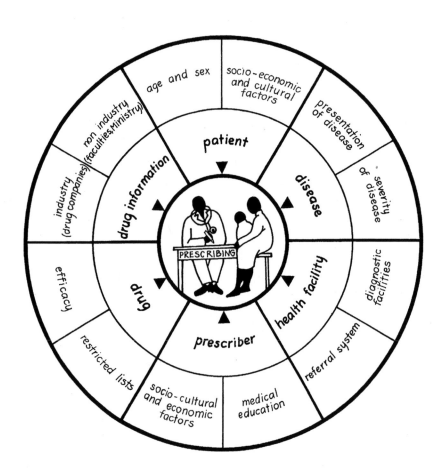

Source: Diwan/Tomson, IHCAR 1988. Reprinted with permission.

1987). The application of the principles has mainly been in post-marketing drug surveillance.

John Graunt represents an important milestone in the history of epidemiology. He introduced quantitative methods into epidemiology and in 1662 published his "Natural and Political Observations on the Bills of Mortality" using the very first life-table. Later, William Farr, an English doctor in charge of the official medical statistics in England and Wales in the 1830s, studied mortality in British prisons. He was able to assess the "population at risk," a basic epidemiological concept (the denominator) as well as the number of deaths (the numerator). William Farr collaborated with John Snow, a doctor in the Soho district of London, where there was an outbreak of cholera in the 1850s. By systematically mapping the cholera deaths in the area, Snow found an uneven distribution, which could be related to contaminated water from certain stand pipes. Basic calculations such as relating a numerator to a denominator is very much what epidemiology is all about. It is, however, imperative that there is no systematic selection of cases for the numerator and that the denominator is representative of the target population. The above mentioned examples should be inspiring also for pharmacoepidemiologists. Large computerized data bases are no prerequisites for well-conducted pharmacoepidemiology studies.

The pioneering study by Snow became a model for epidemiological work from clinical observation to description, hypothesis testing, and intervention, thus working at three levels: characterization, analysis, and intervention. In its early phase, pharmacoepidemiology emerged mainly from an increasing interest in drug issues among epidemiologists, not the least, adverse drug reactions, but gradually, clinical pharmacologists became involved (see Table 21.1). With few exceptions, the studies have not reached beyond the descriptive and analytical level to include the intervention level of epidemiology.

Study Designs

There are three important questions that distinguish among different study designs. The first question is whether the investigator is in control of the action; the second, whether comparisons are based on some randomization procedure; and the third, whether the time perspective is prospective or retrospective. We can also distinguish

TABLE 21.1. Pharmacoepidemiology and Society*

Kinds of information needed to supplement premarketing studies to achieve better knowledge of adverse and beneficial effects:

1. Higher precision

2. For the elderly, CHILDREN, pregnant women, patients not studied prior to marketing

3. As modified by other drugs or diseases

4. Relative to other drugs used for the same indication

Types of information not available from premarketing studies:

1. Uncommon or delayed adverse and beneficial effects

2. Drug utilization

3. Drug overdoses

4. Health economics and drug use

General contributions of pharmacoepidemiology:

1. Drug safety and reassurance

2. Ethical and legal obligations

*Adapted from Strom 1992.

among three different kinds of epidemiological studies. The first one is the prospective cohort study, wherein the investigator classifies one group (cohort) as to exposure and follows the group to the point where disease starts to develop. The second kind of design is the historical or retrospective cohort study, where a cohort is identified in the past and followed up in time to determine whether or not disease developed. The third type of study is called the retrospective case referent (control) study, in which a group of disease cases is compared with a group of referents, usually composed of healthy individuals, to try to find out if the people with the sickness have been exposed to a certain risk factor in the past.

Drug safety studies in children have used these techniques whereas drug utilization studies in children typically are cross-sectional; cohort studies are seldom conducted. However, e.g., the U.S. health insurance system for the disadvantaged (Medicaid) includes large data bases enabling health systems research including drug utilization and drug effects. For example, cohort studies have been conducted on the irrational use of chloramphenicol (Ray, Federspiel, and Schaffner 1967) and tetracycline (Ray, Federspiel and Schaffner 1977) in children. Other similar types of studies that have used cohorts include a sample in a Swedish county (Boethius and Wiman 1977) in which children's asthma therapy was followed. Experiments with randomized clinical trials using the intervention level of epidemiology are surprisingly few. Some have been conducted aiming at improving children's medicine use (Schaffner et al. 1983).

RECOMMENDATIONS

In epidemiology, an increasing emphasis is placed on the importance of people themselves taking an active part in evaluating the health status, as well as the quality and availability of health services, in their own communities (Farquhar et al. 1977). Furthermore, the health problem should be identified by members of the community or by health workers who are there. Furthermore, pharmacoepidemiology also should be developed in a way that enables more active collaboration among researchers, policymakers, and those who prescribe, dispense, or consume drugs. Also, attempts are needed to develop methods for interventions and evaluating their effectiveness (Dayton 1970; Diwan 1992).

From a public health perspective, observed differences in national and international patterns of drug utilization require innovative methods. Pharmacoepidemiology is a useful tool both in analyses and interventions. The discipline has so far not been optimally used to study younger populations. The next step in development should foster collaboration with other disciplines such as social and behavioral sciences in order to come closer to an understanding of why children's medicines are being used in the way they are (Trakas and Sanz 1992).

REFERENCES

Adams, S. 1991. "Prescribing of psychotropic drugs to children and adolescents." *British Medical Journal* 302:217.

Boethius, G. and Wiman, F. 1977. "Recording of drug prescriptions in the county of Jämtland, Sweden. I. Methodological aspects." *Journal of Clinical Pharmacology* 33:7-13.

Bonati, M. 1994. "Epidemiologic evaluation of drug use in children." *Journal of Clinical Pharmacology* 34:300-305.

Bush P. J., Iannotti R. J., and Davidson F. R. 1985. A longitudinal study of children and medicines. *Topics in Pharmaceutical Sciences*, edited by D. D. Breimer and P. Speiser. Amsterdam: Elsevier Sciences, pgs. 391-403.

Cluff, L. E., Thornton, G. F., and Seidl, L. G. 1964. "Studies on the epidemiology of adverse drug reactions. I. Methods of surveillance." *Journal American Medical Association* 188:976-983.

Dayton, C. M. 1970. *The Design of Educational Experiments*. New York: McGraw Hill.

Diwan, V. K. 1992. *Epidemiology in Context. Effectiveness of Health Care Interventions*. (Thesis). Stockholm: Department of International Health Care Research (IHCAR), Karolinska Institutet.

Diwan, V. K. and Tomson G. 1988. (Mimeo). Stockholm: Department of International Health Care Research (IHCAR), Karolinska Institutet.

Engels, A. and Siderius, P. 1968. "The consumption of drugs. Report on a study 1966-1967." WHO Regional Office for Europe (EURO Document 3101).

Farquhar, J. W., Maccoby, N., Wood, P. D., Alexander, J. K., Breitrose, H., Brown, Jr., B. W., Haskell, W. L., McAlister, A. L., Meyer, A. J., Nash, J. D., and Stern, M. P. 1977. "Community education for cardiovascular health." *Lancet* i:1192-1195.

Hardon, A. 1987. "The use of modern pharmaceuticals in a Filipino village: Doctors' prescription and self-medication. *Social Science and Medicine* 25(3):277-292.

Herbst, A. L., Ulfelder, H., and Poskanzer, D. C. 1971. "Adenocarcinoma of the vagina: Association of maternal stilbestrol therapy with tumor appearance in young women." *New England Journal of Medicine* 284:878-881.

Hurwitz, E. S, Bareet, M. J., Bregman, D., Gunn, W. J., Pinsky, P., Schonberger, L. B., Drage. J. S., Kaslow, R. A., Burlington, B., Quinlan, G. V., LaMontagne, J. R., Fairweather, W. R., Dayton, D., and Dowdee, W. R. 1987. "Public Health Service Study of Reye's syndrome and medications: Report of the main study." *Journal American Medical Association* 257:1905-1911.

Lenz, W. 1966. "Malformations caused by drugs in pregnancy." *American Journal Diseases of Children* 112:99-106.

McBride, W. G. 1961. "Thalidomide and congenital abnormalities." *Lancet* ii:1358.

McEwen, J. 1987. "Improving adverse drug reaction monitoring." *Medical Toxicology* 2:398-404.

Ray, W. A., Federspiel, C. F., and Schaffner, W. 1967. "Prescribing of chloramphenicol in ambulatory practice: An epidemiologic study among Tennessee Medicaid recipients." *Annals of Internal Medicine* 84:266-270.

Ray, W. A, Federspiel, C. F., and Schaffner, W. 1977. "Prescribing of tetracycline to children less than 8 years old: A two-year epidemiologic study among ambulatory Tennessee Medicaid recipients." *Journal American Medical Association* 237:2069-2074.

Rylance, G. 1987. *Drugs for Children*. Copenhagen: WHO Regional Office for Europe.

Rylance G. W., Woods, C. G., Cullen, R. E., and Rylance, M. E. 1988. "Use of drugs by children." *British Medical Journal* 297:445-447.

Sachs, L., Sterky, G., and Tomson, G. 1988. "Medicines and society–towards a new perspective." *Journal Social Administrative Pharmacy* 5(3/4):133-140.

Sanz, E. J., Bergman, U., and Dahlstrom, M. 1989. "Paediatric drug prescribing. A comparison of Tenerife (Canary Islands, Spain) and Sweden." *European Journal of Clinical Pharmacology* 37:65-68.

Schaffner, W., Ray, W. A, Federspiel, C. F., and Miller, W. O. 1983. "Improved antibiotic prescribing in office practice. A controlled trial of three educational methods." *Journal American Medical Association* 250:1728-1732.

Sterky, G., Tomson, G., Diwan, V. K., and Sachs, L. 1991. "Drug use and the role of patients and prescribers." *Journal of Clinical Epidemiology* 44 (Suppl. II):67s-72s.

Strom, B. L. 1994. "What is pharmacology?" *Pharmacoepidemiology (2nd edition)*, edited by B. L. Strom. Chichester, England: Wiley, pgs. 3-13.

Strom, B. L. (ed). 1992. *Pharmacoepidemiology*. Chichester, England: Wiley.

Tomson, G., Diwan, V. K., and Angunawela, L. 1990. "Paediatric prescribing in outpatient care." *European Journal of Clinical Pharmacology* 39:469-473.

Trakas, D. J. and Sanz, E.J. (eds). 1992. *Studying Childhood and Medicine use. A Multidisciplinary Approach*. Athens: ZHTA Medical Publications.

World Bank. 1993. *Investing in Health*. World Development Report, World Bank: Washington, DC.

Chapter 22

Drugs for Children:
View from a Pharmacoepidemiologist

Syed Rizwanuddin Ahmad

Nowhere is the concern for proper prescribing as acute as in the pediatric age group (Amhad and Bhutta 1990) since the risk of toxicity is increased by inefficient renal filtration, relative enzyme deficiencies, and rapidly evolving changes in pharmacokinetics (what the body does to a drug) and pharmacodynamics (what the drug does to the body) in the growing patient. The problem of prescribing in children is further aggravated by the fact that most prescription drug products still lack adequate information about their use in the pediatric populations. In pediatrics, probably more than in any other field of pharmacotherapy, we frequently use medications for indications and at doses not present in the official drug labeling (Spielberg 1992). An informal survey done by the American Academy of Pediatrics found that 80 percent of newly approved drugs between 1984 and 1989 had no information on pediatric use in the labeling. The problem of pediatric labeling results from the fact that most drugs are tested by their manufacturers in adults. And only later, if ever, are they tested in children (Kessler 1992). In December 1994, the U.S. Food and Drug Administration (FDA) issued landmark regulations permitting drug companies, in some situations, especially if the disease runs the same course in adults and children, to extrapolate from studies conducted in adults and use that information to provide labeling information on the appropriate use in children (U.S. *Federal Register* 1994).

Despite major strides in the field of pediatric clinical pharmacology (Koren and Macleod 1989), there still exists a large vacuum in our knowledge of various aspects of drug use in children (Soumerai and Ross-Degnan 1990). A recent review of the English language literature pertaining to drug use in children found a substantial lack of systematic attention to this area of drug epidemiology. The author of the review concluded that children can be still considered "methodologic orphans" with respect to the transferable knowledge on the benefit/risk profile of therapies they receive (Bonati 1994).

Under these circumstances, it is very commendable that a multidisciplinary team of anthropologists, epidemiologists, pharmacists, pharmacologists, physicians, sociologists, and others pooled their resources and expertise to examine what people, especially children, do and think about medicines. The authors set out to perform a multinational cross-cultural study of medicine use and pledged to use anthropological and sociological rather than pharmacoepidemiological methods. However, pharmacoepidemiologists can learn many lessons from the findings of this multinational study. After all, pharmacoepidemiology has been defined as the study of the patterns and effects of pharmaceuticals within communities. A pharmacoepidemiologist is able to examine and judge patterns of drug use; to determine how "efficacy" measured in clinical trials translates into "effectiveness" in the community; to see to what extent these gains are offset by adverse effects (Henry 1988).

Unlike adults, appropriate drug use in children often requires the support of a caregiver (usually parents or other family members). *Children, Medicines, and Culture* confirms the important role that parents, notably mothers, play in different societies in the supervision and care of their sick children, especially at the time of medicine intake. This is extremely crucial because the young child left alone may not understand the instructions for taking the medicines, and as a result, may use medicine too frequently or not often enough, or may take the wrong drug at the wrong time and thereby suffer adverse drug experience. Involvement of two or more people, e.g., parent and child, may lead to increased compliance in therapy. However, one author has suggested that the involvement of more than one person may complicate the whole process and increase the chance of medication error (Rylance 1987).

PRESCRIPTIONS OF CONCERN

A rapid review of various chapters of this book revealed few drug use patterns that cannot be considered satisfactory by present standards. The types of irrational drug use that caught my attention include:

- Continued use of aspirin (acetylsalicylic acid or ASA) for fever, which is known to have hazardous side effects in children, in the presence of safer alternatives such as paracetamol (acetaminophen).
- Continued use of antidiarrheal drugs (instead of oral rehydration therapy) such as loperamide and opium extract in children which lack evidence of efficacy and have the potential to cause dangerous side effects.
- Use of antibiotics as decongestants, as "cold" medicines (see Chapter 5).
- Use of aspirin for stomachache in children (see Chapter 14).
- Use of preparations containing iron and cod-liver oil for poor appetite (see Chapter 14).
- Use of vitamins and minerals to avoid fatigue or as stimulants (see Chapter 14).

Aspirin Use in Children

Aspirin was still being used for the treatment of childhood fever in Spain and Finland (see Chapters 6 and 14), Germany (see Chapter 12) and Yugoslavia (see Chapter 13). It is well known that aspirin use in children can result in deleterious effects. A number of pharmacoepidemiological studies have found an association between aspirin intake and Reye's syndrome, a severe but rare disorder occurring exclusively in children and characterized by acute encephalopathy and liver degeneration (Hurwitz et al. 1987; Halpin et al. 1982; Starko et al. 1980; Waldman et al. 1982). Consequently, the use of aspirin in children as a general analgesic or antipyretic is no longer considered justified (Reynolds 1989).

Drug regulatory authorities in a number of countries have taken appropriate actions. In 1986, largely due to the efforts of the consumer advocacy organization Public Citizen Health Research Group (Mortimer 1987), the FDA mandated the following warning label on all products containing aspirin: "Children and teenagers should not use this medicine for chicken pox or flu symptoms before a doctor is consulted about Reye's syndrome, a rare but serious illness reported to be associated with aspirin" (PDR 1995). And in the United Kingdom, the Committee on Safety of Medicines (CSM) banned all pediatric formulations of aspirin and the British National Formulary (BNF) (Prasad 1993) carries the following warning: "Owing to an association with Reye's syndrome the CSM has recommended that aspirin-containing preparations should no longer be given to children under the age of 12 years, unless specifically indicated, e.g., for juvenile arthritis (Still's disease). It is important to advise families that aspirin is not a suitable medicine for children with minor illness."

Drugs for Diarrhea in Children

It was interesting to note that parents in Finland (see Chapter 14) were aware of the fact that diarrhea caused by viral infections does not need to be treated with medicines. However, the use of loperamide or opium extract for the pharmacological treatment of diarrhea in children by some Finnish parents emphasizes the need to educate and inform parents and health care professionals about appropriate therapy for the management of diarrhea.

There is no reason for the continued availability of these potentially dangerous antidiarrheal drugs for children. By contrast, management of diarrhea with Oral Rehydration Solution (ORS) is considered one of the most important medical advances of this century (Anonymous 1978). ORS is a simple, low-cost, and easily obtainable method to prevent or correct the dehydration that accompanies diarrhea (Hirschhorn and Greenough 1991). According to the World Health Organization report entitled "The Rational Use of Drugs in the Management of Acute Diarrhea in Children," (WHO 1990) which is a thorough review of studies on the efficacy and safety of the most commonly used antidiarrheal preparations, "antidiarrheal drugs should never be used. None has any proven value and some are dangerous."

Discussing loperamide, the WHO report concludes that "Loperamide has not been shown to reduce losses of fluid and electrolytes in acute diarrhea. While the drug may have a modest effect on the duration of diarrhea . . . this effect is dose-dependent and of questionable clinical importance . . . . Loperamide has no place in the routine management of diarrhea in children and there is thus no rationale for the production and sale of liquid or syrup formulations for pediatric use."

As a result of loperamide's reported association with six infant and child deaths in Pakistan (Bhutta and Tahir 1990) and potential to cause abdominal distension and fatal paralytic ileus (cessation of the function of the intestines), the drug's leading manufacturer halted the sale of loperamide drops worldwide and has withdrawn the distribution of loperamide syrup in countries where the WHO has a program for control of diarrheal diseases (Gussin 1990). At least a dozen countries have either banned or severely restricted the use of the loperamide in children.

There are multiple problems associated with the widespread use of these drugs in diarrhea. The U.S. Centers for Disease Control and Prevention's (CDC) report (1992) has summarized these succinctly "[S]ide effects of these drugs are well known, including opiate-induced ileus, drowsiness and nausea . . . . In addition, reliance on antidiarrheal agents shifts the therapeutic focus away from appropriate fluid, electrolyte, and nutritional therapy; can interfere with oral therapy; and can unnecessarily add to the economic cost of the illness."

MEDICINES AND CULTURE

Intercultural differences in the prescription and use of medicines because of differences in the knowledge, attitudes, and beliefs have been well described in this book (see Chapter 4). Such a state of affairs is not restricted to use of drugs in children. A recent study done by the Paris-based Research Center for Study and Documentation of Health Economics (CREDES) compared the prescribing habits of physicians in Britain, France, Germany, and Italy. They found that the French doctors prescribe about four times as many defined daily doses (DDDs: the amount of a drug that would be needed by a person weighing 75 kilograms [165 lbs.]) of drugs for anxiety and depression than their British and German counterparts, and two and a half times what was prescribed in Italy. Overall, French physicians prescribe more drugs of all types than their colleagues in the other three countries, except for anti-inflammatory and anti-ulcer drugs (Patel 1995). However, such stark difference does not reflect a change in the prevalence of illnesses in France and therefore illustrates irrational drug use.

Intercultural differences in drug use are not unique to the countries that collaborated in this multinational study. In developing countries, for example, numerous studies point out that injections are preferred over oral medications by patients and healers for a variety of health problems, even when their administration is not medically justified (WHO 1992). In a seven-country UNICEF-supported Children's Medicines Project conducted in Asia, it was noted that family physicians in the private sector derived financial gains from prescribing drugs because they dispensed their own prescriptions, a situation leading to poly-prescribing (Balasubramaniam 1994).

ADVERSE DRUG EXPERIENCE AND CHILDREN

It was a bit surprising to note that almost all children were aware of the fact that medicines have the potential to cause adverse drug experiences. However, Chapter 10 in *Children, Medicines, and Culture* conveys the message that "ADRs [Adverse Drug Reactions] in children are normally mild, self-limiting, preventable, and judged inconsequential by both the parents and the doctor." Nevertheless, we should be extra careful and cautious when prescribing drugs to children, pregnant women, and lactating mothers. A number of therapeutic misadventures in the past have affected the pediatric population and have resulted in major legislation including establishment of programs to monitor ADRs. Examples of such misadventure include: the elixir of sulfanilamide tragedy in 1937 where 104 people died, including 34 children (Calvery and Klumpp 1939); the grey baby syndrome associated with the antibiotic chloramphenicol (Burns, Hodgman, and Cass 1959); kernicturus in association with the antibacterial sulfonamide (Silverman et al. 1956); and phocomelia (limb deformities) associated with the hypnotic thalidomide (McBride

1961). It is important to mention here that between November 1981 when the U.S. CDC forwarded its recommendations to the FDA that aspirin should be avoided to treat fever in acute viral infections in children, and when the warning label was issued in June 1986, it was estimated that 1,700 deaths occurred in children due to Reye's syndrome (Davis and Buffler 1992).

The U.S. FDA received more than 4,000 suspected adverse drug experience (ADE) reports with fatal outcomes in children between 1969 and 1993. This is just the tip of the iceberg because underreporting of ADE reports to the FDA is widespread (personal communication with Franz Rosa, MD, Food and Drug Administration, USA, April 19, 1995).

Given the fact that expired medicines can be harmful to unsuspecting consumers, it was disturbing to note that up to 30 percent of medicines stored in homes had expired (see Chapter 5). Another alarming finding was the storage of medicines in places easily accessible to children (see Chapter 5). Although it may be unrealistic to keep all medicines away from the reach of children in the age group that was studied, we should be aware that such storage practice may lead to devastating consequences where younger children also live in the home. For example, Canadian hospitals reported that more than 20 percent of emergency admissions for poisonings in youngsters involved OTC medications, including colorful, fruit-flavored cough/cold drugs, some of which resulted from children getting into the medicine cabinet (Canadian Broadcasting Corporation Television Newsmagazine *Marketplace.* Feature on "Kids' Medicines," broadcast March 21, 1995).

WHAT IS OUR RESPONSIBILITY?

While practically no drug is free of adverse effects, it is our responsibility to help prevent or minimize unwanted effects, especially in situations where reliable scientific data exists and suggests a cause-and-effect relationship between a drug and an undesirable effect. It is a matter of great concern that children are continually being exposed to medications known to be associated with serious adverse outcomes.

In cases where adverse events are well known and safer alternatives exist, such as the use of paracetamol instead of aspirin to treat fever in children and prevent Reye's syndrome, we need to launch massive and concerted media campaigns to inform and educate both the parents and the health professionals about the appropriate fever therapy. According to the WHO, paracetamol (acetaminophen) is the preferred drug (Rylance 1987), and in the U.S. the drug of choice for the treatment of fever in children. A large randomized double-blind study published recently that compared paracetamol with ibuprofen found that the risk of hospitalization for gastrointestinal bleeding, renal failure, or anaphylaxis was not increased following short-term use of ibuprofen in febrile children (Lesko and Mitchell 1995). And on March 28, 1995, an FDA advisory committee recommended over-the-counter switch for ibuprofen for use as an antipyretic and analgesic in children.

I will conclude with this quotation: "the broad purposes of pharmacoepidemiology are to advance our knowledge of the risks and benefits of medication use in real-world populations, and to foster improved prescribing and patient health outcomes. If, however, physicians and other health practitioners fail to update their knowledge and practice in response to new and clinically important data on the outcomes of specific prescribing patterns, then the 'fruits' of pharmacoepidemiologic research may have little impact on clinical practice" (Soumerai and Lipton 1994).

REFERENCES

Ahmad, S. R. and Bhutta, Z. A. 1990. "A survey of pediatric prescribing and dispensing in Karachi." *Journal of the Pakistan Medical Association* 40:126-130.
Anonymous. 1978. "Water with sugar and salt." *Lancet* ii:300-301.
Balasubramaniam, K. B. 1994. "Rational use of drugs in children." Presentation at the XII Biennial Conference of the Pakistan Pediatric Association. February 2-5, 1994, Lahore.
Bonati, M. 1994. "Epidemiologic evaluation of drug use in children." *Journal of Clinical Pharmacology* 34:300-305.
Bhutta, T. I. and Tahir, K. I. 1990. "Loperamide poisoning in children." *Lancet* 335:363.
Burns, L. E., Hodgman, J. E., and Cass. A. B. 1959. "Fatal circulatory collapse in premature infants receiving chloramphenicol." *New England Journal of Medicine* 261:1318-1321.

Calvery, H. O. and Klumpp, T. G. 1939. "The toxicity for human beings of diethylene glycol with sulfanilamide." *Southern Medical Journal* 32:1105-1109.

Centers for Disease Control and Prevention. 1992. "The Management of Acute Diarrhea in Children: Oral Rehydration, Maintenance, and Nutritional Therapy." *Morbidity and Mortality Weekly Report* 41(RR-16):1-20.

Davis, D. L. and Buffler, P. 1992. "Reduction of deaths after drug labeling for risk of Reye's syndrome." *Lancet* 340:1042.

Gussin, R. Z. 1990. "Withdrawal of loperamide drops." *Lancet* 335:1603-1604.

Halpin, T. J., Holtzhauer, F. J., Campbell, R. J., Hall, L. J., Correa-Villasenor, A., Lanese, R., Rice, J., and Hurwitz, E. S. 1982 "Reye's syndrome and medication use." *Journal of the American Medical Association* 248:687-691.

Henry, D. A. 1988. "Pharmacoepidemiology." *Australian Prescriber* 11:66-67.

Hirschhorn, N. and Greenough III, W. B. 1991. "Progress in oral rehydration therapy." *Scientific American* 264:50-56.

Hurwitz, E. S., Barrett, M. J., Bregman, D., Gunn, W. J., Pinsky, P., Schonberger, L. B., Drage, J. S., Kaslow, R. A., Burlington, B., Quinnan, G. V., LaMontagne, J. R., Fairweather, W. R., Dayton, D., and Dowdle, W. R. 1987. "Public Health Service study of Reye's syndrome and medications: Report of the main study." *Journal of the American Medical Association* 257:1905-1911.

Kessler, D. A. 1992. "Remarks at the Annual Meeting of the American Academy of Pediatrics." October 14, San Francisco, California.

"Kids' Medicines," feature on *Marketplace*, Television newsmagazine. March 21, 1995. Canadian Broadcasting Corporation.

Koren, G. and Macleod, S. M. 1989. "The state of pediatric clinical pharmacology: An international survey of training programs." *Clinical Pharmacology and Therapeutics* 46:489-493.

Lesko, S. M. and Mitchell, A. A. 1995. "An assessment of the safety of pediatric ibuprofen: A practitioner-based randomized control trial." *Journal of the American Medical Association* 273:929-933.

McBride, W. G. 1961. "Thalidomide and congenital abnormalities." *Lancet* ii:1358.

Mortimer, E. A. 1987. "Reye's syndrome, salicylates, epidemiology, and public health policy." *Journal of the American Medical Association* 257:1941.

Patel, T. 1995. "Thank heaven for little pills." *New Scientist* 146:14-15.

Physicians' Desk Reference (PDR). 1995. Montvale, NJ: Medical Economics Data Production Co., pg. 701.

Prasad, A. B. (Ed.). 1993. *British National Formulary (BNF)*. London: British Medical Association and Royal Pharmaceutical Society of Great Britain. No. 26, pgs. 167-168.

Reynolds, J. E. F. (Ed.) 1989. *Martindale: The Extra Pharmacopoeia*. London: The Pharmaceutical Press, pg. 5.

Rylance, G. (Ed.) 1987. *Drugs for Children*. World Health Organization. Copenhagen: WHO Regional Office for Europe, pg. 5.

Silverman, W. A., Anderson, D. H., Blanc, W. A., and Crozier, D. N. 1956. "A difference in mortality rate and incidence of kernicturus among premature infants allotted to two prophylactic antibacterial regimens." *Pediatrics* 18:614.

Soumerai, S. B. and Lipton, H. L. 1994. "Evaluating and improving physician prescribing." *Pharmacoepidemiology,* 2nd ed., edited by B. L. Strom, New York: John Wiley, pgs. 395-412.

Soumerai, S. B. and Ross-Degnan, D. 1990. "Drug prescribing in pediatrics: Challenge for quality improvement." *Pediatrics* 86:782-784.

Spielberg, S. P. 1992. "Pediatrics therapeutics and drug utilization." *Pharmacoepidemiology and Drug Safety* 1 (1):31-32.

Starko, K. M., Ray, C. G., Dominguez, L .B., Stromberg, W. L., and Woodall, D. F. 1980 "Reye's syndrome and salicylate use." *Pediatrics* 248:687-691.

U.S. *Federal Register.* 1994. "Specific requirements on content and format of labeling for human prescription drugs; Revision of 'pediatric use' subsection in the labeling; Final rule." 59 (238):64240-64250.

Waldman, R. J., Hall, W. N., McGee, H., and Amburg, G. V. 1982 "Aspirin as risk factor in Reye's syndrome." *Journal of the American Medical Association* 247: 3089-3094.

World Health Organization. 1990. *The Rational Use of Drugs in the Management of Acute Diarrhea in Children.* Geneva: WHO.

World Health Organization. 1992. *Injection Practices Research.* Action Program on Essential Drugs. WHO/DAP/92.9. Geneva: WHO.

Index

Page numbers followed by "t" indicate tables; page numbers followed by "f" indicate figures.